Nuclear medicine in urology and nephrology

Second edition

Edited by

P. H. O'Reilly, MD, FRCS
Consultant Urologist, Stepping Hill Hospital, Stockport, Cheshire

R. A. Shields, PhD
Chief Physicist, Manchester Royal Infirmary

H. J. Testa, MD, PhD, MRCP
Consultant in Nuclear Medicine, Manchester Royal Infirmary

Butterworths
London · Boston · Durban · Singapore · Sydney · Toronto · Wellington

First edition 1979
Second edition 1986

© Butterworth & Co. (Publishers) Ltd, 1986

British Library Cataloguing in Publication Data

Nuclear medicine in urology and nephrology.—2nd ed.
  1. Urinary organs—Diseases—Diagnosis
  2. Nuclear medicine
  I. O'Reilly, P. H. II. Shields, R. A. III. Testa, H. J.
  616.6'07'575   RC901

  ISBN 0–407–00322–3

Library of Congress Cataloging-in-Publication Data

Nuclear medicine in urology and nephrology.
  Includes bibliographies and index.
  1. Radioisotope scanning. 2. Radioisotopes in
urology. 3. Radioisotopes in nephrology. I. O'Reilly,
P. H. (Patrick Henry), 1947–   . II. Shields,
R. A. III. Testa, H. J. [DNLM: 1. Kidney—radionuclide
imaging. 2. Urinary Tract—radionuclide imaging.
WJ 141 N964]
  RC874.N8 1986   616.6'07575   85-18984

  ISBN 0–407–00322–3

Photoset by Mid-County Press, London SW15
Printed and bound in England by Butler & Tanner, Frome, Somerset

Foreword

The collaboration of the scientist and clinician has significantly advanced non-invasive techniques in nephro-urological investigation. The consequent reduction in morbidity has allowed the surgeon to plan his operation more carefully and to achieve greater success from the selected surgical procedure employed. Nuclear medicine procedures provide information not obtainable by other methods and, when used in combination with other diagnostic modalities, accuracy should be assured.

The greatest contribution of nuclear medicine to urology is the assessment of the dynamism and functional capacity of the urinary tract without submitting the patient to traumatic procedures and high radiation dose. It is readily available to the paediatrician, nephrologist, transplant surgeon and oncologist.

The amalgam of urologists, nephrologists and specialists in nuclear medicine has been essential to the concept of this book, which should be useful to all students and workers in the field of nephro-urology.

The editorial team and many of the authors have gained their experience while working together at the Manchester Royal Infirmary. I think that this concerted approach lends an unusual clarity and consistency to what, in these days of specialization, must inevitabley be a multi-author work. For this second edition they have invited additional contributions from other internationally recognized sources; by thus extending the range of expertise they have produced a most comprehensive volume.

E. Charlton-Edwards

Preface

These days the clinician in every specialty is presented with a bewildering array of diagnostic techniques to assist him in the evaluation and management of his patient. The clinical use of radioisotopes, 'nuclear medicine', is often associated with X-radiology and ultrasound and consequently regarded merely as a branch of 'diagnostic imaging'. This is unfortunate, as it can conceal the unique advantages of radioactive tracer studies in the evaluation of function of organs and systems using the exquisite sensitivity of gamma-ray detectors to minute quantities of tracer material. These advantages are particularly relevant to the investigation of the kidneys and urinary tract, where both nephrologist and urologist require information on the function of every aspect of this dynamic system. The purpose of this work is to describe and explain the applications of nuclear medicine to urology and nephrology, and to evaluate their role in modern clinical diagnosis.

The book is in three parts. The first presents a description of the techniques and their interpretation. The second discusses in depth their application to specific clinical problems. Part 3 deals with basic principles and expands on the relevant theoretical and technical aspects not covered in detail in Part 1.

The clinician interested in the application of the techniques in clinical practice will find most useful the information in Parts 1 and 2. He may wish to use Part 3 only occasionally for reference, but his attention is nevertheless particularly drawn to Chapter 17, on 'Radiopharmaceuticals', wherein lies the key to the successful choice, application and development of nuclear medicine techniques. The remainder of Part 3 may be more useful to the nuclear medicine specialist: diagnostician, physicist or technologist.

In Chapter 18 the reader will find certain passages in small print covering the detailed mathematics involved in nuclear medicine techniques. These passages may be omitted without detracting from an understanding of the principles behind quantification techniques.

Since the publication of the first edition in 1979, there have been significant developments in instrumentation and techniques. Perhaps the most obvious is the greater role played by the gamma camera/computer system in routine clinical studies, so that, whereas in the 1970s the term 'renography' often implied the use of probes and chart recorder, it is now more usually associated with a sequence of images of isotope distribution obtained with a gamma camera. The dynamic information is still presented as a set of curves, but these are interpreted alongside the relevant functional images. The quality of all nuclear medicine images has improved markedly as a result of steady improvements in gamma camera performance, and almost all of the illustrations in this edition are new.

It is interesting to note that the technique of diuresis renography, now widely practised, was mentioned only briefly in the earlier edition. Greater emphasis is also given now to studies of urinary reflux, and a fresh chapter has been added on the diagnosis of lower urinary tract problems.

Many readers of the first edition appreciated the chapter on 'Protocols of procedures'. This has been expanded considerably both in scope and in depth, and includes its own classified contents page.

The chapter on 'Radiation dosimetry' has been updated, not only to take into account improved biological models but also to include estimates of the 'effective dose equivalent' which enables simple comparisons to be made between different procedures involving ionizing radiation.

We hope that the book will be of value to urologists and nephrologists, and also to those working in the fields of nuclear medicine and medical physics.

P. H. O'Reilly
R. A. Shields
H. J. Testa

Note on orientation of illustrations

The radionuclide images in this book are displayed as 'seen' by the gamma camera, i.e. for a posterior view the patient's left is on the left hand side of the picture, whereas for an anterior view the patient's left is on the right hand side. Most renal images are posterior views; this may be assumed unless specifically stated otherwise in the caption.

Radiographs are always displayed in the conventional manner, i.e. with the patient's left on the right hand side of the picture.

Acknowledgements

The editors would like to acknowledge the continuing support of the Manchester and North West Region Kidney Research Association in providing a research fellowship for the study of nuclear medicine in urology and nephrology. This support is now in its ninth consecutive year. Its success can be judged from the fact that four of the contributors to this second edition have been holders of this fellowship.

The cooperation of all the urologists in the Manchester Region is greatly appreciated. Particular thanks are due to Mr Eric Charlton-Edwards, Mr Raymond Carroll and the entire urological department at Manchester Royal Infirmary.

The enthusiasm and dedication of the clinical, scientific, technical and secretarial staff in the departments of nuclear medicine and medical physics at the Manchester Royal Infirmary have been immensely valuable. Miss Wendy Dainty and Miss Wendy-Ann Muirhead deserve particular mention for their hard work in producing the manuscript. This second edition, like the first, is dedicated to the staff of these departments, without whom the task would not have been possible.

Mary and Keith Harrison and the department of Medical Illustration at the University Hospital of South Manchester deserve thanks for their excellent work in preparation of illustrations. We are also grateful to the following for permission to reproduce illustrations:

Dr Richard Johnson, Christie Hospital, for *Figure 9.7*;
Mr Joe Cohen, Booth Hall Children's Hospital, for *Figure 11.5*;
Dr Ralph McCready, Royal Marsden Hospital, for *Figure 9.8*; and
The Editor of *British Journal of Urology* and Longmans Publishers for *Figure 9.3*.
Mr A. R. Constable for *Figure 13.3*.

Contents

Contributors

C. R. A. Bevis, BSc, MB BS, FRCS, MD Senior Registrar in Urology, Freeman Hospital, Newcastle-upon-Tyne

M. Donald Blaufox, MD, PhD Chairman, Department of Nuclear Medicine; Professor of Nuclear Medicine, Medicine, and Radiology, Albert Einstein College of Medicine/Montefiore Medical Center, Bronx, New York, USA

A. R. Constable, MSc, FInstP Hon. Senior Lecturer in Medical Physics, St Paul's Hospital, London

P. J. English, BSc, MB BS, FRCS Senior Registrar in Urology, Edinburgh Royal Infirmary

Eugene J. Fine, MD Assistant Professor of Nuclear Medicine, Department of Nuclear Medicine, Albert Einstein College of Medicine/Montefiore Medical Center, Bronx, New York, USA

D. L. Hastings, PhD Senior Physicist, Manchester Royal Infirmary

D. Holden, MB BS, FRCS Registrar in Urology, Preston Royal Hospital

R. W. G. Johnson, MS, FRCS Senior Lecturer in Surgery, Surgeon in Charge of the Renal Transplant Unit, Manchester Royal Infirmary

R. S. Lawson, PhD Principal Physicist, Manchester Royal Infirmary

E. W. Lupton, MD, FRCS Consultant Urological Surgeon, Department of Urology, University Hospital of South Manchester

P. H. O'Reilly, MD, FRCS Consultant Urological Surgeon, Department of Urology, Stepping Hill Hospital, Stockport, Cheshire

M. C. Prescott, MB ChB, MD Consultant in Nuclear Medicine, Manchester Royal Infirmary

L. Rosenthall, MD Director, Division of Nuclear Medicine, The Montreal General Hospital; Professor of Radiology, McGill University, Montreal, Quebec, Canada

Stephen C. Scharf, MD Chief of Nuclear Medicine, Lenox Hill Hospital, New York; Assistant Clinical Professor of Nuclear Medicine, Albert Einstein College of Medicine, Bronx, New York, USA

Richard Sherman, MD Associate Professor of Medicine, U.M.D.N.J., Rutgers Medical School, New Brunswick, New Jersey, USA

R. A. Shields, PhD Chief Physicist, Manchester Royal Infirmary

H. J. Testa, MD, PhD, MRCP Consultant in Nuclear Medicine, Manchester Royal Infirmary

Part 1

Techniques

1 Introduction

P. H. O'Reilly, R. A. Shields and H. J. Testa

Nuclear medicine is a clinical specialty whose distinctive feature is the use of radioactive materials. It has been defined by the World Health Organization as the branch of medicine 'taken to embrace all applications of radioactive materials in diagnosis, treatment or medical research with the exception of the use of sealed radiation sources in radiotherapy' (WHO, 1972). Its evolution as a scientific discipline has its origin in the development of the atomic theory, whose philosophical basis may be traced back to ancient Greece. In 500 BC Leucippus of Mileto put forward his 'dichotomy theory': if one were to divide anything into two parts, and repeat the process over and over again, there would come a point at which further subdivisions were impossible. At this point one would have obtained the individual *atom*. He also suggested that these atoms were separated by space, correctly recognizing the basis of the structure of matter. These theories were followed up by Democritus of Abdera, who postulated that atoms were distinct in shape and size and that it was this distinction that endowed different elements with their different properties. The atomic theory continued to find followers such as Epicurus in Greece and Lucretius in Rome, who expanded these principles in his didactic masterpiece *De Rerum Natura*. While little of the writing of Leucippus, Democritus or Epicurus survives, the work of Lucretius can be seen to this day, preserving the early atomists' views to modern times.

In the seventeenth century Robert Boyle investigated and defined the elements as substances which could not be broken down into simpler constituents—a modernization of Democritus' ideas—and a century later Lavoisier extended the principle by distinguishing between elements and compounds. In 1808 John Dalton published his *New System of Chemical Philosophy*, which included two fundamentals of our modern understanding of the nature of matter: (*1*) all matter is composed of atoms; and (*2*) chemical combinations take place between atoms. In November 1895 Wilhelm Conrad Röntgen discovered X-rays, and four months later Henri Becquerel made a momentous discovery during his experiments on phosphorescence. He developed a photographic plate which had been left in its wrapping in a drawer together with some uranium salts. To his surprise, he found an intense silhouette of the uranium salts and postulated that they were emitting some rays of unknown nature which had certain properties in common with X-rays (Becquerel, 1896). Shortly afterwards Marie Curie confirmed this postulate and discovered that thorium emitted similar rays to those of uranium, which she called Becquerel rays. This new form of energy was later called radioactivity, and uranium and thorium were termed radioelements. In 1898 Pierre and Marie Curie discovered radium.

At this time Ernest Rutherford began to study radioactivity, first at McGill University, Montreal, and later in the Cavendish Laboratories at Cambridge. In 1911 he proposed his theory that all atoms consist of a small, positively charged nucleus in which practically all the mass is concentrated, surrounded by orbiting electrons. Bohr, working with him in Manchester, further clarified the orbital systems and distinguished between atomic weight and atomic number, so introducing the concept of isotopes as species of an element which are chemically identical but physically different. Out of this pursuit of the atomic theory grew an entirely new branch of physics—nuclear physics.

In 1927 Blumgart and Weiss injected aqueous solutions of radon intravenously and monitored the velocity of blood flow between one arm and the other with a cloud chamber (Blumgart and Weiss, 1927). This was the first recorded nuclear medicine investigation, but the major developments in this field had to await the availability of artificially produced radioactivity. In 1932 Chadwick discovered the neutron, which led to the definition of a nuclide as a particular combination of nuclear particles—protons and neutrons. Two years later Frederick Joliot and Irène Curie bombarded aluminium with alpha particles and produced phosphorus-30 (^{30}P), the first radioactive nuclide to be produced by nuclear transformation. In the same year Ernest Lawrence invented the cyclotron; and in 1942 the world's first nuclear reactor, designed by Enrico Fermi, came into operation. The tremendous flux of neutrons within the reactor provided the possibility for production of large quantities of a wide range of radioactive nuclides which have become available since 1945. Probably the most important of these has been molybdenum-99 (^{99}Mo) because it decays into a short-lived metastable daughter nuclide—technetium-99m (^{99m}Tc)—and has led to the introduction of the technetium generator.

In the early days of medical application of these new tracer materials the only effective radiation detector available was the Geiger–Müller tube. Its efficiency was unfortunately very low when detecting gamma rays—especially the energetic 364 keV gamma ray emitted by iodine-131 (^{131}I), one of the earliest radionuclides produced. In 1947 Kallman, working in Germany, and Coltmann and Marshall, independently in the USA, showed that the radiation-induced scintillations from calcium tungstate crystals could be detected by optically coupled photomultiplier tubes. In 1949 Benedict Cassen explored the possibility of making a sensitive directional gamma ray detector, using a side-window photomultiplier and a calcium tungstate crystal, and was able to detect more than 25% of ^{131}I gamma rays (Cassen, Curtis and Reed, 1950). Later tests showed that rabbit thyroids could be located rapidly and accurately in this way after the administration of 10 mCi of ^{131}I. Once this had been demonstrated, the technique was applied to patients at the Veterans' Administration Hospital in Los Angeles. A detector was set up on a stand and point-by-point counts were made over the thyroid. From 100 to 200 μCi of ^{131}I was administered and the thyroid was mapped completely in 1–1$\frac{1}{2}$ hours. Because of the length of time this took, the system was automated, and thus the first rectilinear scanner came into being. In 1951, calcium tungstate was replaced by thallium-activated sodium iodide crystals, already extensively studied by Hofstadter (1948). The scanner was further refined by employing focused multichannel collimators and developing data-presentation and processing techniques. In 1957 Hal Anger introduced a further significant advance in nuclear medicine instrumentation: the position-sensitive scintillation detector system and its incorporation into the 'gamma camera' (Anger, 1958). This device is able to produce an image of distribution of radioactivity with greater efficiency and more operational simplicity than the scanner.

The artificial production of radioactive tracers and the availability of equipment for their detection was followed quickly by attempts to put them to use in the clinical field, including the investigation of patients with diseases of the kidneys and urinary tract. In

1952 Oeser and Billion devised a method for measuring renal function by injecting ^{131}I-labelled Uroselectan B or Iopax intravenously and measuring the elimination by determining an activity–time curve from the excreted urine. However, they failed to recognize the potential value of measuring the radioactivity over the renal areas. This was attempted for the first time by Kimbel (1956), who generated an activity–time curve from the region of the kidneys after the injection of ^{131}I-Perabrodil M and ^{131}I-Urografin. It was left to Taplin to put renography on a firm clinical footing when he used two collimated scintillation detectors, two ratemeters and two chart recorders to measure the changes in renal activity following the injection of ^{131}I-Urokon. Although this was unsuccessful, the procedure was repeated with ^{131}I-Diodrast, which gave a pattern closely resembling the present-day renogram (Taplin *et al.*, 1956; Winter and Taplin, 1958). All these agents suffered from slow renal clearance and accumulation in extrarenal tissues, but these disadvantages were overcome in 1960 with the introduction of ^{131}I-labelled ortho-iodohippurate (OIH) by Tubis, Posnick and Nordyke (1960). OIH had already been used in urography (Swick, 1933), and its rapid uptake and elimination by the kidneys had been shown to be similar to that of para-aminohippuric acid (Smith, 1951). Labelled with ^{131}I, it proved an invaluable agent for the investigation of renal function, and probe renography became a widely adopted technique for screening in nephro-urological practice.

The first attempt to produce renal images using radionuclides is said to have been made by Goodwin, who labelled the radiographic contrast agent Diodrast with ^{131}I; Winter also tried this technique, but both attempts were unsuccessful (Winter, 1963). Hanie and colleagues (1960) demonstrated renal infarcts in dogs using a continuous infusion of ^{131}I-OIH with some success, but because of the large radiation dose involved with the infusion, the application of this technique in the clinical field was unacceptable. In 1956 the mercurial diuretic Chlormerodrin was labelled with mercury-203 ([203]Hg), and this was later used successfully in clinical renal imaging (McAfee and Wagner, 1960). In 1964 Sodee introduced mercury-197 ([197]Hg), which has a shorter half-life than [203]Hg and was thus a more suitable agent. More recently the ^{99m}Tc agents have been widely adopted. The most commonly used compounds to which this radionuclide is labelled are currently diethylene triamine pentaacetic acid (DTPA) (Hauser *et al.*, 1970), gluconate (Boyd *et al.*, 1973) and dimercaptosuccinic acid (DMSA) (Englander, Weber and dos Remedios, 1974). Any technetium compound, or indeed technetium in its ionic form of pertechnetate as eluted from a generator, may be used for first-circulation studies of renal perfusion.

In recent years the probe renogram has been replaced largely by the gamma camera renogram in which a sequence of images is obtained in addition to the functional curves. In many centres this is performed with ^{99m}Tc-DTPA. The use of the gamma camera has been further justified and emphasized by the introduction of ^{123}I-OIH. [123]I is a cyclotron-produced isotope which emits gamma rays of 159 keV and has a half-life of 13 hours. These excellent physical characteristics permit the production of renal images of high quality, while giving a low radiation dose to the patient (O'Reilly *et al.*, 1977). Furthermore, ^{123}I-OIH has been successfully used to measure effective renal plasma flow (Chisholm, Short and Glass, 1974); when available it is the radio-pharmaceutical of choice for functional renal studies.

Another important development in recent years has been the introduction of the technique of diuresis renography. This addresses the problem, common in urology, of assessing the significance of dilatation of the upper urinary tract. Obstruction of this tract will be evident at both low and high urine flow rates whereas a dilated, but non-obstructed, system may yield to diuretic provocation and demonstrate washout of urine previously retained by a reservoir effect. This modification has been rapidly accepted by clinicians, and diuresis renography is now considered a standard investigation in the practice of nephro-urology.

A further notable development of interest to the urologist was the introduction of suitable radiopharmaceuticals for skeletal imaging. A number of agents have been used, and the ^{99m}Tc-labelled phosphate compounds have achieved widespread popularity in the detection of metastatic disease and in metabolic and other benign skeletal disorders. The detection of bone metastases in carcinoma of the prostate is the main indication for the procedure in urological practice.

The techniques of renography, renal scanning, clearance studies and bone scanning described in this book have developed as a result of the multidisciplinary inspiration, dedication and research of physicists, chemists, pharmacists, biochemists, mathematicians and clinicians. They have reached a point where a wealth of information is available to the clinician conversant with their capabilities and limitations. The procedures are simple, rapid and safe and allow the acquisition of information often unavailable from other sources. This book describes the techniques currently available, the direction in which nuclear medicine is developing in the nephro-urological field, and the value of the procedures to the clinician in the management of his patients.

References

ANGER, H. O. (1958) Scintillation camera. *Review of Scientific Instruments*, **29**, 27–33

BECQUEREL, H. (1896) Sur les radiations invisibles émises par les corps phosphorescents. *Comptes rendus des séances de l'Académie des Sciences*, **122**, 501–502

BLUMGART, H. L. and WEISS, S. (1927) Studies on the velocity of blood flow. *Journal of Clinical Investigation*, **4**, 15–31

BOYD, R. E., ROBSON, J., HUNT, F. C., SORBY, P. J., MURRAY, I. P. C. and McKAY, W. J. (1973) ^{99m}Tc-Gluconate complexes for renal scintigraphy. *British Journal of Radiology*, **46**, 604–660

CASSEN, B., CURTIS, L. and REED, C. (1950) A sensitive directional gamma ray detector. *Nucleonics*, **6**, 78–88

CHISHOLM, G. D., SHORT, M. D. and GLASS, H. J. (1974) The measurement of individual renal plasma flow using ^{123}I-hippuran and the gamma camera. *British Journal of Urology*, **46**, 591–600

COLTMAN, J. W. and MARSHALL, F. W. (1947) Some characteristics of the Photomultiplier radiation detector. *Physical Review*, **73**, 528

DALTON, J. (1808) *New System of Chemical Philosophy*

ENGLANDER, D., WEBER, P. M. and DOS REMEDIOS, L. V. (1974) Renal cortical imaging in 35 patients. Superior quality with ^{99m}Tc-DMSA. *Journal of Nuclear Medicine*, **15**, 743–749

HAUSER, W., ATKINS, H. L., NELSON, K. G. and RICHARDS, P. (1970) ^{99m}Tc-DTPA: a new radiopharmaceutical for brain and kidney scanning. *Radiology*, **94**, 679–684

HANIE, T. P., NAFAL, M., CARR, E. A. Jr and BEIERWALTES, W. H. (1960) Scintillation scanning of the kidneys and radioiodinated contrast media. *Clinical Research*, **8**, 288

HOFSTADTER, R. (1948) Alkali halide scintillation counters. *Physical Review*, **74**, 100

KALLMAN, H. (1947) *Naturwissenschaft und Technik in Lehre*

KIMBEL, K. H. (1956) Discussion of paper by W. Schlungbaum and H. Billion. In: *Radioaktif Isotope in Klinik und Forschung, Vortrage am Gasteiner Internationalen Symposium*, Vol. 2. Berlin: Urban and Schartzenburg.

McAFEE, J. G. and WAGNER, H. N. Jr (1960) Visualisation of renal parenchyma: scinti-scanning with ^{203}Hg Neohydrin. *Radiology*, **75**, 820

OESER, H. and BILLION, H. (1952) Functionelle Strahlendiagnostik durch ettiketierte Röntgen Kontrastmittel. *Fortschritte auf dem Gebiete Röntgenstrahlen*, **76**, 431–437

O'REILLY, P. H., HERMAN, K. J., LAWSON, R. S., SHIELDS, R. A. and TESTA, H. J. (1977) 123-iodine: a new isotope for functional renal scanning. *British Journal of Urology*, **49**, 15–21

SMITH, H. W. (1951) *The Kidney, Structure and Function in Health and Disease*. London: Oxford University Press

SODEE, D. B. (1964) A new scanning isotope ^{197}Hg Neohydrin. *Journal of Nuclear Medicine*, **51**, 74

SWICK, M. (1933) Excretion urography by means of the i.v. and oral administration of sodium ortho-iodohippurate with some physiological considerations. *Surgery, Gynecology and Obstetrics*, **56**, 62

TAPLIN, G. V., MEREDITH, O. M., KADE, H. and WINTER, C. C. (1956) The radioisotope renogram. *Journal of Laboratory and Clinical Medicine*, **48**, 886

TUBIS, M., POSNICK, N. and NORDYKE, R. A. (1960) The preparation and use of ^{131}I-labelled sodium ortho-iodohippurate in kidney function tests. *Proceedings of the Society of Experimental Biology and Medicine*, **103**, 498

WINTER, C. C. and TAPLIN, G. V. (1958) A clinical comparison and analysis of radioactive Diodrast, Hypaque, Miokon and Urokon renograms as tests of renal function. *Journal of Urology*, **79**, 573

WINTER, C. C. (1963) Discussion. *Journal of Urology*, **90**, 658

WORLD HEALTH ORGANIZATION (1972) The Medical Uses of Ionising Radiation. *Technical Report Series* No. 492. WHO, Geneva

2 Renography

P. H. O'Reilly, R. A. Shields and H. J. Testa

The radionuclide renogram and its variations should be as familiar to the urologist as the electrocardiogram is to the cardiologist. The physiological determinants of renogram responses mean that the procedure reflects accurately both individual renal function and urine transport. Renography monitors the arrival, uptake, transit and elimination of a radiopharmaceutical by the kidneys following its intravenous injection. This radiopharmaceutical can be detected externally only if it contains a gamma-emitting nuclide. Renography was performed at first using probe detectors; now the gamma camera is used in the majority of centres. The current radio-pharmaceuticals of choice are ^{123}I-orthoiodohippurate (OIH) or ^{99m}Tc-diethylene triaminepentaacetic acid (DTPA).

^{123}I-OIH is an ideal compound combining a good radionuclide (half-life of 13 hours and monoenergetic gamma emission at 159 keV) with an agent handled almost exclusively by tubular secretion. Eighty per cent of the amount supplied to the kidney is actively secreted by the renal tubules, and only a small proportion is filtered. This results in fast and efficient extraction from the blood and passage through the kidneys. Maximum renal concentration is reached within 5 minutes of injection. It is cleared from the parenchyma and collecting system of normal kidneys within 30 minutes. It gives an assessment of individual effective renal plasma flow (ERPF).

In contrast ^{99m}Tc-DTPA combines an ideal radionuclide (half-life of 6 hours and monoenergetic gamma emission at 140 keV) with a *filtered* compound which has negligible tubular secretion or reabsorption and gives an assessment of glomerular filtration rate (GFR). Following injection, peak concentration is reached within 5 minutes at which time about 5% of the injected dose can be found in the kidneys. Its renal handling is similar to that of radiographic contrast media and inulin.

Gamma camera renography

The only patient preparation required is to ensure that an adequate state of hydration is maintained during the test, i.e. the patient should be instructed not to abstain from fluid. It may be appropriate (e.g. during hot weather) to give a 500-ml drink on arrival. It is important to avoid an oliguric state, since the result can mimic an obstructive pattern to a misleading degree owing to sluggish urine flow. It is unwise to perform renography on the same day as intravenous urography, since many centres insist on a period of dehydration before this investigation. In addition, hyperosmolar contrast

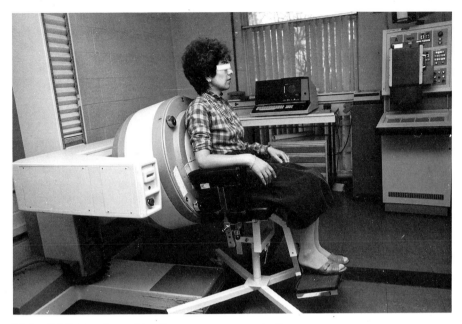

Figure 2.1 Patient in position for gamma camera studies

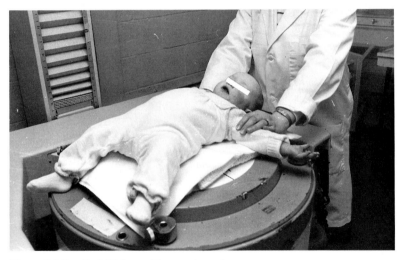

Figure 2.2 Small child in position on top of gamma camera

media used in this and other radiographic procedures can themselves exaggerate anatomical obstruction to give misleading renogram appearances (Kaude and Nordenport, 1973). The bladder is emptied immediately before the examination, and the patient is then placed in a sitting position with the gamma camera in contact with the patient's back. This is more representative of the patient's everyday waking posture than supine or prone positions although, in certain circumstances, these may be necessary. The field of view of the gamma camera should include both kidneys and bladder. Ideally both seat and camera should be tilted back 10–20 degrees so that the patient can lean back against the camera and maintain the same posture comfortably

TABLE 2.1. Adult doses for renography

Radiopharmaceutical	Administered dose			
	Gamma camera		Probe	
	(MBq)	(µCi)	(MBq)	(µCi)
¹²³I-OIH	12	300	2	50
¹³¹I-OIH	4	100	1	25
⁹⁹ᵐTc-DTPA	75	2000	6	150

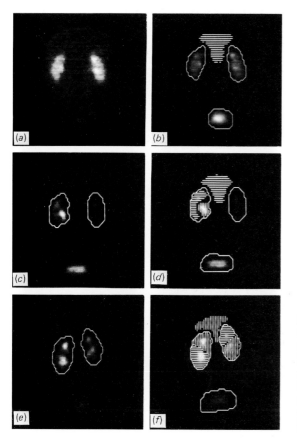

Figure 2.3 Regions of interest: (*a*) and (*b*) image of kidneys summed for 1 to 5 minutes and standard regions of interest over kidneys, background and bladder superimposed upon composite image (1–5 minutes plus 15–20 minutes); (*c*) and (*d*) separate identification of parenchymal and pelvic regions superimposed upon 10–15 minute image with kidneys outlined; (*e*) and (*f*) separate identification of intrarenal areas in a case of bilateral duplication

for up to 40 minutes. A foot-rest is essential. Several 'imaging chairs' have been designed to facilitate positioning, and *Figure 2.1* shows one in use for renography. It is helpful, particularly for children, if the sides of the chair are adjusted to prevent lateral motion of the patient during the test. Small children may be lain on top of the camera (*Figure 2.2*).

The appropriate dose of radiopharmaceutical (*see Table 2.1*) is drawn up into a syringe and measured in an isotope calibrator. It is injected intravenously, taking care to avoid any extravasation or contamination. Acquisition of images is started immediately: 20-second frames are stored in a computer system for a period of 20–40 minutes. It is also desirable to acquire analogue images of high quality every 5 minutes.

At the end of the procedure the patient again empties his bladder. This reduces radiation dose to the bladder wall, and measurement of the voided volume will permit calculation of the urine production rate during the test. This should be between 1 and 3 ml/minute to avoid dehydration effects.

The study is analysed by producing a clear summed computer image and defining regions of interest over each kidney and the bladder. A region of interest must also be defined for blood/tissue background; the area most suitable is an irregular region between and above the kidneys (*Figures 2.3a* and *b*). Curves are then obtained of detected count rate against time for each region, and the kidney and bladder curves are corrected for background by subtracting the background activity on a count-rate-per-unit-area basis. Each corrected curve is plotted with the ordinate expressed as a percentage of injected dose (*see*, for example, *Figure 2.6*). (For detailed protocol, *see* Chapter 7).

Such operator-interactive computer analysis permits many variations to the standard procedure. In particular it is sometimes useful to identify renal parenchyma and pelvic regions separately (*Figures 2.3c* and *d*) and to obtain renogram curves for each. Furthermore, individual intrarenal areas of interest may be identified (*Figures 2.3e* and *f*) and selective renograms obtained.

Probe renography

It is possible to obtain renogram curves without imaging by the use of a dual or multiple probe detector system such as that shown in *Figure 2.4*. One detector is positioned behind each renal area, and additional information may be obtained from further detectors over the bladder and over the right infraclavicular area (for measuring blood background activity). After the patient and detectors have been positioned, an injection of the appropriate radiopharmaceutical is given (*see Table 2.1*); for classic

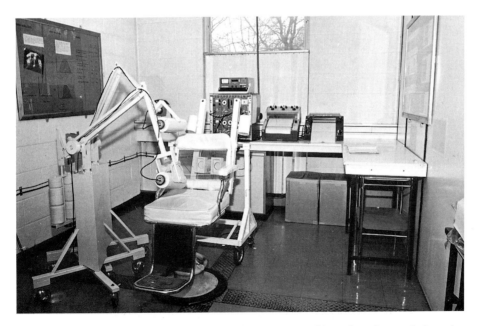

Figure 2.4 Detectors used for probe renography incorporated into dental-type chair and linked to scintillation detector channels and chart recorder

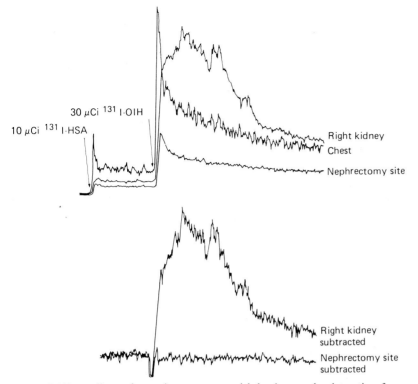

30 µCi ^{131}I-OIH

10 µCi ^{131}I-HSA

Right kidney
Chest
Nephrectomy site

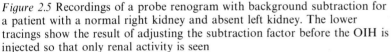

Right kidney
subtracted
Nephrectomy site
subtracted

Figure 2.5 Recordings of a probe renogram with background subtraction for
a patient with a normal right kidney and absent left kidney. The lower
tracings show the result of adjusting the subtraction factor before the OIH is
injected so that only renal activity is seen

probe renography this would be ^{131}I-OIH. Each scintillation detector channel is
connected to a chart recorder: the output from the two channels representing each
kidney constitutes a raw, or uncorrected, renogram. With this system it is not possible
to do a simple subtraction for blood background correction, as the field of view of each
detector is ill-defined. One approach to this problem is to perform 'analogue blood
background subtraction renography' which involves a preliminary injection of an
intravascular tracer such as ^{131}I human serum albumin (HSA) so that circuitry may be
adjusted to subtract a proportion of the background count rate from each kidney count
rate (*Figure 2.5*). Another approach is to perform more complex mathematical analysis
of the raw renograms (*see* below, and Chapter 18).

Accurate positioning obtained by using the patient's anatomical landmarks to locate
the renal areas is more important if the probe system is used than with gamma camera
renography.

The detectors used for the probe system are fitted with collimators giving a field of
view of 17 cm (vertical) by 9 cm depth (*see* Chapter 16).

Interpretation of the renogram

The gamma camera renogram comprises a series of images and a set of derived blood-
background subtracted curves (*Figure 2.6*). The normal renogram curve shows three
classic phases. The first phase is a rapid rise immediately following the intravenous

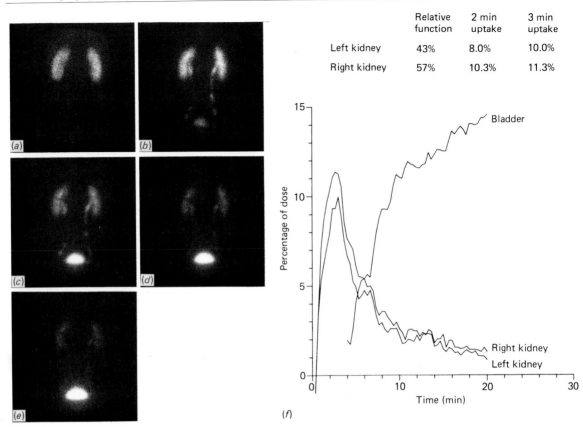

	Relative function	2 min uptake	3 min uptake
Left kidney	43%	8.0%	10.0%
Right kidney	57%	10.3%	11.3%

Figure 2.6 Normal gamma camera renogram: (*a*) to (*e*) analogue images at $0-2\frac{1}{2}$, $2\frac{1}{2}-5$, 5–10, 10–15 and 15–20 minutes after injection; (*f*) derived renogram curves with ordinate expressed as percentage of dose injected

injection of radiopharmaceutical which reflects the speed of injection and the vascular supply to the kidney. After a few seconds this gives way to a more gradual slope—the second phase—which corresponds to the renal handling of the OIH as it is taken up by the kidney and passed through the tubular cells to the lumen of the nephrons. The shape and duration of this part of the curve are dependent on several factors including supply rate, extraction efficiency, intraluminal transit and excretion. The rising curve represents a period when more OIH is being extracted by the kidney from the circulation, while none has yet left the kidney. If no activity were excreted, for example because of an obstructive process, this second phase would continue (*Figure 2.7*). In the normal kidney, however, at 2–5 minutes, the curve reaches a peak and activity starts to leave the renal area—the beginning of the third phase. This point corresponds to the time at which activity first appears in the bladder. The peak can be delayed by a variety of conditions, such as an obstructive process preventing excretion of tracer, renal artery stenosis causing a more prolonged, gradual supply of tracer to the kidney, low urine flow rate, or parenchymal disease (*Figure 2.8*); these conditions can also influence the slope of both second and third phases. The third phase of the curve is predominantly, but not exclusively, excretory; it reflects the balance achieved between the amount of OIH arriving at the kidney and that leaving it. If the kidney has no function, the corrected curve will be zero because the uncorrected curve will resemble that of blood background activity (*Figure 2.9*).

The gamma camera technique has the advantage over the use of probes for

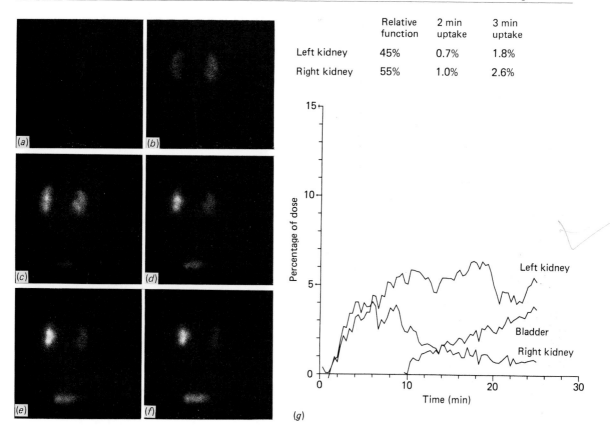

	Relative function	2 min uptake	3 min uptake
Left kidney	45%	0.7%	1.8%
Right kidney	55%	1.0%	2.6%

Figure 2.7 Renogram showing an obstructive pattern on left side: (*a*) to (*f*) analogue images at 0–2½, 2½–5, 5–10, 10–15, 15–20 and 20–25 minutes; (*g*) derived renogram curves

renography as it produces pictures of the urinary system and gives useful morphological information which complements that available from intravenous urography and other imaging techniques. However, it is the functional and urodynamic data rather than structural images which are the dominant features of renography. If the detector is equally sensitive to activity in each kidney (i.e. assuming the same depth for each kidney), then during the second phase of the renogram the ratio of background-corrected uptakes between left and right will be equal to the ratio of their renal plasma flow (or their GFRs if DTPA is used). A useful practical method is to evaluate the mean uptake for each kidney by calculating the area under each background-corrected renogram between 1 minute after injection and an end-point defined as 20 seconds before the first peak or 3 minutes, whichever occurs earlier. Individual relative renal function is then expressed in percentage terms as the ratio of the mean uptake for each kidney to the sum of the two.

Estimates of relative function can be vital to patient management in unilateral disease such as that caused by stones, reflux, pelvi-ureteric junction obstruction, etc. The use of OIH for this purpose has been widely evaluated, while in recent studies DTPA has shown similar accuracy (Dubovsky and Russell, 1982). There is no evidence to show that it is an advantage to measure individual ERPF rather than GFR in the majority of clinical conditions requiring divided studies, although OIH has been seen to produce clearer images and more accurate results at reduced levels of function because of higher target-to-background ratios (Jewkes and Jayasingh, 1981).

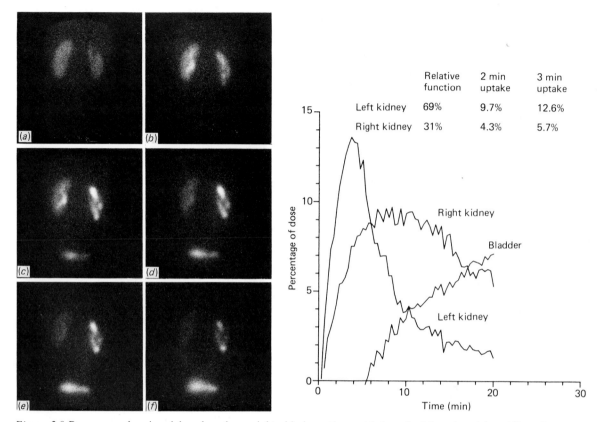

	Relative function	2 min uptake	3 min uptake
Left kidney	69%	9.7%	12.6%
Right kidney	31%	4.3%	5.7%

Figure 2.8 Renogram showing delayed peak on right side in patient with impaired function: (*a*) to (*f*) analogue images at 0–$2\frac{1}{2}$, $2\frac{1}{2}$–5, 5–10, 10–15, 15–20 and 20–25 minutes; (*g*) derived renogram curves

For accurate, reproducible results, attention to detail is vital. The first 2 minutes of the test may influence a clinical decision on conservation or nephrectomy. A moving patient, inaccurate mapping of regions of interest, or variations in kidney position, depth and size may all affect the ultimate values.

The shape of the curve after the peak will reflect the urodynamic behaviour of the kidney and the transit through the pelvicalyceal systems to the ureters and bladder. The third phase is highly sensitive to abnormalities in the outflow tract, and a normal pattern excludes the presence of even trivial degrees of obstruction. It is not uncommon for elimination to proceed stepwise (*Figure 2.10*). The cause for this is not clear. Elimination is efficient and complete, and there is nothing to suggest it is an obstructive phenomenon. It may represent a variation in the volume and speed of bolus formation and peristaltic rate. Another finding is saw-tooth waves on the downslope. These may be gross (*Figure 2.11*) and, if occurring in a patient with urinary tract duplication or suspected reflux, they may be indicative of abnormalities of transport such as yo-yoing or vesico-ureteric reflux (*see* Chapter 4). Occasionally minor degrees of saw-tooth can be seen in the renogram performed in ureteric stone disease. Here the explanation may lie in retrograde peristalsis. This occurs as a bolus hits the obstructed ureteric segment causing delay in its progress and a localized, acute dilatation; a weak retrograde peristaltic wave is induced delaying excretion or even causing a tiny amount of reflux of activity.

Severe degrees of impeded flow will be reflected in the shape of the curve (*Figure*

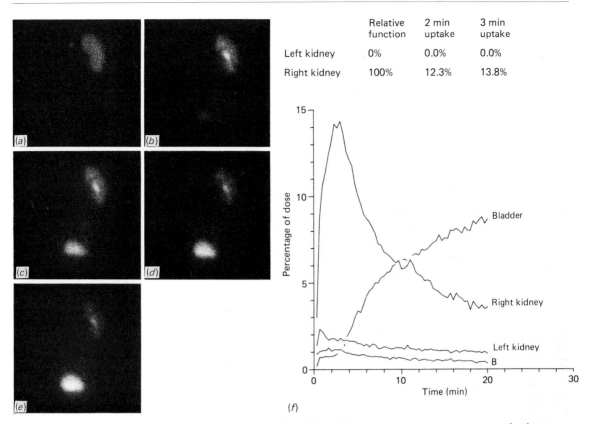

	Relative function	2 min uptake	3 min uptake
Left kidney	0%	0.0%	0.0%
Right kidney	100%	12.3%	13.8%

Figure 2.9 Renogram in patient with non-functioning left kidney: (*a*) to (*e*) analogue images at 0–2½, 2½–5, 5–10, 10–15 and 15–20 minutes; (*f*) uncorrected derived renogram curves showing left kidney trace similar to background trace (B)

2.12). In complete obstruction, no peak occurs and the second phase simply persists. It is vital when interpreting this pattern to appreciate that delay in elimination may also be caused by retention of activity in the renal areas for reasons other than obstruction. Thus dehydration will mimic obstruction while dilatation of the outflow tract without obstruction will often be indistinguishable from genuine obstruction on the standard renogram. It is for this reason that the modification of diuresis renography was introduced.

Diuresis renography

This technique is based on the phenomenon that an obstructed dilated upper urinary tract will be obstructed at low and high flow rates. A non-obstructed, dilated tract may appear obstructed at low flow rates due to stasis, but high flow rates induced by a diuretic will eliminate stasis and produce unimpeded washout from the upper tract. The technique is simple. If renography is to be performed in a patient with suspected obstruction or a dilated upper tract, 0.5 mg/kg of frusemide should be given intravenously 20 minutes after the radiopharmaceutical to observe its effect on the curve and particularly on any retained tracer. Alternatively the procedure can be performed giving the frusemide before the radiopharmaceutical to ensure a high flow rate during

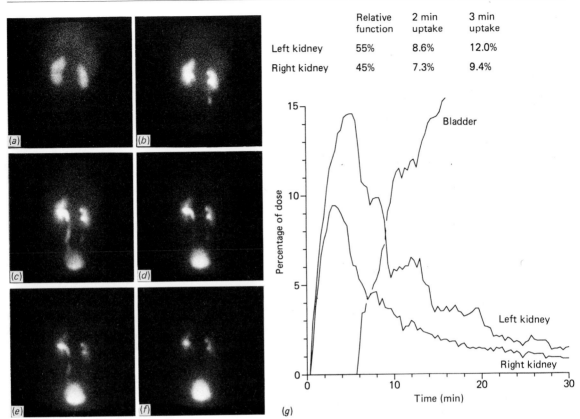

	Relative function	2 min uptake	3 min uptake
Left kidney	55%	8.6%	12.0%
Right kidney	45%	7.3%	9.4%

Figure 2.10 Renogram showing stepwise elimination on left kidney curve: (*a*) to (*f*) analogue image at $0–2\frac{1}{2}$, $2\frac{1}{2}–5$, 5–10, 10–15, 15–20 and 20–25 minutes; (*g*) derived renogram curves

the whole test (*Figure 2.13*). In practice, the former method is often more useful, demonstrating the curve before and after the diuretic stimulus and permitting estimates of relative function unaffected by the diuretic. If diuretic techniques are to be employed their use must include knowledge of their effects and responses in states of altered renal function. The patient must be well- or even hyperhydrated to ensure a good response to the diuretic. Frusemide has a greater maximum potency than other diuretics. Its effect is usually unimpaired down to GFRs between 15 and 20 ml/minute. At these levels its effects may vary while remaining broadly proportional to the clearance values. Below a GFR of 10 ml/minute however, it becomes less predictable and efficient. Even when a good diuresis is achieved a response may be delayed by many minutes and may be more drawn out and prolonged than in the normal kidney. Increasing the administered dose will not improve this immediate response, and it is a rapid, brisk diuretic response upon which the rationale of the diuresis renogram depends—a sudden and significant increase in the urine flow rate to test the outflow tract. Despite this problem, the vast majority of cases of urinary tract dilatation will be categorized easily by the procedure. An obstructive curve which remains obstructive during diuresis indicates obstruction (*Figure 2.14*). An obstructive curve which suddenly gives way to rapid elimination under diuresis indicates a dilated non-obstructed tract (*Figure 2.15*). Equivocal responses will require further clarification. The clinical applications of diuresis renography are fully discussed in Chapter 8.

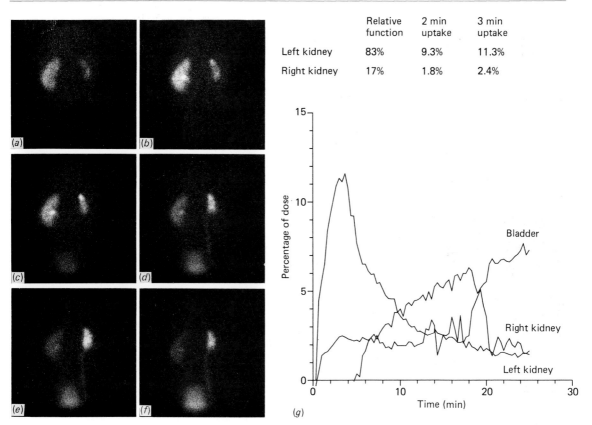

	Relative function	2 min uptake	3 min uptake
Left kidney	83%	9.3%	11.3%
Right kidney	17%	1.8%	2.4%

Figure 2.11 Gross saw-tooth waves on right kidney curve in patient with vesico-ureteric reflux: (*a*) to (*f*) analogue images at 0–2½, 2½–5, 5–10, 10–15, 15–20 and 20–25 minutes; (*g*) derived renogram curves

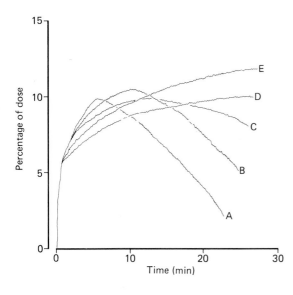

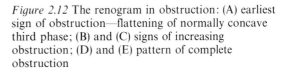

Figure 2.12 The renogram in obstruction: (A) earliest sign of obstruction—flattening of normally concave third phase; (B) and (C) signs of increasing obstruction; (D) and (E) pattern of complete obstruction

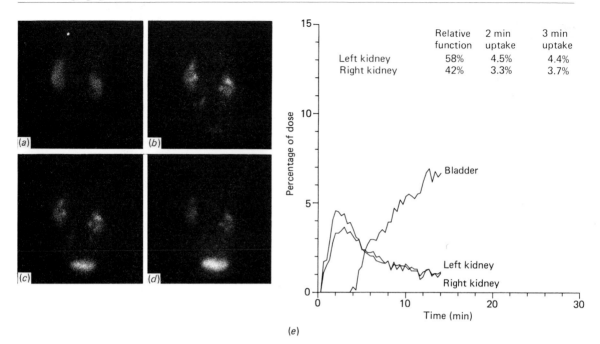

	Relative function	2 min uptake	3 min uptake
Left kidney	58%	4.5%	4.4%
Right kidney	42%	3.3%	3.7%

Figure 2.13A Standard gamma camera renogram in patient prior to diuresis study: (*a*) to (*d*) analogue images at 0–2½, 2½–5, 5–10, 10–15 minutes after injection; (*e*) derived renogram curves

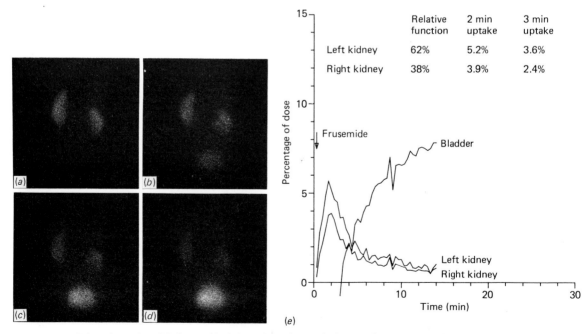

	Relative function	2 min uptake	3 min uptake
Left kidney	62%	5.2%	3.6%
Right kidney	38%	3.9%	2.4%

Figure 2.13B Diuresis study with frusemide injected 3 minutes before radiopharmaceutical; normal response: (*a*) to (*d*) analogue images at 0–2½, 2½–5, 5–10, 10–15 minutes after injection of radiopharmaceutical; (*e*) derived renogram curves

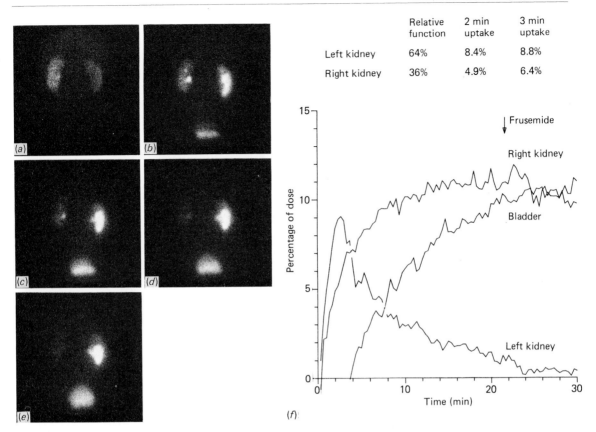

	Relative function	2 min uptake	3 min uptake
Left kidney	64%	8.4%	8.8%
Right kidney	36%	4.9%	6.4%

Figure 2.14 Gamma camera diuresis renogram in case of dilated obstructed right renal pelvis; frusemide injected 20 minutes after radiopharmaceutical: (*a*) to (*e*) analogue images at 0–2½, 5–10, 15–20, 20–25 and 25–30 minutes; (*f*) derived renogram curves. Note persistent retention of tracer in right kidney images and lack of response to frusemide in derived curve

Deconvolution of the renogram

The renogram curves obtained by either the probe or gamma camera methods described above represent the response of the kidney to an arterial input of labelled compound which is changing in time: the arterial concentration rises suddenly initially and then gradually falls during the test, as indicated by the blood background curve. Many workers have asked what the shape of the renogram would be if it were possible to give a single bolus injection into the aorta proximal to the renal arteries, and to eliminate any recirculation. The resulting kidney activity time curve would be an 'impulse retention function': the response of the kidney to an impulse input.

It is possible to calculate an estimate of this curve from a knowledge of the observed renogram together with simultaneous measurement of the blood activity. The latter gives the actual 'input function' to the kidney, and the mathematical technique whereby the impulse retention function is derived from these two curves is known as 'deconvolution', or unfolding. This is described in detail in Chapter 18. Note that the blood activity curve used for the input function should indicate activity entering the renal arteries and that this implies a different region of interest from that used to measure blood and tissue background subtraction—as the contribution of tissue background is clearly separate on the impulse retention function (*see* below).

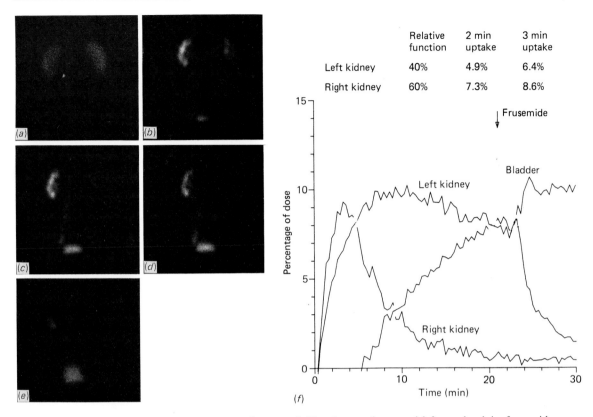

Figure 2.15 Gamma camera diuresis renogram in case of dilated, non-obstructed left renal pelvis; frusemide injected 20 minutes after radiopharmaceutical: (*a*) to (*e*) analogue images at 0–2½, 5–10, 15–20, 20–25 and 25–30 minutes; (*f*) derived renogram curves. Note rapid washout of tracer from left kidney images and rapid response to frusemide in derived curve

Figure 2.16 shows a typical result from a normal patient. The first few points represent blood/tissue background; bearing in mind the hypothetical conditions of arterial bolus input and no recirculation, any activity in non-renal tissues would be eliminated rapidly. There is then a plateau representing tracer which has entered the kidney. The height of this plateau is proportional to the individual renal clearance. This method does not yield a value for clearance in absolute units, but the relative heights for the two kidneys may be used to assess individual percentage function.

The length of the plateau indicates the shortest transit time of tracer through the kidney, and the point at which the function falls to zero indicates the longest transit time. Thus the slope of the fall-off in retention function indicates the spread of transit times. The parameter most often quoted in association with this analysis is the mean transit time, and *Table 2.2* gives normal values measured using ^{123}I-OIH and ^{99m}Tc-DTPA.

Unfortunately there may be a difference between theory and practice in this difficult field; the effects of statistical noise and physiological fluctuations can be compounded by the mathematical analysis to produce results which are often 'noisy' and difficult to interpret—particularly if renal function is impaired. Nevertheless the method can be used diagnostically (*see Figure 2.17*).

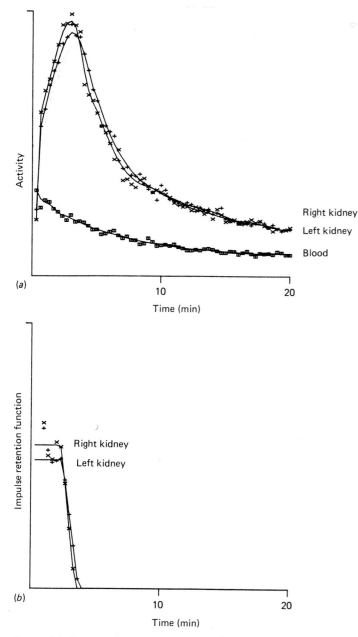

Figure 2.16 Deconvolution applied to a normal renogram. The
kidneys have nearly equal uptake and normal mean transit times of
2.8 minutes: (*a*) standard activity–time curves. The points indicate
the raw data and the solid lines the smoothed curves used for
deconvolution; (*b*) impulse retention functions. The first two points
in each curve, which include the background contribution, are off
the top of the scale, and points beyond the time at which the curve
reaches zero have been suppressed for clarity. The solid line
indicates the retention function after having been trimmed to
remove background and constrained to be a monotonically
decreasing function

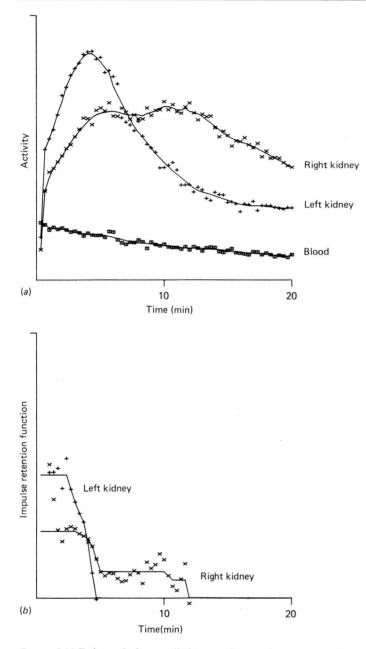

Figure 2.17 Deconvolution applied to an abnormal renogram. The left kidney has a mean transit time of 3.5 minutes, within normal limits. The right kidney is contributing 38% of total renal function and has a prolonged mean transit time of 7.0 minutes due to retention of tracer in a dilated renal pelvis: (*a*) standard activity–time curves—same format as *Figure 2.16a*; (*b*) impulse retention functions—same format as *Figure 2.16b*

TABLE 2.2. Transit times of OIH and DTPA

Radiopharmaceutical	Region	Transit times (minutes) (mean ± s.d.)		
		Minimum	Maximum	Mean
^{123}I-OIH	Whole kidney	2.0 ± 0.6	4.1 ± 1.8	3.1 ± 1.1
	Parenchyma	1.8 ± 0.4	2.7 ± 1.1	2.2 ± 0.7
^{99m}Tc-DTPA	Whole kidney	1.9 ± 0.3	4.2 ± 1.1	3.4 ± 1.1
	Parenchyma	1.9 ± 0.3	3.3 ± 0.7	2.6 ± 0.5

Each figure is the mean and estimated standard deviation of results obtained from deconvolution analysis of renograms of 12 normal kidneys.

In conclusion, gamma camera renography will provide the clinician with information unavailable from any other procedure, that is an estimate of individual renal function combined with synchronous information on urodynamic transport through each renal outflow tract. It will be demonstrated in Part 2 how valuable this investigation can be in practice and how the procedure can be tailored to particular clinical situations by employing various modifications. It is no exaggeration to state that the modern practice of urology and nephrology is incomplete without the availability of facilities for quantitative gamma camera renography.

References

DUBOVSKY, E. V. and RUSSELL, C. D. (1982) Quantification of renal function with glomerular and tubular agents. *Seminars in Nuclear Medicine*, **12**, 4

JEWKES, R. F. and JAYASINGH, K. (1981) Comparison of ^{123}I-hippuran and ^{99m}Tc DTPA. *Nuclear Medicine Communications*, **2**, 278–288

KÅUDE, J. and NORDENPORT, J. (1973) Influence of nephroangiography on ^{131}I-hippuran renography. *Acta Radiologica*, **14**, 69

3 Radionuclide renal imaging

P. H. O'Reilly, R. A. Shields and H. J. Testa

This chapter describes those radionuclide imaging procedures, other than renography, which may be used to obtain further information on aspects of renal function or structure, particularly the integrity of the renal parenchyma. Such procedures are of value in the investigation of tumours, cysts, pseudotumours, infarcts, infections and scars; the results are complementary to those obtained by other imaging modalities.

Several radiopharmaceuticals may be used for renal imaging; the ^{99m}Tc-labelled agents are the most popular because of the excellent physical properties of the radionuclide. Compounds such as DTPA, gluconate and DMSA are all useful and have their own specific advantages and disadvantages.

The renal scan is performed in two parts, referred to as the vascular and the parenchymal studies. The vascular study gives a visual representation of aortic flow and renal perfusion, while the parenchymal images reflect renal morphology and early excretory events. The vascular study is usually carried out in the posterior projection— that is, with the patient sitting or prone and the camera resting against his back (*see Figure 2.1*, p. 10). Young babies may be examined lying on top of the collimator (*see Figure 2.2*, p. 10). In some situations (e.g. horseshoe kidney, pelvic kidney, renal transplant, trauma) the anterior projection will be more appropriate. The technique of injection is vital to obtain a rapid first circulation of the tracer. An intermittent infusion needle (butterfly cannula) is inserted into a suitable antecubital vein and taped into position. Two syringes are prepared, one containing 10 ml normal saline and the other 400 MBq (10 mCi) of the radiopharmaceutical (200 MBq (5 mCi) if DMSA is used). Flow is established by injecting a few millilitres of the saline, after which this injection is stopped momentarily. At this point the radiopharmaceutical is injected, keeping just enough pressure on the saline plunger to prevent backflow. Immediately after this, the remainder of the saline is injected rapidly as a bolus to force the scanning agent into the vascular system. One-second frames are collected and stored in the computer for 60 seconds, commencing at 5 seconds after the injection, and at the same time analogue pictures are obtained at 5-second intervals. Following this, 2-minute static images are collected for the parenchymal study, at the same time producing analogue pictures. An anterior view should also be taken, and if this demonstrates a region of reduced uptake not seen on the posterior view, the vascular study should be repeated in the anterior position. The static images give information on the parenchymal concentration of the tracer and its subsequent elimination. An example of the normal renal scan performed in this way using ^{99m}Tc-gluconate is shown in *Figure 3.1*. These studies permit the

27

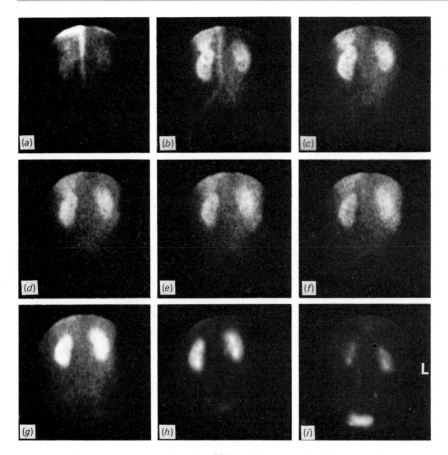

Figure 3.1 Gamma camera study using ^{99m}Tc-gluconate showing normal kidneys: (*a*) to (*f*) 5-second images of first circulation, showing transit through aorta and renal perfusion; (*g*) and (*h*) 2- and 5-minute images of parenchymal uptake; (*i*) anterior view at 9 minutes. Note that in the anterior view only, patient's left is on the right

detection of areas of abnormal flow such as tumours, inflammatory lesions, arteriovenous malformations, avascular regions (renal infarcts, abscesses, cysts), vascular anomalies (aneurysms, aortic stenoses, bifurcation grafts), transplanted kidneys and congenital abnormalities (e.g. pelvic kidneys, horseshoe kidneys; *see Figures 3.2–3.6*).

Investigation of space-occupying lesions

A space-occupying lesion of the kidney may be discovered incidentally at routine intravenous urography or may be suspected and investigated in patients who present with symptoms such as haematuria and loin pain.

If a tumour or cyst is present, areas of renal parenchyma will be replaced by non-functioning renal tissue. This can be demonstrated by the lack of uptake of the radiopharmaceutical in the affected area; the vascular phase of the study will demonstrate whether or not the lesion is perfused (*Figures 3.7–3.9*).

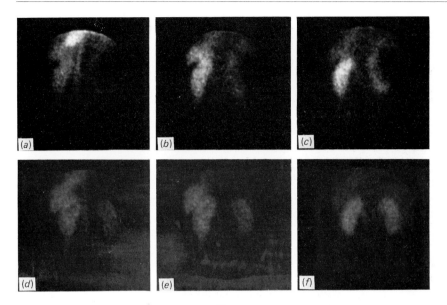

Figure 3.2 Gamma camera study using ^{99m}Tc-gluconate in a case of renal carbuncle: (*a*) and (*b*) 5-second images of first circulation; (*c*) 2-minute image of parenchymal uptake, showing non-vascular space-occupying lesion involving upper and middle regions of right kidney; (*d*) to (*f*) corresponding images after treatment showing complete return to normal

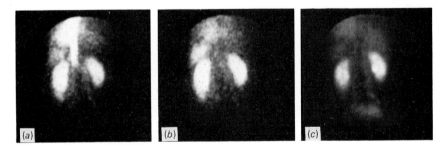

Figure 3.3 Gamma camera study using ^{99m}Tc-gluconate in a case of aortic stenosis: (*a*) and (*b*) 5-second images of first circulation; (*c*) 2-minute image of parenchymal uptake. Note sharp cut-off to aortic flow with preserved renal perfusion and uptake

The clinical value of radionuclide scanning in the detection of space-occupying lesions has to be considered against other available imaging modalities. The intravenous urogram is usually the first procedure to be performed, but in many cases more information is required to establish the nature of renal space-occupying lesions. In studies in which radiographic and tissue diagnoses have been compared the false negative rate (cancer being misdiagnosed as benign) has been over 10% (Clayman, Williams and Fraley, 1979). After urography, therefore, further investigation of renal mass lesions is necessary, and this may be done by ultrasound, radionuclide studies, computed tomography, arteriography or digital radiography. These tests reflect different physiological and physical characteristics of the kidneys and are complementary rather than competitive. They are discussed in detail in Chapter 9.

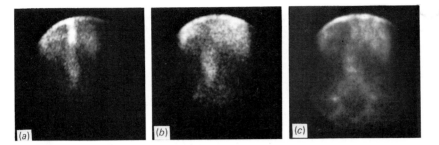

Figure 3.4 Gamma camera study using ^{99m}Tc-gluconate in a case of aortic aneurysm: (*a*) and (*b*) 5-second images of first circulation; (*c*) 2-minute image of parenchymal uptake. Note aortic dilatation and absent renal perfusion and uptake

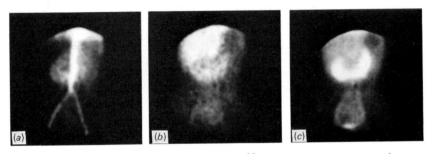

Figure 3.5 Anterior gamma camera study using ^{99m}Tc-gluconate in a case of horseshoe kidney: (*a*) and (*b*) 5-second images of first circulation; (*c*) 5-minute image of parenchymal uptake. Note perfusion and uptake in isthmus

Investigation of inflammatory disease

Several radionuclide procedures are now available to study patients with pyelonephritis. These include the assessment of renal parenchyma using ^{99m}Tc-DMSA or ^{99m}Tc-gluconate, and the investigation of infection using ^{67}Ga-gallium citrate.

Chronic pyelonephritis

In chronic pyelonephritis the detection of renal scarring by radionuclide scanning using ^{99m}Tc-DMSA has been reported to have sensitivity and specificity significantly better than urography (Merrick, Uttley and Wild, 1980).

The studies are carried out by injecting 200 MBq (5 mCi) of ^{99m}Tc-DMSA intravenously. The only patient preparation required is adequate hydration. Images of at least 200 000 counts are obtained and stored in the computer in anterior, posterior and oblique views, 2–6 hours after injection (*Figures 3.10–3.12*). Uptake by the renal parenchyma is visualized clearly since activity is retained by the cortical tubules reaching a plateau at 6 hours and remaining constant for 24 hours. During this period approximately 30% of the dose is excreted in the urine, reducing significantly the background activity and consequently enhancing the kidney-to-background ratios.

Quantitative analysis of the renal uptake allows the calculation of relative renal function and, indeed, absolute individual renal function (*see* Chapter 18). Morales, Evans and Gordon (1984) showed that the uptake is approximately 17% of the injected

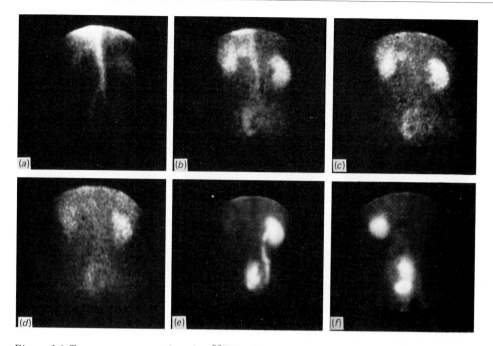

Figure 3.6 Gamma camera study using ^{99m}Tc-gluconate in a case of pelvic kidney: (*a*) to (*d*) 5-second images of first circulation; (*e*) 5-minute image of parenchymal uptake; (*f*) 7-minute *anterior* image of parenchymal uptake

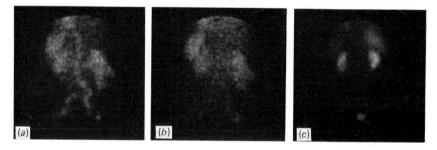

Figure 3.7 Gamma camera study using ^{99m}Tc-gluconate in a case of hypernephroma of the right kidney: (*a*) and (*b*) 5-second images of first circulation; (*c*) 5-minute image of parenchymal uptake. Note tumour circulation in lower pole of right kidney and lack of uptake in corresponding area on parenchymal image

dose in each kidney. Abnormal function may be detected by decreased uptake, while increased uptake may be seen in compensatory hypertrophy. Recent work using rotating gamma cameras (single photon emission tomography) permits functioning renal volume to be estimated by summing the ^{99m}Tc-DMSA distribution volumes of the transaxial slices in the whole kidney (Tauxe *et al.*, 1983; Kawamura *et al.*, 1984). The dimensions of the kidneys compared well with those obtained with ultrasound studies. There is also close agreement between renal volume and DMSA renal uptake. The clinical application of emission tomography needs further evaluation but its usefulness is envisaged in the diagnosis of early graft rejection and of glomerulonephritis.

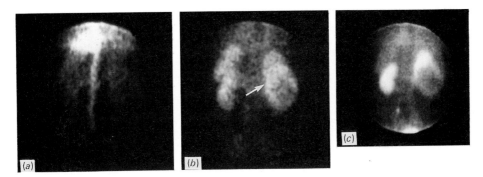

Figure 3.8 Gamma camera study using ^{99m}Tc-gluconate in a case of right hypernephroma:
(*a*) and (*b*) 5-second images of first circulation; (*c*) 5-minute image of parenchymal uptake.
Note tumour circulation in middle region of the right kidney (arrow) corresponding to
lack of uptake in corresponding area on parenchymal image, but also note cold areas on
vascular and parenchymal images in lower pole indicating necrotic tumour

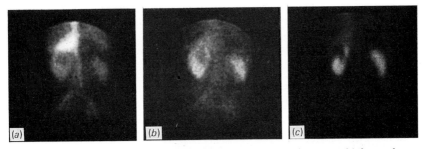

Figure 3.9 Gamma camera study using ^{99m}Tc-gluconate in a case of left renal
cyst: (*a*) and (*b*) 5-second images of first circulation; (*c*) 5-minute image of
parenchymal uptake. Note non-vascular area in upper pole of left kidney
corresponding to lack of uptake in corresponding area on parenchymal image

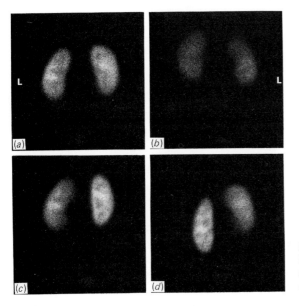

Figure 3.10 Gamma camera study using ^{99m}Tc-
DMSA showing normal kidneys: (*a*) posterior; (*b*)
anterior; (*c*) right posterior oblique; (*d*) left posterior
oblique

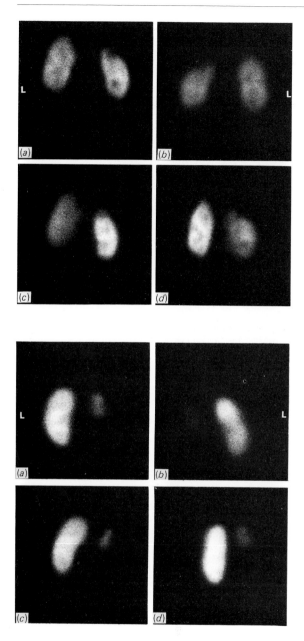

Figure 3.11 Gamma camera study using ^{99m}Tc-DMSA in case of renal scarring: (*a*) posterior; (*b*) anterior; (*c*) right posterior oblique; (*d*) left posterior oblique. Note parenchymal defect in upper pole of right kidney corresponding to cortical scar

Figure 3.12 Gamma camera study using ^{99m}Tc-DMSA, in case of end-stage reflux nephropathy of right kidney: (*a*) posterior; (*b*) anterior; (*c*) right posterior oblique; (*d*) left posterior oblique

Acute pyelonephritis

In acute pyelonephritis cortical imaging agents such as ^{99m}Tc-DMSA give information on regional and global parenchymal function and morphology, and are also useful to monitor the response to treatment; these studies may be complemented using ^{67}Ga-gallium citrate (*Figure 3.13*) to localize areas of focal bacterial infection (Handmaker, 1982).

Gallium citrate is injected intravenously in doses of 80–160 MBq (2–4 mCi) and reduced in relation to body weight in children. Images are obtained using a gamma

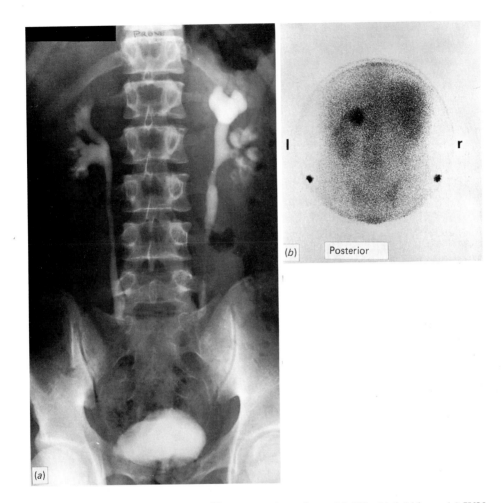

Figure 3.13 Gamma camera study using ^{67}Ga citrate in patient with TB of left kidney: (*a*) IVU showing gross clubbing, particularly involving upper pole calyces; (*b*) 48-hour gallium image showing increased uptake of gallium in upper pole of left kidney

camera after 24–48 hours in order to achieve good target-to-background ratios. Gallium localizes in polymorphonuclear leucocytes and in areas of high tissue concentration of lactoferrin, which is a major component of the soluble protein fraction of neutrophilic leucocytes (Hoffer, Huberty and Khayam-Bashi, 1977). This may explain its localization at sites of infection.

Unfortunately normal concentrations of gallium by the kidneys may interfere with interpretation of pathological uptake (Frankel *et al.*, 1975). Difficulties also arise because it is impossible to distinguish between intrarenal and extrarenal infections. However, gallium studies have been shown to have an accuracy of 86% in differentiating between upper and lower tract infection, and this compares well with other procedures used to detect acute pyelonephritis (Hurwitz *et al.*, 1976; Schardijn *et al.*, 1984). When a parenchymal abnormality is detected with a ^{99m}Tc-DMSA study, increased uptake of gallium in that area will be a clear indicator of infection (Handmaker, 1982) (*see* Chapter 14).

Investigation of reflux

Traditionally, the investigation of this problem and its follow-up has been by micturating cystourethrography (MCU), using radiographic contrast media instilled into the bladder through a urethral catheter. This procedure is of great value, although it has two main disadvantages: it is invasive, requiring the introduction of a catheter into the bladder; and it delivers a high radiation dose to the patient, estimated to be of the order of 1 cGy (1 rad) (Fendel, 1970). Reflux of radioactive urine was first reported by Winter (1959). Since that time indirect methods, avoiding the need for urethral catheterization, and direct methods of *radionuclide* cystography have both been developed. These are considered in detail in the next chapter.

References

CLAYMAN, R. V., WILLIAMS, R. D. and FRALEY, E. E. (1979) The pursuit of the renal mass. *New England Journal of Medicine*, **300**, 72–74

FENDEL, H. (1970) Radiation exposure due to urinary tract disease. *Progress in Pediatric Radiology*, **3**, 116–120

FRANKEL, R. S., RICHMAN, S. O., LEVENSON, S. M. and JOHNSTON, G. S. (1975) Renal localisation of gallium-67 citrate. *Radiology*, **114**, 393–397

HANDMAKER, H. (1982) Nuclear renal imaging in acute pyelonephritis. *Seminars in Nuclear Medicine*, **12**, 246–253

HOFFER, P. B., HUBERTY, J. and KHAYAM-BASHI, H. (1977) The association of Ga-67 and lactoferrin. *Journal of Nuclear Medicine*, **18**, 713–717

HURWITZ, S. R., KESSLER, W. D. and ALAZRAKI, N. P. (1976) Gallium-67 imaging to localise urinary tract infections. *British Journal of Radiology*, **49**, 156–160

KAWAMURA, J., ITOH, H., YOSHIDA, O., FUJITA, T. and TORIZUKA, K. (1984) In vivo estimation of renal volume using a rotating gamma camera for ^{99m}Tc-dimercaptosuccinic acid renal imaging. *European Journal of Nuclear Medicine*, **9**, 168–172

MERRICK, M. V., UTTLEY, W. S. and WILD, M. B. (1980) The detection of pyelonephritic scarring in children by radioisotope imaging. *British Journal of Radiology*, **53**, 544–546

MORALES, B., EVANS, K. and GORDON, I. (1984) Absolute quantitation of ^{99m}Tc-DMSA in paediatrics. *Nuclear Medicine Communications*, **5**, 212 (abstract)

SCHARDIJN, G. H. C., STATIUS VAN EPS, L. W., PAUW, W., HOEFNAGEL, C. and NOOYEN, W. J. (1984) Comparison of reliability of tests to distinguish upper from lower urinary tract infection. *British Medical Journal*, **289**, 284–287

TAUXE, W. N., TODD-POKROPEK, A., SOUSSALINE, F., RAYNAUD, C. and KELLERSHOHN, C. (1983) Estimates of kidney volume by single photon emission tomography: A preliminary report. *European Journal of Nuclear Medicine*, **8**, 72–74

WINTER, C. C. (1959) A new test for vesico-ureteric reflux: an external technique using radioisotopes. *Journal of Urology*, **81**, 105–111

4 Reflux studies

C. R. A. Bevis

The function of the urinary tract is to transport urine from the collecting ducts of the kidney via the calyces, renal pelvis, ureter and bladder to the exterior. The bladder is the only storage organ along this route. Pacemaker-induced contractions, assisted by hydrostatic pressure and nephron pressure, propel urine from the minor calyces to the distal renal pelvis and ureter where a bolus is formed. Peristaltic contractions then transport successive boluses towards the bladder at a rate of 2–6 per minute. The terminal 2 cm of ureter enters the bladder at an angle to take an oblique intramural course to the ureteric meatus—an arrangement which prevents the retrograde passage of urine from bladder to ureter when the intravesical pressure rises during micturition.

The retrograde passage of urine against this one-way system is always abnormal. The most common form is vesico-ureteric reflux. This can occur through a normally situated ureteric orifice or ureterocele draining a single kidney and ureter, but it is more common in complete ureteric duplication. It may be present in both duplicated ureters, but is more likely in the one draining the lower renal moiety. It may also result from damage to a ureteric orifice during such procedures as transurethral resection of bladder tumours, ureteric meatotomy or Dormia basket stone extraction. Reflux may also occur between the two moieties of an incomplete duplication, when the ureters join somewhere along their course to empty into the bladder by a common stem.

Reflux may have several consequences. It may cause renal damage due to the passage of infected urine from the bladder to the kidney, and the presence of a 'functional residual urine' in the upper tracts may lead to dilatation, stasis, infection, and stone formation. Reflux nephropathy is probably the commonest cause of chronic renal failure in children (Bailey, 1981); however, reflux can be expected to cease spontaneously in approximately 50% of affected ureters before the age of 12 years (Baker *et al.*, 1966; Rolleston *et al.*, 1970; Lenaghan *et al.*, 1976; Edwards *et al.*, 1977).

The importance of this condition has emphasized the need for investigations to determine the presence and severity of reflux, so that either corrective surgery or conservative management may be undertaken and subsequently reviewed. In the assessment of treatment, failure of kidney growth, the development of further scarring, deterioration in renal function and the incidence of urinary tract infections will all need to be considered. Both intravenous urography and radiographic micturating cystography are used and will allow the assessment of anatomical changes and of the presence of reflux (*Figure 4.1*). However, neither will detect minor changes in renal function, and the radiation dose will be high, particularly if frequent assessment is

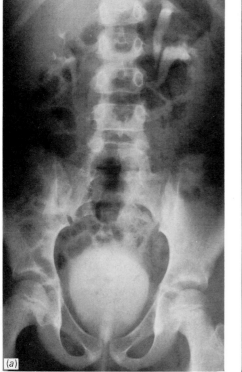 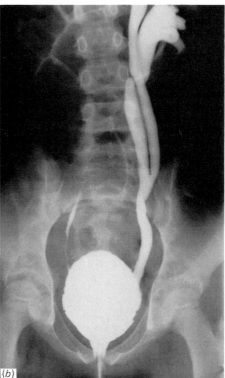

Figure 4.1a IVU showing duplication of left upper urinary tract

Figure 4.1b Radiographic micturating cystogram showing vesico-ureteric reflux into duplicated left upper urinary tract

required. Alternative methods have therefore been developed utilizing radionuclides.

Winter (1959) first reported the detection of vesico-ureteric reflux by instilling ^{131}I into the bladder and placing probe detectors over the kidney and bladder regions. Dodge (1963) described an indirect technique using the intravenous injection of ^{131}I-OIH. However, it was not until the later development of shorter half-life isotopes and the gamma camera that radionuclide studies became more widespread. Today most radionuclide reflux studies rely on the visual display of radioactivity using gamma camera computer systems rather than on the graphic record of probe detectors over the kidneys.

Direct radionuclide cystography

Direct radionuclide cystography (RNC) requires catheterization and thus shares one of the disadvantages of radiographic micturating cysto-urethrography (MCU). There is evidence, however, that the technique may be more accurate than the radiological procedures (Conway *et al.*, 1972; Conway *et al.*, 1975; Nasarallah *et al.*, 1982). The commonly used method involves the instillation of 20–40 MBq (0.5–1 mCi) ^{99m}Tc pertechnetate into the empty bladder. A gamma camera is positioned, with the patient supine, to obtain posterior views of the kidneys and bladder. Saline is instilled through a urethral catheter into the bladder at low pressure by a drip infusion, under continuous monitoring on a display oscilloscope. Simultaneous images are obtained at 5-minute

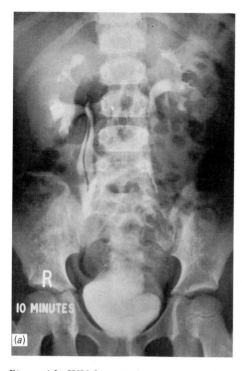 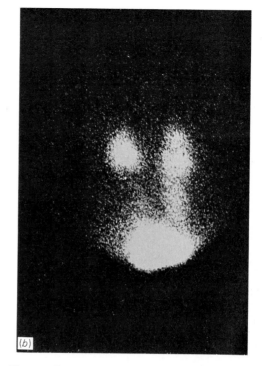

Figure 4.2a IVU from patient with complete duplication of right upper urinary tract

Figure 4.2b Radionuclide cystogram from same patient showing bilateral vesico-ureteric reflux

intervals. The saline instillation continues until the patient complains of severe urgency to void or the bladder is judged to be full. The catheter is then clamped and the patient instructed to strain as if to void. Several pictures are taken during straining. The patient is then placed either standing, or sitting on a commode, with the camera again positioned to give posterior views, and asked to void as imaging continues. An example of a radionuclide cystogram is given in *Figure 4.2*.

It is important to appreciate that the rate of urine flow can modify the presence and severity of vesico-ureteric reflux. By inducing a diuresis it is possible to reduce the severity of, or even abolish, reflux as detected by MCU (Eckman *et al.*, 1966; Fairley and Raysmith, 1977). Some standardization of the rate of urine production, possibly by preliminary fluid restriction, would therefore appear to be wise during micturating cystography.

Reflux may occur during bladder filling, straining, voiding or all three. The phenomenon tends to be intermittent and may be missed unless continuous monitoring is employed. This is impractical with radiographic techniques since the large amount of radiation involved would be unacceptable, especially in children. Fendel (1970) estimated the dose in radiographic micturating cystography to range from several mGy (several hundred mrad) in spot films, to several cGy (rad) when fluoroscopy or cine was used. In contrast, during the average 30-minute exposure to 40 MBq of ^{99m}Tc pertechnetate, the radiation dose to the bladder is approximately 0.3 mGy (30 mrad) and the gonad dose only 0.04 mGy (4 mrad) (Blaufox *et al.*, 1971; Conway *et al.*, 1972). Furthermore, continuous monitoring is performed without any increase in the radiation dose.

A major disadvantage of direct RNC is the poor resolution, as compared with MCU.

Thus co-existing abnormalities such as bladder diverticula and ureteroceles cannot be detected with certainty; also, minor reflux into the lower third of the ureter may be masked by the bladder activity, especially in children. For structural bladder information the first investigation in the patient with suspected reflux should therefore remain radiographic MCU.

Neither MCU nor direct RNC provides information about renal function or anatomy, both of which should be considered in the evaluation of treatment. For this reason indirect RNC has been considered an attractive alternative to direct RNC. Not only can it detect reflux, it will also allow the estimation of renal function, and indicate the presence of obstruction which is occasionally overlooked during the initial evaluation.

Indirect radionuclide cystography

A standard gamma camera renogram is performed with either ^{123}I-OIH or ^{99m}Tc-DTPA, as seen in *Figure 4.3*. When the radionuclide has accumulated in the bladder and renal activity is low enough to permit evaluation of voiding reflux (approximately 60 minutes after the injection), the patient is positioned either standing or sitting and posterior images of the bladder are obtained. Continuous imaging

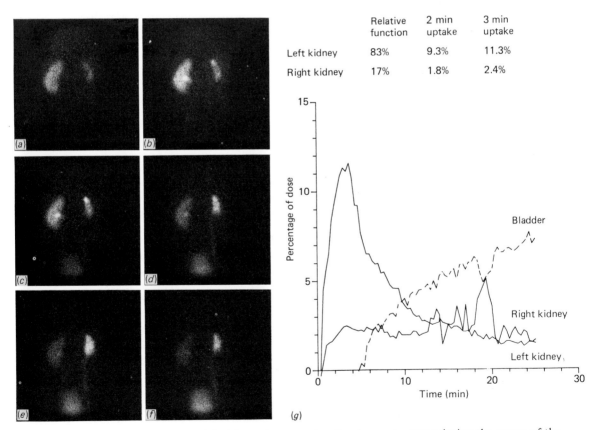

	Relative function	2 min uptake	3 min uptake
Left kidney	83%	9.3%	11.3%
Right kidney	17%	1.8%	2.4%

Figure 4.3A Standard renogram in which right vesico-ureteric reflux is seen to occur during the course of the study: (*a*) to (*f*) analogue images at $0-2\frac{1}{2}$, $2\frac{1}{2}-5$, 5–10, 10–15, 15–20 and 20–25 minutes; (*g*) derived renogram curves. Note complementary fluctuations in activity between right kidney and bladder

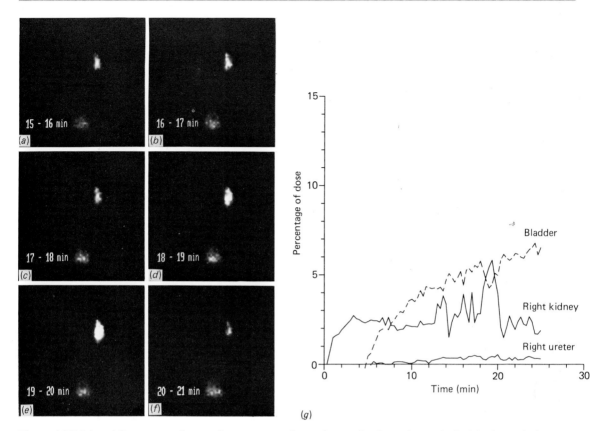

Figure 4.3B (*a*) to (*f*) computer images from same patient taken at 1-minute intervals during the period when reflux was noted; (*g*) derived curves from right kidney, right ureter and bladder

proceeds as the patient voids, and 5-second exposures are obtained (*Figure 4.4*). While the possibility of evaluating renal function and anatomy makes indirect RNC attractive, and the avoidance of catheterization abolishes the attendant risk of introducing infection, the technique has several shortcomings. It requires considerable co-operation from the patient, who must attempt to retain urine until the radionuclide has cleared from the renal areas, and then void on command. Many children can do neither. Furthermore, the presence of impaired renal function and/or hydronephrosis can lead to the retention of tracer in the kidneys for long periods and may mask small degrees of reflux. Finally, reflux during the bladder-filling phase may be missed unless continuous monitoring is employed throughout. This is impractical, due to the length of time involved. For these reasons it is likely that direct RNC is more reliable than the indirect technique in the diagnosis of reflux (Conway and Kruglik, 1976; Rothwell, Constable and Albrecht, 1977). The indirect method may still have a role in infected patients and in follow-up studies.

Maizels *et al.* (1979) performed cystometric studies in conjunction with direct RNC and were able to diagnose voiding abnormalities in some children who were suspected of having reflux. They concluded that it was useful to combine the two techniques to detect both neurological deficit and abnormal voiding patterns in the absence of neurological deficit in refluxers.

Radionuclide cystography has an important part to play in the management of vesico-ureteric reflux. Following the initial radiographic study to establish bladder

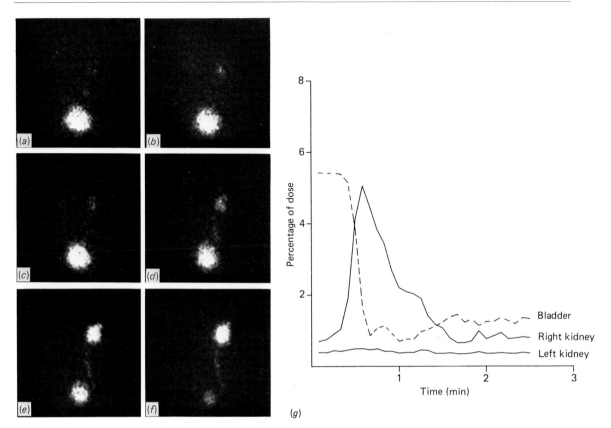

Figure 4.4 (*a*) to (*f*) 5-second computer images during voiding showing gross right vesico-ureteric reflux; (*g*) derived curves from left kidney, right kidney and bladder

morphology and the degree of reflux, direct RNC is the method of choice for follow-up, given its sensitivity and low radiation dose. Renography combined with indirect RNC will be useful in some cases.

A further radionuclide investigation which is of value to assess the consequences of reflux is the ^{99m}Tc-DMSA scan. This will complement these studies by detecting and following the progression of renal scarring (Merrick, Uttley and Wild, 1980; *see* Chapter 11).

Uretero-ureteric reflux

Duplication of the upper urinary tract is the commonest congenital abnormality of the genito-urinary system (Nordmark, 1948). Thompson and Amar (1958) reported its incidence as 6% of urological cases admitted to hospital. Unilateral duplication is three to four times more common than bilateral duplication (Nation, 1944; Nordmark, 1948). When duplication is incomplete the confluence of the ureters occurs equally in the middle and lower thirds, and least often in the upper third (Lenaghan, 1962; Kaplan and Elkin, 1968).

Vesico-ureteric reflux, which is so common in complete duplication, is unusual in the incomplete form, but there may be abnormal reflux from one pelvicalyceal system to the other (Campbell, 1967). The incidence and magnitude of such reflux increases with

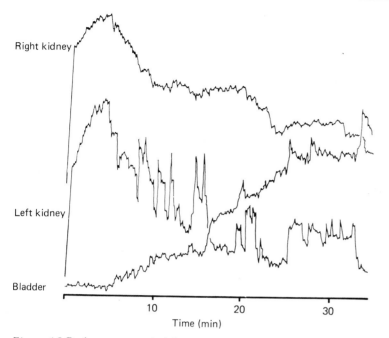
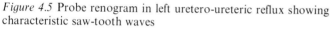

Figure 4.5 Probe renogram in left uretero-ureteric reflux showing characteristic saw-tooth waves

the distance from the ureteropelvic junction to the confluence of the bifid ureter (Amar, 1968). The treatment of urinary tract disease associated with incomplete duplication depends on knowledge of the presence or absence of this reflux. High dose intravenous urography combined with cine fluoroscopy has been the investigation commonly employed for the assessment of this phenomenon, but this entails a high radiation dose. Probe renography has been shown to be a sensitive detector of the presence of uretero-ureteric reflux, demonstrating rapid saw-tooth waves as activity passes away from the

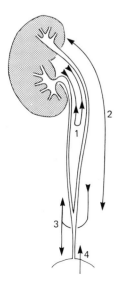

Figure 4.6 Possible urodynamic abnormalities which may occur in incomplete duplication of the upper urinary tract: (*1*) seesaw reflux; (*2*) up-and-down reflux between one moiety and ureteric confluence; (*3*) up-and-down reflux from one moiety to the other and from there to bladder; (*4*) vesico-ureteric reflux

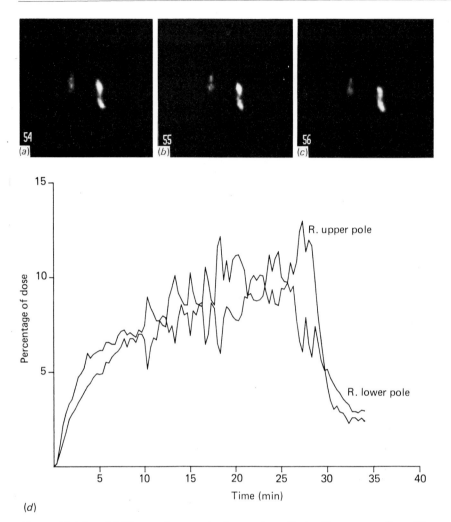

(d)

Figure 4.7 (a) to (c) 20-second computer images in patient with seesaw reflux; (d) derived renogram curves. Note decrease in concentration in upper moiety and increase in concentration in lower moiety of right kidney when comparing frame image (a) with (c). Note also gross complementary fluctuations in activity between upper and lower moieties of right kidney on derived renogram

region of the detector and back again (O'Reilly *et al.*, 1978), as shown in *Figure 4.5*. More recently gamma camera renography has been used (*see* Chapter 2). Areas of interest are defined over the upper and lower moieties of the duplication and a renogram derived for each. From these curves, periods of time are identified when activity in each of the two moieties is significantly different. The data within these periods may be summed and the new images used to define the two moieties even more accurately. Renograms are then re-derived from these newly defined regions. At the same time, indices of differential function are obtained for both kidneys and for each moiety of the duplication by comparing the individual background subtracted counts between 1 and 3 minutes for each region of interest. Time–activity curves are also derived from the bladder and the area of the ureteric confluence, where many of the urodynamic abnormalities originate.

The possible abnormalities which may occur in incomplete duplication of the upper urinary tract are shown in *Figure 4.6*.

1. Reflux may occur from one moiety via the ureteric confluence up to the other and then back again—so-called *seesaw* reflux (*Figure 4.7*).
2. Reflux may be limited to one moiety. Urine passes from the kidney down to the ureteric confluence then back up to the same moiety again, without involving the other part of the duplication, small amounts negotiating the confluence at each pass to reach the bladder. This may be called *up-and-down reflux type 1* (*Figure 4.8*).
3. Reflux may occur from one dominant moiety via the ureteric confluence up to the other and from there down to the bladder. This may be called *up-and-down reflux type 2* (Tresidder, Blandy and Murray, 1970).
4. *Vesico-ureteric* reflux may occur from the bladder up to one or both moieties of the duplication.

The radionuclide method described here will clearly demonstrate and discriminate each of these possible urodynamic abnormalities.

The incidence of reflux in incomplete ureteric duplication has not yet been

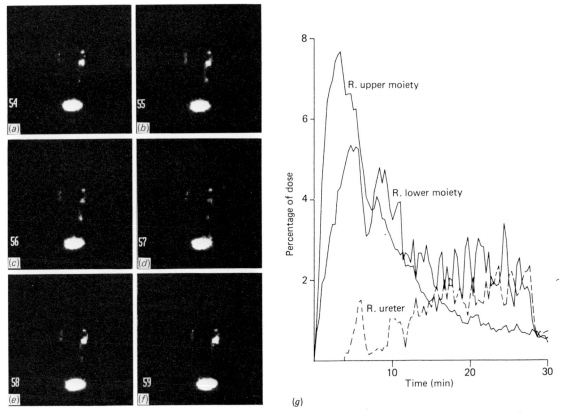

Figure 4.8 (*a*) to (*f*) 20-second computer images in patient with up-and-down reflux type 1; (*g*) derived renogram curves. Note decrease in concentration in lower moiety of right kidney with simultaneous increase in concentration of ureteric confluence between frames (*a*) and (*c*). This is followed by a decrease in concentration at the confluence and with simultaneous increase in concentration in lower moiety between frames (*d*) and (*f*). Note also complementary fluctuations in activity between lower moiety and ureteric confluence on derived renogram

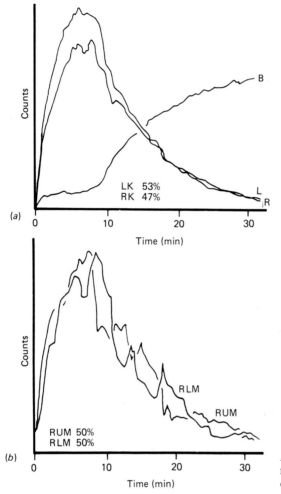

Figure 4.9 (*a*) Initial renogram showing apparently normal appearances; (*b*) moiety study clearly demonstrating seesaw reflux

established. In the Manchester series it occurred in 8 of 28 consecutive cases (O'Reilly *et al.*, 1984). This series also emphasized the necessity to perform such moiety studies in all cases where the condition is suspected clinically. In some patients the degree of seesaw reflux between the two renal pelves may be so equal and symmetrical that whole kidney curves are smooth with no suspicious saw-tooth waves, yet the study described here discloses marked urodynamic abnormalities (*Figure 4.9*). These studies are considerably quicker, easier and less radiotoxic than fluoroscopic methods (O'Reilly *et al.*, 1978) and are now recommended in patients with symptomatic upper tract duplication.

References

AMAR, A. D. (1968) Reflux in duplicated ureters. *British Journal of Urology*, **40**, 385–401

BAILEY, R. R. (1981) End stage reflux nephropathy. *Nephron*, **27**, 302–306

BAKER, R., MAXTED, W., MAYLATH, J. and SHUMAN, I. (1966) Relation of age, sex and infection to reflux: Data indicating high spontaneous cure rate in paediatric patients. *Journal of Urology*, **95**, 27–32

BLAUFOX, M. D., GRUSKING, A., SANDLER, P., GOLDMAN, H., OGWO, J. E. and EDELMANN, C. M. (1971) Radionuclide scintigraphy for detection of vesico-ureteral reflux in children. *Journal of Pediatrics*, **79**, 239–246

CAMPBELL, J. E. (1967) Ureteral peristalsis in duplex renal collecting systems. *American Journal of Roentgenology, Radium Therapy and Nuclear Medicine*, **99**, 577–580

CONWAY, J. J., KING, L. R., BELMA, A. B. and THORSEN, T. (1972) Detection of vesico-ureteral reflux in radionuclide cystography: A comparison study with roentgenographic cystography. *American Journal of Roentgenology, Radium Therapy and Nuclear Medicine*, **115**, 720–727

CONWAY, J. J., BELMA, A. B., KING, L. R. and FILMER, R. B. (1975) Direct and indirect radionuclide cystography. *Journal of Urology*, **113**, 689–693

CONWAY, J. J. and KRUGLIK, G. D. (1976) Effectiveness of direct and indirect radionuclide cystography in detecting vesico-ureteral reflux. *Journal of Nuclear Medicine*, **17**, 81–83

DODGE, E. A. (1963) Vesico-ureteric reflux: Diagnosis with iodine-131 sodium ortho-iodohippurate. *Lancet*, **1**, 303–304

ECKMAN, H., JACOBSON, B., KOCK, N. G. and SUNDIN, T. (1966) High diuresis—a factor in preventing vesico-ureteral reflux. *Journal of Urology*, **95**, 511–515

EDWARDS, D., NORMAND, I. C. S., PRESCOD, N. and SMELLIE, J. M. (1977) Disappearance of vesico-ureteric reflux during long term prophylaxis of urinary tract infection in childhood. *British Medical Journal*, **2**, 285–288

FAIRLEY, K. F. and RAYSMITH, J. (1977) The forgotten factor in the evaluations of vesico-ureteric reflux. *Medical Journal of Australia*, **2**, 10–12

FENDEL, H. (1970) Radiation exposure due to urinary tract disease. *Progress in Paediatric Urology*, **3**, 116–135

KAPLAN, N. and ELKIN, M. (1968) Bifid renal pelves and ureters. Radiological and cinefluoroscopic observations. *British Journal of Urology*, **40**, 235–244

LENAGHAN, D. (1962) Bifid ureters in children: An anatomical, physiological and clinical study. *Journal of Urology*, **87**, 808–817

LENAGHAN, D., WHITAKER, J. G., JENSEN, F. and STEPHENS, F. D. (1976) The natural history of reflux and long term effects of reflux on the kidney. *Journal of Urology*, **115**, 728–730

MAIZELS, M., WEISS, S., CONWAY, J. J. and FIRLIT, C. F. (1979) The cystometric nuclear cystogram. *Journal of Urology*, **121**, 203–205

MERRICK, M. V., UTTLEY, M. S. and WILD, S. R. (1980) The detection of pyelonephritic scarring in children by radioisotope imaging. *British Journal of Radiology*, **53**, 544–556

NASARALLAH, P. F., NARA, S. and CRAWFORD, J. (1982) Clinical applications of nuclear cystography. *Journal of Radiology*, **51**, 550–553

NATION, F. E. (1944) Duplication of the kidney and ureter: A statistical study of 230 new cases. *Journal of Urology*, **51**, 456–465

NORDMARK, B. (1948) Double formation of pelves of kidneys and ureters: Embryology, occurrence and clinical significance. *Acta Radiologica*, **30**, 267–278

O'REILLY, P. H., LAWSON, R. S., SHIELDS, R. A., TESTA, H. J., CHARLTON EDWARDS, E. and CARROLL, R. N. P. (1978) A radioisotope method of assessing uretero-ureteric reflux. *British Journal of Urology*, **50**, 164–168

O'REILLY, P. H., SHIELDS, R. A., TESTA, H. J., LAWSON, R. S. and CHARLTON EDWARDS, E. (1984) Uretero-ureteric reflux. A pathological entity or physiological phenomenon? *British Journal of Urology*, **56**, 159–164

ROLLESTON, G. L., SHANNON, F. T. and UTLEY, W. L. F. (1970) Relationship of infantile vesico-ureteric reflux to renal damage. *British Medical Journal*, **1**, 460–463

ROTHWELL, D. L., CONSTABLE, A. R. and ALBRECHT, M. (1977) Radionuclide cystography in the investigation of vesico-ureteric reflux in children. *Lancet*, **1**, 1072–1074

THOMPSON, L. M. and AMAR, A. D. (1958) Clinical importance of ureteral duplication and ectopia. *Journal of the American Medical Association*, **168**, 881–886

TRESIDDER, G. C., BLANDY, J. P. and MURRAY, R. S. (1970) Pyelo-pelvic and uretero-ureteric reflux. *British Journal of Urology*, **42**, 728–735

WINTER, C. C. (1959) A new test for vesico-ureteral reflux: An external technique using radioisotopes. *Journal of Urology*, **81**, 105–111

5 Clearance studies

R. A. Shields

The concept of clearance is fundamental to an understanding of renal function, and its measurement or estimation can be of great value in the management of renal or urological disease.

Radionuclide techniques offer, in addition to greater simplicity of laboratory procedures and patient-handling protocols, one unique potential advantage over classic methods—the assessment of clearance by individual kidneys.

Theory and terminology

Figure 5.1 represents the function of the kidney by a single nephron. Any substance may be found to have a concentration of P_A mg/ml in the plasma of a renal artery and to appear in the urine with a concentration of U mg/ml. If the urine is being produced at a rate of $\dot{V}$ ml/min, it may be deduced that the substance is excreted at a rate of $U\dot{V}$ mg/min. In each minute, therefore, the volume of plasma from which all the substance might have been cleared is equal to $(U\dot{V}/P_A)$ ml, and this quantity is known as the *renal clearance* of that specific substance:

$$\text{Clearance} = \frac{U\dot{V}}{P_A} \qquad (1)$$

If the substance is filtered by the glomerulus as efficiently as water and if it subsequently passes through the tubular system without further exchange with plasma, then its clearance is a measurement of the *glomerular filtration rate* (GFR). These conditions imply that the substance be neither reabsorbed nor secreted by the tubules, that it remain free of plasma protein binding, and that it be not metabolized within the kidney. Normal values of GFR are 124 ± 26 ml/min for adult males and 109 ± 13 ml/min for adult females (Smith, 1951). If the substance is not metabolized by the kidney, it may be deduced that any amount passing through the renal artery must, under equilibrium conditions, be equal to the total amount leaving via the renal vein and the urine (the Fick principle). Let the total renal plasma flow be F ml/min and the renal venous concentration be P_V mg/ml. Then

$$FP_A = FP_V + U\dot{V}$$

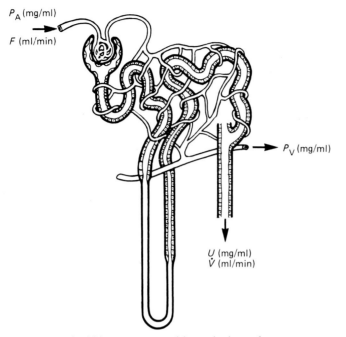

P_A (mg/ml)

F (ml/min)

P_V (mg/ml)

U (mg/ml)
$\dot{V}$ (ml/min)

Figure 5.1 The kidney represented by a single nephron

or

$$F = \frac{U\dot{V}}{P_A - P_V} \tag{2}$$

A substance which was completely eliminated from the plasma in one pass (for which P_V would be zero) would therefore have a clearance equal to the renal plasma flow. This would imply elimination by tubular secretion in addition to, or instead of, glomerular filtration. In practice, no substance has been found to have such ideal characteristics and it is therefore useful to define the *extraction ratio, E*, as

$$E = \frac{P_A - P_V}{P_A} \tag{3}$$

an indicator of the efficiency of extraction of the substance by the kidney from arterial plasma. Substituting for P_V in equation (2) gives

$$F = \frac{1}{E} \cdot \frac{U\dot{V}}{P_A} = \frac{\text{Clearance}}{E} \tag{4}$$

so that the renal plasma flow can be calculated by dividing the clearance of a substance by its extraction ratio. A substance whose extraction ratio approaches unity exhibits a clearance nearly equal to the renal plasma flow, and this is often referred to as the *effective renal plasma flow* (ERPF).

Traditional methods

In the 1930s inulin—a fructose polysaccharide—was found to satisfy the conditions outlined above for an indicator of glomerular filtration rate. Its concentration can be measured in samples of plasma and urine, and it can safely be infused intravenously. The clearance of inulin, as measured from plasma and urine samples taken while a constant plasma concentration is maintained by continuous infusion, has therefore become a reference standard for the measurement of glomerular filtration rate.

Endogenous creatinine may be analysed chemically in plasma and urine samples, and its clearance is also used as a measure of GFR. This has been criticized (Berlyne, 1965; Kim *et al.*, 1969) because of suspicions of significant tubular secretion and non-specificity of the chromogen test used, but the method has been shown to correlate well with inulin clearance (Bennett and Porter, 1971).

The classic substance used for measurement of ERPF is *p*-aminohippuric acid (PAH), and the normal clearance values obtained are $623 \pm 112 \, \text{ml/min}$ (Smith, 1951). The extraction ratio of this compound has been measured by sampling renal arterial and venous blood or by sampling peripheral venous and renal venous blood (Maher, Strong and Elveback, 1971) to be 0.8–0.9.

The traditional methods of measurement of clearance of inulin or PAH involve continuous intravenous infusion, multiple venous sampling, bladder catheterization in order to obtain complete urine collections during successive time intervals, and difficult chemical determinations. They are too time consuming for routine diagnostic tests and do not lend themselves to simplification. Techniques using tracer doses of radioactive pharmaceuticals have, however, brought the routine measurement of clearance within the time schedules and technical capabilities of many hospitals. The ease and sensitivity with which samples of gamma-emitting radionuclide may be measured in a scintillation well counter has enabled the continuous infusion method to be replaced by the simpler techniques described below, all of which have been validated by correlation with the chemical methods.

Radionuclide techniques for clearance measurement

The choice of radiopharmaceuticals for measurement of glomerular filtration rate and effective renal plasma flow is fully discussed in Chapter 17. A number of measurement techniques may be employed, and these may be classified as follows:

1. Constant infusion methods;
2. Single-injection methods: urine and plasma sampling;
3. Single-injection methods: plasma sampling only;
4. The single sample method;
5. External monitoring: (a) vascular; (b) vesical; (c) renal.

Constant infusion methods

If the appropriate radiopharmaceutical is administered by constant intravenous infusion, the concentration of radioactivity in plasma will build up until the rate of infusion of activity is equal to its rate of excretion. The level of activity in the plasma must be monitored, either by taking sequential samples or, less accurately, by external detection, until this equilibrium is attained. During any period while this equilibrium persists all the urine produced and passed via a bladder catheter may be collected and a representative plasma sample taken. The clearance is then calculated as UV/PT, where V is the volume of urine produced during time T, and U and P are the concentrations in urine and plasma, which may be measured in any convenient units provided that they are identical—for example, counts per minute per ml.

It may be noted that if the tracer is excreted only by the kidneys, then the rate at which it is excreted (UV/T) is equal to the rate at which it is being infused, which is equal

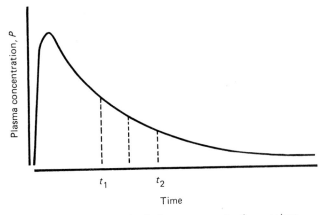

Figure 5.2 Typical graph of plasma concentration against time after a single injection of radiopharmaceutical

to the concentration of the infusate (I cpm/ml) multiplied by the infusion rate (R ml/min). The use of a calibrated infusion pump will therefore permit instantaneous measurements of clearance (during equilibrium) as IR/P. This method has been used experimentally by Gragnon and colleagues (Gragnon *et al.*, 1970).

In general, the constant infusion methods fail to exploit the main advantages of the use of radioactive tracers, and they find a place only in the validation of simpler techniques or in research or experiment.

Single-injection methods: urine and plasma sampling

After a single injection of radiopharmaceutical the concentration in plasma will change with time in a manner such as is shown in *Figure 5.2*. The equation for calculation of clearance should now strictly be applied to a short interval of time, δt, during which the plasma concentration, P, is sensibly constant. If the volume of urine produced during this short time is δV and it has, as before, a concentration of tracer U, then

$$\text{Clearance} = \frac{U \, \delta V}{P \, \delta t} \tag{5}$$

Integrating both numerator and denominator gives

$$\text{Clearance} = \frac{UV}{\int_{t_1}^{t_2} P \, dt} \tag{6}$$

where V is the volume of urine produced between sampling times t_1 and t_2. The denominator may be computed from a graph fitted to measured plasma concentrations; or an acceptable approximation may be obtained by taking a plasma sample at the time mid-way between urine sampling times and multiplying the measured concentration by the urine collection time.

A technique used for measurement of GFR is as follows: 3 MBq (80 μCi) of ^{51}Cr-EDTA is given intravenously at time zero. Heparinized blood samples (10 ml) are taken at times 90, 150, 210 and 270 minutes. The patient empties his bladder at 60 minutes, and complete urine collections are taken at 120, 180 and 240 minutes. The volume of each urine collection is measured, the blood samples are centrifuged, and 2 ml samples of plasma and urine are counted in a scintillation well counter. The best fit of the plasma concentrations after 90 minutes to a single-exponential decay curve is calculated and a value of clearance is obtained by the method indicated above for each of the three urine sampling periods.

It is difficult and less accurate to apply this method directly to the measurement of ERPF because of the much shorter times available for urine and plasma sampling.

Single-injection methods: plasma sampling only

Equation (6) showed how the clearance might be calculated as the quantity of tracer excreted during a given time interval divided by the area under the plasma concentration curve for that time interval. Considering the entire, infinite time 'interval' from the injection onwards, if it is assumed that all the tracer is excreted and that the only route is renal, then the total amount of tracer excreted will be equal to the quantity injected (say Q_0).

$$\text{Clearance} = \frac{Q_0}{\int_0^\infty P \, dt} \tag{7}$$

Initial measurement of the dose and mathematical analysis of the plasma disappearance curve should therefore allow calculation of renal clearance without recourse to urine sampling. In order to calculate the area under the plasma curve up to infinite time, the data available must be fitted to a suitable equation. It has been shown (Cohen, 1974) that the data usually fit a double exponential: an equation of the type

$$\text{Plasma concentration} = C_1 \, e^{-\lambda_1 t} + C_2 \, e^{-\lambda_2 t} \tag{8}$$

where C_1, C_2, λ_1, λ_2 are constants.

Calculating the integral of this to infinity and inserting it into equation (8) leads to

$$\text{Clearance} = \frac{Q_0 \lambda_1 \lambda_2}{C_1 \lambda_2 + C_2 \lambda_1} \tag{9}$$

Equations (8) and (9) correspond exactly to equations (8) and (10) of Chapter 18 because the double-exponential plasma disappearance curve is precisely what is predicted by the three-compartment mamillary system analysed there.

A method suitable for the measurement of ERPF is therefore summarized as follows. A dose of pure ^{131}I-OIH is dispensed and *calibrated*. This is accurately done by comparing either its total activity or its weight with that of another 'standard' aliquot, diluting this standard to 1 litre and taking a sample of the diluted standard to count with the plasma samples. The dose is injected intravenously and eight plasma samples are taken during 1 hour. All samples are counted in a scintillation well counter, and the plasma concentration is plotted on a logarithmic scale against time, as shown in *Figure 5.3*. The best straight line through the later part of the curve gives one exponential component; subtraction or *peeling* of this from the observed values gives new data points to which the other exponential component is fitted. Two straight lines are thus obtained whose intercepts give C_1 and C_2 and whose slopes give λ_1 and λ_2. The latter are conveniently calculated by measuring the half-times ($t_{1/2}$) and using the formula

$$\lambda = \frac{0.693}{t_{1/2}} \tag{10}$$

Results obtained with this method have been shown to correlate very well with classically determined PAH clearance (Tauxe, Maher and Taylor, 1971).

Many workers have settled for an approximation to this technique in which only a

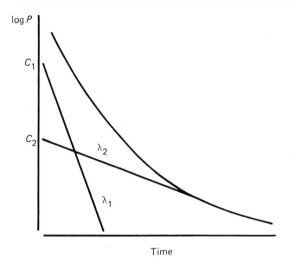

$\log P$

C_1

C_2

λ_2

λ_1

Time

Figure 5.3 Double exponential analysis of a plasma disappearance curve

single exponential is fitted to the plasma disappearance curve. If the curve fitted is

Plasma concentration $= C\, e^{-\lambda t}$

then

$$\text{Clearance} = \frac{Q_0 \lambda}{C} \qquad (11)$$

It is worth noting that Q_0/C, the dose injected divided by the concentration at time zero, is equal to the apparent volume of dilution of the tracer. This simple technique thus establishes clearance as the product of the volume of dilution and the decay constant of the fitted exponential—the '$V\lambda$ method'. It may be routinely applied, concurrently with the urine sampling technique (*see* pp. 52–53), in the measurements of GFR, the only additional physical requirement being the calibration of the dose. The $V\lambda$ method, despite its theoretical inadequacy, has been shown to give respectable results for GFR, correlating well with the more established methods (Chantler *et al.*, 1969).

It has been shown by Veall and Gibbs (1982) that the elegance of calculation by the continuous infusion method may be combined with the practicality of the single injection with plasma sampling. The continuous infusion is simulated mathematically as a repeated sequence of input impulses, and the plasma response is computed by convolution of this input function with the measured plasma response to a single injection. The digital computer is thus used to replace the continuous infusion pump. An iterative procedure also enables the simulation of a suitable 'priming dose' in order to achieve a true equilibrium plasma concentration.

The single sample method

The methods for measurement of clearance described thus far have been developed from physiological research techniques and are not necessarily suitable for the busy clinical diagnostic unit. An expedient approach, and one which is receiving much attention currently, is to reduce the number of samples and measurements from a given patient to the absolute minimum, and to correlate a single parameter obtained with the required parameter as measured 'properly' on a sufficiently large initial trial population. For clearance studies, this means the measurement of one plasma sample taken at a specific time after the administration of a calibrated dose. Dividing the dose by the plasma concentration gives an apparent volume of distribution, and this volume should correspond to a particular clearance value.

Tauxe and colleagues (1971) described the fitting of a quadratic equation to the relationship between this apparent volume and ERPF and investigated the effect of sampling time upon accuracy. When correlating with ^{131}I-OIH clearance they found an optimum sampling time at 44 minutes, and ERPF could be determined from the volume of distribution indicated by the 44-minute sample (V_{44}) with an estimated standard error of 31 ml/min. This was more accurate than the classic determination of clearance using PAH. In later work (Tauxe et al., 1982) they extended the initial database to 68 patients with a wider range of clearance values and suggested an exponential fit with best values expressed in the regression equation:

$$ERPF = 1126[1 - e^{-0.008(V_{44} - 7.9)}] \, ml/min \tag{12}$$

where V_{44} is the volume of distribution (in litres) indicated by the 44-minute sample. The errors obtained using this formula were approximately 50% less than those using slope/intercept methods (Tauxe, Dubovsky and Kidd, 1984).

Constable and colleagues (1979) also used a 44-minute plasma sample and obtained the following regression equation for prediction of ERPF based upon a study of 30 patients:

$$ERPF = 120(V_{44} + 56)^{1/2} - 936 \, ml/min \tag{13}$$

In the author's department these formulae have been noted and a much simpler relationship adopted which correlates well both with them and with observed data:

$$ERPF = 5.5V_{44} \tag{14}$$

This is the relationship given in the routine protocol in Chapter 7.

A similar approach may be made to the estimation of glomerular filtration rate. Fisher and Veall (1975) used a single sample at 3 hours following the injection of ^{51}Cr-EDTA and correlated the apparent volume of distribution with GFR measurement by the single exponential plasma disappearance method. The method was found to be accurate, although not valid for clearance below 30 ml/min. This method was also evaluated by Constable and colleagues (1979) who found the regression equation:

$$GFR = 24.5(V_3 - 6.2)^{1/2} - 67 \, ml/min \tag{15}$$

where V_3 litres is the apparent volume of the distribution of the 3-hour sample. They showed that a reliable estimate of GFR could be obtained in non-oedematous patients, and furthermore that the reliability was maintained even when the patient did not maintain a constant state of rest during the test period. The technique is therefore well suited to attendances at an out-patient clinic.

It is possible to administer a combination of radiopharmaceuticals by simultaneous injection, and thus to determine both ERPF and GFR by sampling, at 44 minutes and 3 hours for example, using dual isotope counting techniques for the measurement of quantity at each agent in each sample (Morgan et al., 1977; Constable et al., 1979). This works well for ^{125}I-OIH and ^{51}Cr-EDTA, whose gamma emissions are well separated in energy. It also applies to the combination of ^{125}I-OIH and ^{99m}Tc-DTPA, with the added advantage that, if the samples are kept for a few days, the ^{99m}Tc will have decayed and the ^{125}I may be counted without interference.

Given the initial effort in validation by individual laboratories, these single-sample techniques are an important development in practical diagnostic method. They are faster and simpler than, for example, the measurement of endogenous creatinine clearance, which requires a 24-hour urine collection.

External monitoring

Vascular

The principle of obtaining measurements of clearance from the rate of disappearance from plasma after a single injection of tracer may be exploited by the use of a scintillation detector probe to monitor vascular radioactivity externally. A site must be chosen for the detector which will permit it to see a significant volume of blood with as little contribution as possible from activity in the tissues or any other 'compartment'. Many workers measure over the head. After the injection of the patient, such a detector coupled to a ratemeter and chart recorder will produce a plasma disappearance curve similar to that shown in *Figure 5.3*. The slope of this curve may be measured to evaluate λ_1 and λ_2 (or a single λ) exactly as described in the previous section, but the ordinate of the curve is now in arbitrary units, because the response of the external detector depends upon a number of intangible (but hopefully constant) anatomical and physical factors. In order to obtain a value for clearance, the intercepts C_1 and C_2 (or one intercept in the case of the single exponential) need to be evaluated in the same units as those used to measure the injected dose. Thus at least one blood sample must be taken in order to calibrate the curve.

Blaufox and colleagues (1967) describe a technique for measurement of ERPF based on these principles. Injection of a calibrated dose of 2.7 MBq pure ^{131}I-OIH is followed by external monitoring of the patient with a scintillation detector directed as the zygomatic arch of the skull. A chart record is produced for 60 minutes, and blood samples are taken at 3 minutes and 60 minutes. The activity of the plasma of the samples is measured in the same counter as the diluted standard against which the dose has been calibrated. The two slopes, λ_1 and λ_2, are obtained from the chart record replotted on semi-logarithmic paper. A third graph is then constructed as shown in *Figure 5.4*—also on a log scale. The plasma concentration at 60 minutes is plotted as a

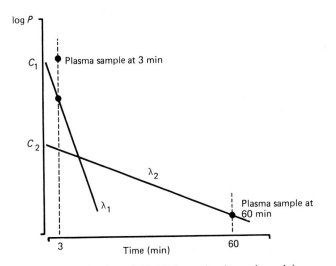

Figure 5.4 Derivation of ERPF from the slopes λ_1 and λ_2 determined by external monitoring and two plasma sample measurements. *See* text for details

single point, and a straight line drawn through it of slope λ_2. The 3-minute concentration is plotted and replotted after subtraction of the contribution from the longer exponential. A straight line is now drawn through this point having slope λ_1. In this way the two intercepts C_1 and C_2 are obtained in the correct units.

Vesical

External monitoring may also be used to measure urinary concentration of tracer in order to diminish errors due to incomplete collection of urine in the application of a '*UV/P*' technique. The same problem of calibration pertains. Bianchi (1972) describes such a method for GFR: 80 minutes after administration of the tracer the patient empties his bladder and then lies under an external scintillation detector directed at the bladder. The rise in activity during the next 30 minutes is taken as '*UV*', to be compared with the radioactive concentration of a plasma sample (*P*) taken at the mid-time. The value of '*UV*' is calibrated by taking external measurements before and after bladder voiding and measuring the concentration of activity in the voided urine.

Kidney

Paradoxically, perhaps, more difficulties are found in the calculation of clearance from the renogram than from measurements over extrarenal sites. The problems are discussed in detail in Chapter 18, but it is appropriate here to summarize their relevance to the calculation of clearance.

First, the activity measured over the kidney site must be corrected for background activity. The uptake phase of this background-corrected renogram may then be used as an indicator of relative individual renal clearances (q.v.), but for absolute quantification the 'uptake constant' is calculated from the values of the renogram and the sums of blood background measurements as described on page 256. A blood sample is needed in order to obtain the volume of dilution by which to multiply this parameter. In Chapter 18 deconvolution of the renogram curve is used to evaluate *relative* renal plasma flow, but the derivation of absolute value of clearance would require unknown information about detector sensitivity.

In summary, although the characteristics of the renogram are principally determined by renal plasma flow (RPF), the various factors are too confused to permit direct absolute quantification in terms of ERPF and GFR from the kidney curve.

An empirical approach, analogous to that of the previous section on the single sample method, may be made, however, by correlating the uptake measured over kidney and bladder at a certain time with clearance measured 'properly' in an initial trial population. It has been described for the estimation of GFR from a 22-minute gamma camera image using ^{99m}Tc-DTPA and correcting the calibrated uptakes for attenuation by measuring the kidney and bladder depths from lateral images (Lee, Constable and Cranage, 1982).

Individual kidney clearances

There are many diagnostic situations in which we need to establish the relative contribution to renal function from each kidney. In such cases it may often be sufficient to evaluate a ratio of clearances rather than two absolute values, although the latter may be obtained by combination of the results with overall clearance as measured by one of the standard methods.

How and why the background-corrected OIH renogram may be used for this purpose is described in Chapter 18. If the sensitivities to the two kidneys are identical, then, during the second phase of the renogram, the ratio of left to right heights is equal to the ratio of their RPFs. This ratio is usually evaluated by counting over a 1-minute period from 1–2 minutes or 2–3 minutes. In a more sophisticated approach the uptake constant may be evaluated for each kidney.

If the renogram is deconvolved then the relative RPF is given by ratio of the heights of the first points on the deconvolved curves (*see* Chapter 18). Whichever method is chosen, it will be appreciated that the renogram, while not an absolute measurement, can be used for estimation of relative renal plasma flow.

Depending on the radiopharmaceutical used, the renal scan may depict the distribution of the filtration function. Analysis of the counts over individual kidneys during the early stages may be used in a manner analogous to that of quantitative renography to establish individual relative GFRs (Britton, 1975). Of course, a background correction must be similarly applied, and it should be noted that depth dependence effects may be significant for ^{99m}Tc.

Correction for the different attenuation of gamma rays from kidneys at different depths may be made by taking additional lateral views, measuring the depths of each kidney and applying correction factors. In this way the calibrated ^{99m}Tc-DTPA gamma camera renogram may be used to estimate individual kidney GFRs (Duffy, Casey and Barker, 1982).

References

BENNETT, W. M. and PORTER, G. A. (1971) Endogenous creatinine clearance as a clinical measure of glomerular filtration rate. *British Medical Journal*, **4**, 84–86

BERLYNE, G. M. (1965) Endogenous creatinine clearance and the glomerular filtration rate. *American Heart Journal*, **70**, 143–144

BIANCHI, C. (1972) Measurement of glomerular filtration rate. *Progress in Nuclear Medicine*, **2**

BLAUFOX, M. D., POTCHEN, E. J. and MERRILL, J. P. (1967) Measurement of effective renal plasma flow in man by external counting methods. *Journal of Nuclear Medicine*, **8**, 77

BRITTON, K. E. (1975) Renal function studies with radioisotopes. In: *Dynamic Studies with Radioisotopes in Medicine 1974: Proceedings of a Symposium in Knoxville*, Vol. 2, Vienna: International Atomic Energy Authority, pp. 216–217

CHANTLER, C., GARNETT, E. S., PARSONS, V. and VEALL, N. (1969) Glomerular filtration rate measurement in man by the single injection method using ^{51}Cr-EDTA. *Clinical Science*, **37**, 169–180

COHEN, M. L. (1974) Radionuclide clearance techniques. *Seminars in Nuclear Medicine*, **4**(1), 23–38

CONSTABLE, A. R., HUSSEIN, M. M., ALBRECHT, M. P., THOMPSON, F. D., PHILALITHIS, P. E. and JOEKES, A. M. (1979) Single sample estimates of renal clearances. *British Journal of Urology*, **51**, 84–87

DUFFY, G. J., CASEY, M. and BARKER, F. (1982) A comparison of individual kidney GFR measured by Tc-99m DTPA gamma camera renography and by direct collection of creatinine from each kidney. *Radionuclides in Nephrology*, A. M. Joekes, A. R. Constable, N. J. G. Brown and W. N. Tauxe (eds.), London: Academic Press; New York: Grune and Stratton, pp. 101–106

FISHER, M. and VEALL, N. (1975) Glomerular filtration rate estimation based on a single sample. *British Medical Journal*, **2**, 542

GRAGNON, J. A., MAILLOUX, L. U., DOLITTLE, J. E. and TESCHAN, P. E. (1970) An isotopic method for instantaneous measurements of effective renal blood flow. *American Journal of Physiology*, **218**, 180–186

KIM, K. E., ONESTI, G., RAMIREZ, O., BREST, A. N. and SWARTZ, C. (1969) Creatinine clearance in renal disease: a reappraisal. *British Medical Journal*, **4**, 11–14

LEE, T. Y., CONSTABLE, A. R. and CRANAGE, R. W. (1982) A method for GFR determination without blood samples in routine renal scintigraphy with Tc-99m-DTPA. In: *Radionuclides in Nephrology*, A. M. Joekes, A. R. Constable, N. J. G. Brown and W. N. Tauxe (eds.), London: Academic Press; New York: Grune and Stratton, pp. 107–112

MAHER, F. T., STRONG, C. G. and ELVEBACK, L. R. (1971) Renal extraction ratios and plasma binding studies of radioiodinated o-iodohippurate and iodopyracet and of p-aminohippurate in man. *Mayo Clinic Proceedings*, **46**, 189–192

MORGAN, W. D., BIRKO, J. L., SIVYER, A. and GHOSE, R. R. (1977) An efficient technique for the simultaneous estimation of GFR and ERPF involving a single injection and two blood samples. *International Journal of Nuclear Medicine and Biology*, **4**, 79–82

SMITH, M. W. (1951) *The Kidney: Structure and Function in Health and Disease*, London: Oxford University Press

TAUXE, W. N., MAHER, F. T. and TAYLOR, W. F. (1971) ERPF: estimation from theoretical volumes of distribution of intravenously injected ^{131}I-orthoiodohippurate. *Mayo Clinic Proceedings*, **46**, 524–531

TAUXE, W. N., DUBOVSKY, E. V., KIDD, T. E. Jr., DIAZ, F. and SMITH, C. R. (1982) New formulas for the calculation of effective renal plasma flow. *European Journal of Nuclear Medicine*, **7**, 51–54

TAUXE, W. N., DUBOVSKY, E. V. and KIDD, T. E. Jr. (1984) Comparison of measurement of effective renal plasma flow by single plasma sample and plasma disappearance slope/volume methods. *European Journal of Nuclear Medicine*, **9**, 443–445

VEALL, N. and GIBBS, G. P. (1982) The accurate determination of tracer clearance rates and equilibrium distribution volumes from single injection plasma measurements using numerical analysis. In: *Radionuclides in Nephrology*, A. M. Joekes, A. R. Constable, N. J. G. Brown and W. N. Tauxe (eds.), London: Academic Press; New York: Grune and Stratton, pp. 125–130

6　Bone scintigraphy

A. R. Constable

The reliable management of diseases which give rise to bone metastases depends on the early detection of functional abnormalities of the skeleton. Anatomical abnormalities of the bone, such as enlargement, high- or low-density structures and fracture, are well suited to conventional radiographic investigation. However, the density changes which occur in metastatic bone lesions, and the enlargements associated with Paget's disease, are a consequence of functional abnormalities which in many cases will have commenced a long time before any radiographic abnormality can be detected. Active metabolic turnover at a metastatic site causes new bone formation or resorption with eventual changes of bone density, and it has been estimated that 30–50% of the substance of a human vertebra has to be removed before a distinctly recognizable lesion appears on the radiograph (Borak, 1942). Furthermore, the active osteoblastic phase of metastatic disease may be indistinguishable radiographically from the healed osteosclerotic condition.

Nuclear medicine imaging methods are sensitive in the exploration of functional abnormalities and, in such a widely distributed organ as the human skeleton, do not lag far behind the methods of radiography in providing morphological and spatial information. Radiography, while capable of considerable specificity when a lesion is detected, completely lacks the sensitivity required for the early detection of metastatic disease of the skeleton or in following its changing condition. The superior sensitivity of bone scintigraphy was not immediately obvious in the early days of rectilinear scanning and during the early development period of the gamma camera. However, despite the poor resolution of the primitive gamma cameras of the 1960s and the low bone-to-soft-tissue contrast obtained with the radioactive imaging agents then in use, systematic comparisons of the two imaging methods eventually revealed quite convincingly the improvements in detection efficiency available with radionuclides (Faber *et al.*, 1967; Morgan and Mills, 1968; Galasko, 1969). Radiographic skeletal surveys remained the principal method of screening for metastatic bone disease until better quality imaging agents and gamma cameras came into use in the early 1970s.

Bone imaging agents have progressed from the radionuclide forms initially in use— ^{47}Ca, ^{85}Sr, ^{87m}Sr, ^{18}F—to the labelled pharmaceuticals developed in the 1970s (^{99m}Tc polyphosphates, pyrophosphates and diphosphonates). These labelled phosphate compounds, introduced by Subramanian and McAfee (1971), immediately increased the credibility of bone scintigraphy and, indirectly, the whole of nuclear medicine. The first of the commercially available technetium-labelled compounds was polyphosphate. The principal compounds in current use are hydroxyethylidene disphosphonate (EHDP) and methylene diphosphonate (MDP). Phosphate compounds are incorporated into normal bone by chemisorption, possibly at kink and dislocation sites on the apatite crystal surface. Their heavier concentration in osteoblastic and osteolytic lesions is accounted for by the larger number of binding sites available on the surfaces of immature, growing or resorbing apatite crystal. Thus bone scintigraphy of the normal skeleton will have a generally uniform appearance (*Figure 6.1*) in which the high- and low-density regions can be accounted for largely in terms of skeletal geometry and variations in bone thickness. The avidity of metabolically active sites, whether osteolytic or osteoblastic, benign or malignant, will give rise to regions, more or less well defined, of varying degrees of increased tracer uptake against a normal skeletal background (*Figure 6.2*). Lytic lesions may sometimes show as photon deficiencies as do avascular regions or sites of surgical bone removal (Sy *et al.*, 1977; Spencer *et al.*, 1981).

The chosen bone-seeking agent is administered to the patient intravenously and is distributed throughout the body by blood-flow. Although blood-flow is the essential

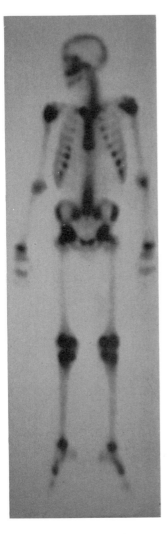

Figure 6.1 A normal bone appearance obtained with a scanning gamma camera

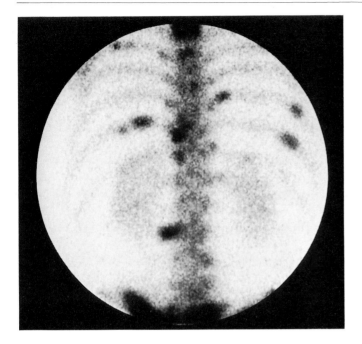

Figure 6.2 A single gamma camera image extending from the
mid-thoracic spine to the sacrum. The several focal regions of
heavy tracer uptake mark the sites of prostatic metastases

mechanism for delivering the tracer to the sites of deposition, there is no direct
proportionality between blood-flow and tracer uptake (Charkes, Makler and Philips,
1978). A localized reduction in bone blood-flow due to infarction or any other cause
will be observed as a region of photon deficiency. The increased blood-flow which
occurs at the site of a metastatic lesion or other focal abnormality is insufficient to
account for the high concentration of tracer frequently encountered in the abnormal
bone scintigram (Lavender, Khan and Hughes, 1979; Charkes, 1980). The reactive
immature bone plays the dominant role of gathering high concentrations of tracer at
the lesion site from whatever is available through existing vascular pathways.

A useful five-compartmental model has been proposed by Charkes and his co-
workers for the kinetics of distribution of bone-seeking agents whether of the ionic
exchange form, such as ^{18}F and ^{87m}Sr (Charkes, Makler and Philips, 1978), or of the
chemisorption form, such as ^{99m}Tc-MDP (Makler and Charkes, 1980). This model is
illustrated in *Figure 6.3*. Following the injection of tracer, rapid distribution takes place
into the extra-cellular fluid space (ECF) and, by way of renal uptake and excretion, into
the urine. The model proposes a non-bone-ECF and a bone-ECF. The presence of the
bone-ECF acts as a buffer space between the blood and bone and accounts for the
insensitivity of rate of bone uptake in response to changes of blood-flow. The model is
appealing and has been successful in accounting for most of the experimental and
clinical observations of bone scintigraphy.

During the first 3 hours following the administration of ^{99m}Tc-MDP about 60%
of the dose is excreted (Subramanian *et al.*, 1975a). *Figure 6.4* shows the relative
distribution of tracer (^{99m}Tc-MDP) in plasma and urine as a function of time. The
difference between the dose and the combined contents of these two compartments (the
remainder curve in *Figure 6.4*) represents the fraction of tracer already taken up by the
skeleton plus tracer being presented to the skeleton in the bone-ECF plus tracer

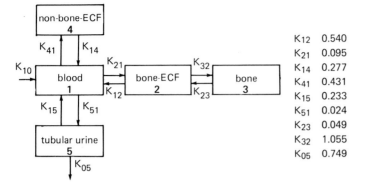

K_{12}	0.540
K_{21}	0.095
K_{14}	0.277
K_{41}	0.431
K_{15}	0.233
K_{51}	0.024
K_{23}	0.049
K_{32}	1.055
K_{05}	0.749

Figure 6.3 The five-compartmental model showing the manner and rates of distribution of ^{99m}Tc-MDP. Note the total independence of the bone ECF from the non-bone ECF. The buffer effect of the bone ECF can be appreciated by studying the values of the rate constants associated with it. The rate constants were derived from experimental data by an iterative, least-squares method (Makler and Charkes, 1980)

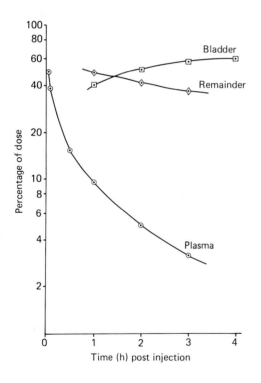

Figure 6.4 The rate of plasma disappearance and bladder accumulation of ^{99m}Tc-MDP taken from the data of Subramanian *et al.* (1975). The difference between the dose and the combined contents of the plasma and bladder gives the remainder curve which represents the percentage of the dose in bone-ECF, non-bone-ECF and skeleton

currently languishing in the non-bone-ECF. A more detailed analysis of the five-compartmental model (Makler and Charkes, 1980), combined with experimental and clinical observations (Subramanian *et al.*, 1975b; Rosenthall *et al.*, 1977; Fogelman *et al.*, 1979), shows that the bone-to-soft-tissue ratio increases progressively during the first five or more hours after dose administration. However, optimum imaging time may not be best selected from a simple consideration of target-to-background ratio.

Figures of merit may be derived from more detailed statistical considerations (Beck and Harper, 1968) which, in theoretical combination with the five-compartmental model, suggest that a 1- or 2-hour delay time is optimum. In practice, however, it is generally found that better quality images are obtained at 3–4 hours post injection than at 1–2 hours. In the daily routine of a busy nuclear medicine department more trivial considerations often prevent an exactly timed protocol, and imaging generally takes place with a delay time of between 2 and 4 hours. Although longer delay times will produce images with better contrast, efficiency of lesion detection does not improve substantially.

Practical methods

Patients attending hospital for bone scintigraphy need no special preparation. If several patients are to attend on a single day, and are to be imaged on the same camera, it may be possible to give them staggered appointments. The time taken under the gamma camera typically may be 20 minutes, and, if injection times are so staggered, similar delay times will be achieved by all patients giving rise to an inherent consistency and allowing the interpretation of variable results to be ascribed to other causes. Experience shows that the organization of patients in this manner is often easier said than done.

Following an intravenous injection of about 400–550 MBq of ^{99m}Tc-labelled compound the patient is encouraged to remain well hydrated and to empty his bladder frequently to avoid unnecessary radiation from the excreted fraction. Immediately before imaging commences the patient is again asked to empty his bladder as completely as possible so that bladder activity does not interfere with the pelvic images. The patient is also asked to remove metallic objects such as coins, buckles and medallions to avoid unnecessary photon-deficient image artefacts.

In some departments a whole-body scanning gamma camera is used to image the skeleton from head to foot (see Figure 6.1). Abnormal areas can then be re-taken as spot views if enlargement is required.

It rarely takes much time, however, to cover the skeleton adequately with spot views. The axial skeleton can usually be imaged completely with five posterior views (left and right shoulders including thoracic spine, lumbar spine, pelvis and femora) and two anterior views (sternum and pelvis). The protocol should also include two skull views, making a total of nine images. Gamma camera image formatters often provide nine images on a standard 20 × 25 cm X-ray film. Thus a single film is adequate for a complete set of spot views (Figure 6.5). If there are any clinical indications for including images of the extremities this should be done. When screening for metastatic bone disease of urological interest, particularly when arising from prostatic carcinoma, the above protocol will provide a clear diagnosis if negative and allow accurate staging if positive.

As about 60% of the administered dose is excreted by the kidneys in the presence of normal kidney function and not too drastically abnormal skeletal uptake, it may be expected that renal images will appear on the scintigrams. Commenting on aspects of renal function from these images can present serious interpretation problems. If the patient's clinical condition suggests that some information on renal function would be of value, then the protocol should be extended to include images from the moment of bolus injection and for the following 20 or 30 minutes as for conventional gamma camera renography. The renal perfusion data from this study will be as valid as for any of the specialized renal function radiopharmaceuticals. The accumulation and excretion phases of the study will also provide valid renal functional data which could

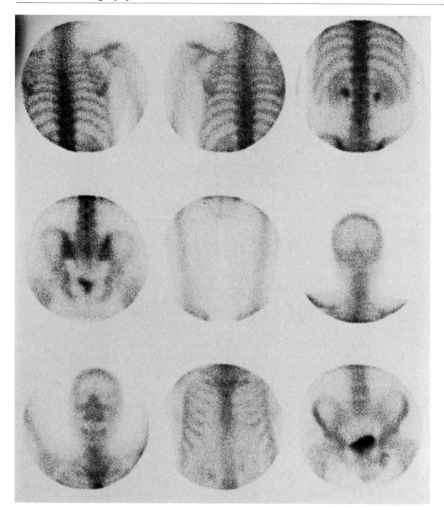

Figure 6.5 The nine single views taken with the gamma camera to cover the skeleton adequately in routine bone scintigraphy

lead the clinician to investigate this aspect of the patient's condition more fully. Early imaging of the kidneys is rarely included in routine bone scintigraphy protocols but should not be overlooked as an additional option.

Prostatic carcinoma

Of all tumours metastatic to bone normally dealt with by the urologist, prostatic carcinoma is the most common. The metastases are generally osteoblastic, but osteolytic lesions are not at all unusual. Bone scintigraphy is now totally accepted as the standard method of screening such patients for metastatic bone disease on presentation and for routine follow-up studies for the duration of the patient's treatment.

Several studies have concentrated on this application of bone scintigraphy in establishing its superiority to the previously routine radiographic skeletal survey, comparing one imaging agent with another, relating radionuclide bone imaging to the full gamut of prostatic cancer staging procedures and evaluating its ability to assess the response to treatment (Faber *et al.*, 1967; Morgan and Mills, 1968; Konturi and Kivinitty, 1971; Roy *et al.*, 1971; Robinson and Constable, 1973; Shearer *et al.*, 1974; O'Donoghue *et al.*, 1978; Fitzpatrick *et al.*, 1978). These and other workers have brought the investigation of prostatic carcinoma firmly into the nuclear medicine department, where early functional disorders of the skeletal organ can be detected and monitored for change.

As regions of increased bone uptake can result from a variety of causes, both malignant and benign, it must be remembered that sometimes it will be necessary to follow a positive scintigraphic finding with radiographic investigation, thereby raising the specificity of the overall imaging protocol. When the radionuclide images show multiple, well-defined focal lesions in a patient known to have prostatic carcinoma, the interpretation of multiple secondaries is in little doubt. Radiography at this stage would be unlikely to add anything of real diagnostic value.

A single, well-defined focal defect could arise from other causes, such as fracture, inflammatory disease, Paget's disease and degenerative bone changes. Normal radiography will strongly favour an interpretation of metastatic disease while an abnormal radiograph should enable a specific interpretation to be applied to the isolated (and therefore equivocal) scintigraphic defect. However, modern gamma camera equipment is better able to resolve the single focal lesion than hitherto. With experience and good equipment it should be possible to extend the range of scintigraphic interpretation. Now it is unlikely that either Paget's disease or degenerative disease would be misinterpreted as prostatic metastatic disease. In general Paget's disease presents as an extensive involvement of single bones (*Figure 6.6*), in contrast with the compact focal appearance of metastatic bone disease. Degenerative joint uptake (*Figure 6.7*) is distinguished by its patchy, sometimes asymmetrical uptake with a tracer density that is rarely as intense or as compactly localized as in metastatic deposits. Nevertheless caution in the scintigraphic interpretation of single lesions still suggests that radiography should be called upon, at the very least to confirm these cases.

A negative finding in prostatic bone scintigraphy is consistent with complete absence of active bone metastases. Radiography is rarely necessary in such cases; if undertaken it may reveal a sclerotic lesion missed by the radionuclide study owing to its non-

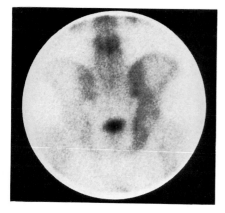

Figure 6.6 Paget's disease, showing the total involvement of the right pelvis and the fourth lumbar vertebra

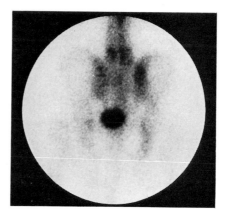

Figure 6.7 Degenerative disease at L5 and the right sacrum

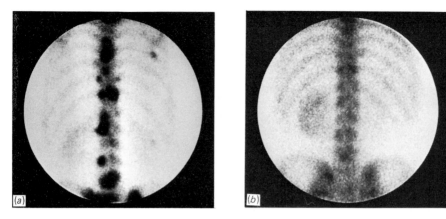

Figure 6.8
(*a*) clearly visible focal lesions seen on presentation
(*b*) the same patient after 15 months of chemotherapy

reactivity. A sclerotic lesion would generally indicate the site of a previously active lesion but may be radiographically indistinguishable from an active osteoblastic secondary. The negative scintigraphic finding had already clinched the only relevant clinical interpretation: no active lesions.

Following an initial positive diagnosis of prostatic metastases, and the selection of an appropriate treatment regimen, one of the urologist's main concerns is to be aware of changes in the patient's condition as they occur. Bone scintigraphy performed at regular intervals—between 3 and 12 months, depending on the patient's condition—enables the changing status of the metastases to be followed with some confidence, though not with quite as much certainty as would be hoped. When a great reduction in the number of observed lesions is seen on follow-up scintigraphy (*Figure 6.8*), regression may be safely assumed, and the general clinical condition of the patient will rarely contradict such a finding.

A large increase in the number of dense focal defects will signify progression of disease, and, again, the patient's clinical condition will probably confirm the interpretation (*Figure 6.9*). But all changes in the number, size and intensity of the focal

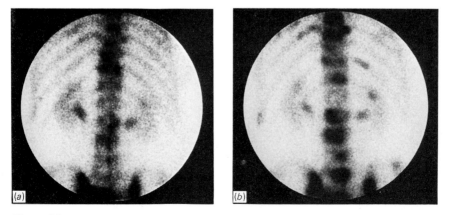

Figure 6.9
(*a*) initial bone scan
(*b*) scan after 16 months of chemotherapy. The increase in number, size and
      intensity of the focal abnormalities strongly suggests progression of the disease

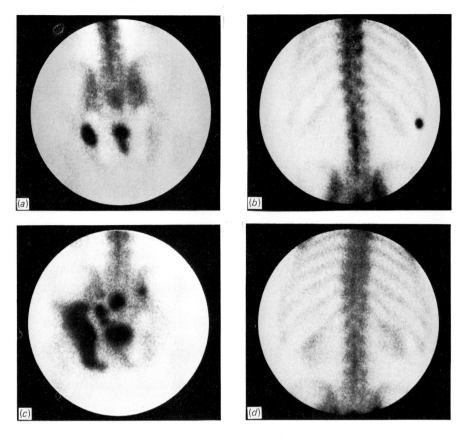

Figure 6.10
(a) distinct lesion demonstrated in the left ischium
(b) lesion in right 11th rib
(c) and (d) images produced 2 years later showing considerably heavier pelvic
   uptake and total disappearance of the rib lesion

lesions should be interpreted with caution and dealt with in the overall context of the patient's clinical condition and treatment regimen. Small changes in either direction may have to be considered uninterpretable. The appearance of increasing tracer uptake in a given lesion may be related to progression, but it may also be a consequence of the increased osteoblastic response in an osteolytic lesion as it passes into a healing phase. The total disappearance of a focal defect usually signifies healing, but there may be other interpretations. The failure of a previously observed focal defect to appear at follow-up could be the result of a very aggressive osteolytic lesion having destroyed normal bone to such an extent that no osteoblastic response is possible. Thus a dense defect may change to normal or to a photon deficiency (Condon *et al.*, 1981). Local infarction may also give rise to a reduction in the intensity of a focal defect or to its reappearance as a photon deficiency (Spencer *et al.*, 1981). It should also be borne in mind that, when one lesion has disappeared as a result of genuine healing, others may have appeared or be about to appear to more than counterbalance the single disappearance (*Figure 6.10*).

Even when all evidence of previously outstanding lesions disappears (*see Figure 6.8*), continued monitoring should not be neglected. Such a patient can often return to his

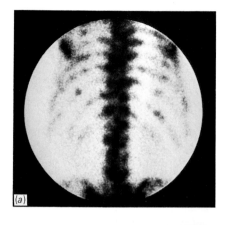

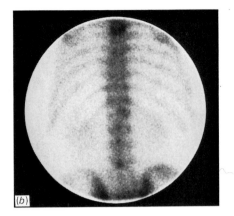

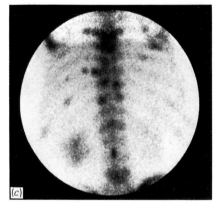

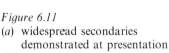

Figure 6.11
(a) widespread secondaries demonstrated at presentation
(b) ten months later, bone scintigraphy is almost normal
(c) six months later, however, the patient returned with bone pain and the images strongly suggest progression of the disease

original condition or worse (*Figure 6.11*). This unhappy state of affairs may demand urgent changes in treatment regimen with the obvious and repeated inference that sensitive methods of follow-up monitoring are essential. Bone scintigraphy in prostatic carcinoma provides the best that is available.

Objective criteria

The high degree of quantification that is now available with the data processing equipment usually attached to gamma cameras should give rise to the widespread use of objective criteria for the assessment of bone scintigrams. However, despite much published work on the subject (Castronovo *et al.*, 1973; Lurye *et al.*, 1977; Bollack *et al.*, 1980; Citrin *et al.*, 1981; De Luca *et al.*, 1983), no technique has been accepted sufficiently to have found its way into routine bone scintigraphy. True quantification in such a large and widely distributed organ as the skeleton presents many problems for the nuclear medicine computer specialist. To the complexity of skeletal geometry must be added the variable and often unpredictable factor of renal uptake and excretion. The patient with normal renal function may excrete 60% or more of the dose between administration and imaging. As renal function diminishes (for whatever reason), more tracer becomes available for skeletal incorporation. Thus quantification methods which attempt to measure the fraction of the administered dose taken up by the skeleton or retained by the body should perhaps apply a correction based on the patient's glomerular filtration rate (GFR) at the time of the study. Although whole-body retention methods of bone scintigraphy quantification have proved moderately successful, it is possible that they could become more so if the retention and GFR variables were both taken into consideration.

Other methods of quantification depend on the determination of various ratios such as: normal bone-to-soft tissue, pathological bone-to-normal bone, pathological bone-to-soft tissue and so on. Bone-to-soft-tissue ratios are also affected by variations of renal function as the amount of tracer remaining in the soft tissue at the time of imaging is usually more dependent on renal function than on bone uptake.

Notwithstanding these comments, it is possible to make broad distinctions of patient categories using either the whole-body retention method (Fogelman et al., 1978) or the bone-to-soft-tissue method (Rosenthall and Kaye, 1975). A bone-to-soft-tissue ratio in which the bone selected does not include a site of heavy uptake will not distinguish between patients with and without metastases. It will, however, separate out very distinctly those patients with excessively heavy but uniform uptake, images which have been described as *superscans* (Osmond et al., 1975). Such patients handle bone imaging agents quite differently from patients in all other categories. The images can often look normal (*Figure 6.12*) but the high bone-to-soft-tissue ratio usually results in very clear, low background images, while the renal images are fainter than usual and sometimes completely absent. Superscan patients excrete considerably less of the injected dose than normal (as shown in *Figure 6.13*, cf. *Figure 6.4*). Bone-to-soft tissue ratios can be five times greater than either normals or patients with discrete metastases. They can also be two or three times higher even when the ratio used in the latter group is obtained from involved bone (Constable and Cranage, 1981).

However, apart from this minority of cases, the bone-to-soft-tissue ratio is not usually helpful, either in the separation of patient categories or in following the progress of metastatic disease.

The response to treatment in patients initially presenting with widespread diffuse bone metastases from prostatic cancer has been followed using an index of quantification based on the fraction of the dose taken up by unit area of bone image (Perkins et al., 1982). In this study the authors noted a variable response between sites in some patients, with the previously uniform appearance resolving into focal deposits.

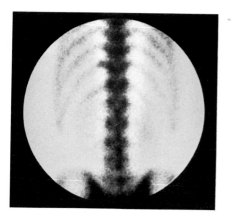

Figure 6.12 The almost uniformly distributed tracer in this patient may look normal at first glance, but the faint renal images and high spine-to-soft tissue contrast are characteristic of widespread diffuse metastases. The gamma camera images obtained are often called superscans

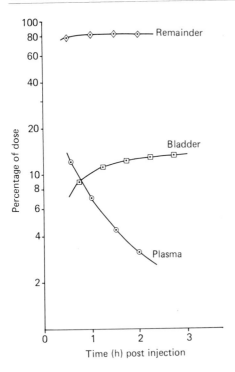

Figure 6.13 The plasma and bladder activity–time curves obtained from a superscan patient. Compared with the normal patient (*Figure 6.4*) considerably less dose is excreted and considerably more tracer is taken up by, or is potentially available to, the skeleton (the remainder curve)

The whole-body retention (WBR) over 24 hours is capable of a higher degree of discrimination between normals and the various metabolic bone disease categories (Fogelman *et al.*, 1978). The use of a 24-hour **WBR** has many applications in quantitative bone scintigraphy but is far from ideal as a method for objectively assessing the severity or the response to treatment of prostatic skeletal metastases.

Non-objective assessment of bone images relies on observing the number and intensity of the various focal lesions. The intensity of a lesion is judged by comparing it visually with the surrounding normal bone. Measurement of this ratio of pathological to normal bone is a cumbersome method but it is sometimes capable of accurately charting response to treatment. The changes observed can vary greatly from patient to patient on the same treatment regimens. The changes can also vary from one lesion to another in the same patient, which is compatible with the visual observation that regression and progression of different metastatic sites can occur simultaneously. However, if the images are analysed lesion by lesion, the method provides useful objective criteria (Bollack *et al.*, 1981). One advantage of this method over methods which use, directly or indirectly, the soft tissue is its comparative independence of renal function variations.

The quantity of tracer available for skeletal incorporation depends on renal function, and the quantity incorporated depends on the intrinsic avidity of normal and abnormal bone. The renal handling of the bone-seeking agent compared with a glomerular-filtered agent could provide an additional index of skeletal uptake to aid objective interpretation. Attempts are in progress to make use of the ratio of the renal clearance of ^{99m}Tc-MDP to that of ^{99m}Tc-DTPA as an index of skeletal uptake (Nisbet *et al.*, 1983). The method is showing itself capable of some degree of specificity in distinguishing the various patient categories and in following treatment response.

Some other aspects

The active renal handling of ^{99m}Tc-labelled diphosphonate compounds results in the renal images we are accustomed to seeing on bone scintigrams. However, as previously indicated, the interpretation of renal images seen between 2 and 4 hours after tracer administration is fraught with problems. Fainter than usual renal images, intense intra-renal concentrations, images with bilateral, uniformly distributed, heavy residual activity should all be interpreted with circumspection and are often best left with no comment. The reasons for these observed slight variations in kidney appearance often have little to do with clearly understood renal causes, though the subject can give rise to considerable speculative argument. Recent work (Buxton-Thomas and Wraight, 1983), however, suggests that dense renal images may be a sign of hypercalcaemia. This could be a worthwhile suggestion at the time of reporting but other possible explanations (e.g. cirrhosis and prior chemotherapy) should be considered.

Certain gross kidney appearances (*Figure 6.14*), such as extreme right/left asymmetry, grossly dilated renal pelvis, distinct parenchymal filling defects suggestive of cysts or tumours or clear visualization of the ureter suggestive of obstruction, could lead to positive comments when reporting bone images. Conventional renal gamma camera studies would then probably be undertaken. If more were known about the

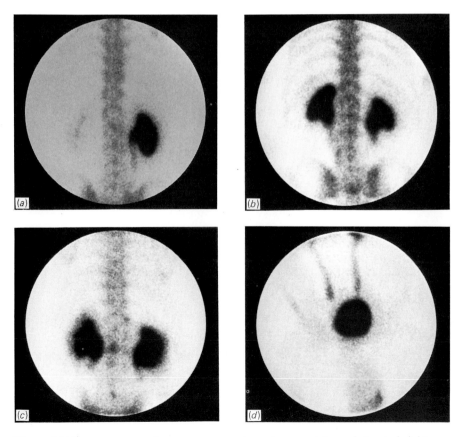

Figure 6.14 Some gross renal appearances on bone images: (*a*) an obstructed right kidney; (*b*) bilateral PUJ obstruction; (*c*) and (*d*) bilateral dilated renal pelvis with visualization of both ureters characteristic of persistent bladder retention

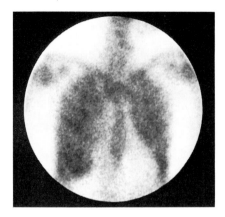

Figure 6.15 The anterior chest view of a chronic dialysis patient with severe uraemic pulmonary calcification

renal handling of ^{99m}Tc-labelled disphosphonates, perhaps the late images on bone scintigrams, particularly in combination with DTPA or DMSA scintigraphic studies, might be capable of adding usefully to the range of renal diagnostic capability.

On the other hand, early images acquired immediately following the injection of the bone imaging agent can be of considerable use. As indicated on p. 65, the perfusion phase is as valid as with any of the conventional renal imaging agents. The early uptake phase will provide a good broad assessment of comparative and individual renal function, and all the usual observations of filling and emptying in the upper and lower urinary tracts can be made during excretion. The bone scintigraphy protocol could, without much additional complication, include a micturition study. The large quantity of activity present in the bladder at any convenient time between 30 minutes post-injection and bone imaging time provides an opportunity to measure residual urine volume (*see* p. 171) and the maximum achievable rate of voiding (O'Reilly *et al.*, 1981). Such data are not at all out of place when dealing with prostatic disease.

The use of bone scintigraphy in monitoring patients in renal failure and on dialysis is of some value in detecting early bone abnormalities such as renal osteodystrophy. But, in the presence of poor or zero renal function, where a greater fraction of the injected tracer dose is available for bone incorporation, care should be taken interpreting data (Ølgaard *et al.*, 1979). Uraemic pulmonary calcification, where severe, shows up clearly on bone scintigrams (*Figure 6.15*) but is usually a late stage finding (de Graaf *et al.*, 1979) when the patient's condition has already been diagnosed.

For the urologist, prostatic carcinoma remains the commonest reason for requesting bone scintigraphy. Patients with renal, bladder or urethral carcinoma may also develop skeletal metastases and can be referred to the nuclear medicine department, where the bone imaging protocol will be essentially the same as for patients with prostatic cancer.

Bone scintigraphy is a well-established routine, and perhaps lacks some of the glamour enjoyed by the newer, less routine, work of the department. However, like most nuclear medicine procedures, bone scintigraphy investigates a very functional aspect of the body. It does so with high sensitivity for bone abnormalities and increasing sensitivity to treatment response. It offers rewarding prospects for those wishing to study the development of acceptable methods of quantitative assessment and more specific diagnosis.

References

BECK, R. N. and HARPER, P. V. (1968) Criteria for evaluating radioisotope imaging system. In: *Fundamental Problems in Scanning*, A. Gottschalk and R. N. Beck (eds.), Springfield, Illinois: Charles C. Thomas, pp. 348–382

BORAK, J. (1942) Relationship between the clinical and roentgenological findings in bone metastases. *Surgery, Gynecology and Obstetrics*, **75**, 599–604

BOLLACK, C., METHLIN, G., OLIVEUX, A., GROB, J. C. and CARLOZ, I. (1981) Quantitative bone scanning and the supervision of metastases in prostatic cancer. In: *Advances in Diagnostic Urology*, C. C. Schulman (ed.), Berlin: Springer-Verlag, pp. 239–245

BUXTON-THOMAS, M. S. and WRAIGHT, E. P. (1983) High renal activity on bone scintigrams. A sign of hypercalcaemia? *British Journal of Radiology*, **56**, 911–914

CASTRONOVO, F. P. Jr., POTSAID, M. S. and PENDERGRASS, H. P. (1973) Effects of radiation therapy on bone lesions as measured by Tc-99m-diphosphonate. *Journal of Nuclear Medicine*, **14**, 604–605

CHARKES, N. D., MAKLER, P. T. and PHILIPS, C. (1978) Studies of skeletal tracer kinetics. I. Digital computer solution of a five-compartment model of (^{18}F) fluoride kinetics in humans. *Journal of Nuclear Medicine*, **19**, 1301–1309

CHARKES, N. D. (1980) Skeletal blood flow: Implications for bone-scan interpretation. *Journal of Nuclear Medicine*, **21**, 91–98

CITRIN, D. L., HOUGE, C., ZWEIHEL, W., SCHLISE, S., PRUITT, B., ERSHLER, W., DAVIS, T. E., HARBERG, J. and COHEN, A. I. (1981) The use of serial bone scans in assessing response of bone metastases to systematic treatment. *Cancer*, **47**, 680–685

CONDON, B. R., BUCHANAN, R., GARVIE, N. W., ACKERY, D. M., FLEMMING, J., TAYLOR, D., HAWKES, D. and GODDARD, B. A. (1981) Assessment of progression of secondary bone lesions following cancer of the breast or prostate using serial radionuclide imaging. *British Journal of Radiology*, **54**, 18–23

CONSTABLE, A. R. and CRANAGE, R. W. (1981) Recognition of Superscan in prostatic bone scintigraphy. *British Journal of Radiology*, **54**, 122–125

DE GRAAF, P., SCHICHT, I. M., PAUWELS, E. K. J., SOUVERIJN, J. H. M. and DE GRAEF, J. (1979) Bone scintigraphy in uremic pulmonary calcification. *Journal of Nuclear Medicine*, **20**, 201–206

DE LUCA, S. A., CASTRONOVO, F. P. and RHEA, J. T. (1983) The effects of chemotherapy on bone metastases as measured by quantitative skeletal imaging. *Clinical Nuclear Medicine*, **8**, 11–13

FABER, D. D., WAHMAN, G. E., BAILEY, T. A., FLOCKS, R. H., CULP, D. A. and MORRISON, R. T. (1967) An evaluation of the strontium-85 scan for the detection and localization of bone metastases from prostatic carcinoma: A preliminary report of 93 cases. *Journal of Urology*, **97**, 526–532

FITZPATRICK, J. M., CONSTABLE, A. R., SHERWOOD, T., STEVENSON, J. J., CHISHOLM, G. D. and O'DONOGHUE, E. P. N. (1978) Serial bone scanning: The assessment of treatment response in carcinoma of the prostate. *British Journal of Urology*, **50**, 555–561

FOGELMAN, I., BESSENT, R. G., TURNER, J. G., CITRIN, D. L., BOYLE, I. T. and GREIG, W. R. (1978) The use of whole body retention of Tc-99m diphosphonate in the diagnosis of metabolic bone disease. *Journal of Nuclear Medicine*, **19**, 270–275

FOGELMAN, I., CITRIN, D. L., MCKILLOP, J. H., TURNER, J. G., BESSENT, R. G. and GREIG, W. R. (1979) A clinical comparison of Tc-99m HEDP and Tc-99m MDP in the detection of bone metastases. *Journal of Nuclear Medicine*, **20**, 98–101

GALASKO, C. S. (1969) The detection of skeletal metastases from mammary cancer by gamma scintigraphy. *British Journal of Surgery*, **56**, 757–764

KONTTURI, M. and KIVINITTY, K. (1971) Radiostrontium in the early diagnosis of bone metastases in patients with prostate carcinoma. *Scandinavian Journal of Urology and Nephrology*, **5**, 210–214

LAVENDER, J. P., KHAN, R. A. A. and HUGHES, S. P. F. (1979) Blood flow and tracer uptake in normal and abnormal canine bone: Comparisons with Sr-85 microspheres, Kr-81m and Tc-99m MDP. *Journal of Nuclear Medicine*, **20**, 413–418

LURYE, D. R., CASTRONOVO, F. P. and POTSAID, M. S. (1977) An improved method for quantitative bone scanning. *Journal of Nuclear Medicine*, **18**, 1069–1073

MAKLER, P. T. Jr. and CHARKES, N. D. (1980) Studies of skeletal tracer kinetics. IV. Optimum time delay for Tc-99m (Sn) methylene diphosphonate bone imaging. *Journal of Nuclear Medicine*, **21**, 641–645

MORGAN, C. and MILLS, P. (1968) Radioactive bone scans in carcinoma of the prostate. *Southern Medical Journal*, **61**, 785–790

NISBET, A. P., EDWARDS, S., MASHITER, G., WINN, P., HILSON, A. J. W. and MAISEY, M. N. (1983) Quantitation of Tc-99m MDP retention during bone scanning. *Nuclear Medicine Communications*, **4**, 67–71

O'DONOGHUE, E. P. N., CONSTABLE, A. R., SHERWOOD, T., STEVENSON, J. J. and CHISHOLM, G. D. (1978) Bone scanning and plasma phosphates in carcinoma of the prostate. *British Journal of Urology*, **50**, 172–177

ØLGAARD, K., MADSEN, S., HEERFORDT, J., HAMMER, M. and JENSEN, H. (1979) Scintigraphic skeletal changes in non-dialysed patients with advanced renal failure. *Clinical Nephrology*, **12**, 273–278

O'REILLY, P. H., LAWSON, R. S., SHIELDS, R. A., TESTA, H. J. and EDWARDS, E. C. (1981) Radionuclide studies of the lower urinary tract. *British Journal of Urology*, **53**, 266–269

OSMOND, J. D., PENDERGRASS, H. P. and POTSAID, M. S. (1975) Accuracy of Tc-99m diphosphate bone scans and roentgenograms in the detection of prostate, breast and lung carcinoma metastases. *American Journal of Roentgenology*, **125**, 972–977

PERKINS, A. C., HARDY, J. G., WASTIE, M. L. and CLIFFORD, K. M. A. (1982) Serial radionuclide imaging during treatment of patients with diffuse bone metastases from carcinoma of the prostate. *European Journal of Nuclear Medicine*, 7, 322–323

ROBINSON, M. R. G. and CONSTABLE, A. R. (1973) Strontium-87m and the gamma camera in the study of bone metastases from carcinoma of the prostate. *British Journal of Urology*, 45, 173–178

ROSENTHALL, L. and KAY, M. (1975) Technetium-99m-pyrophosphate kinetics and imaging in metabolic bone disease. *Journal of Nuclear Medicine*, 16, 33–39

ROSENTHALL, L., ARZOUMANIAN, A., LISBONA, R. and ITOH, K. (1977) A longitudinal comparison of the kinetics of ^{99m}Tc-MDP and ^{99m}Tc-EHDP in humans. *Clinical Nuclear Medicine*, 2, 232–234

ROY, R. R., NORTHAM, B. E., BEALES, J. S. and CHISHOLM, G. D. (1971) 18 Fluorine total body scans in patients with carcinoma of the prostate. *British Journal of Urology*, 43, 58–64

SHEARER, R. J., CONSTABLE, A. R., GIRLING, M., HENDRY, W. F. and FERGUSSON, J. D. (1974) Radioisotope bone scintigraphy with the gamma camera in the investigation of prostatic cancer. *British Medical Journal*, 2, 362–365

SPENCER, R. P., SZIKLAS, J. J., ROSENBERG, R., YOO, J-H. and WEIDNER, A. (1981) Hemivertebral 'disappearance' on bone scan. *Journal of Nuclear Medicine*, 22, 454–456

SUBRAMANIAN, G. and MCAFEE, J. G. (1971) A new complex of ^{99}Tc^m for skeletal imaging. *Radiology*, 99, 192–196

SUBRAMANIAN, G., MCAFEE, J. G., BLAIR, R. L., KALLFELZ, F. A. and THOMAS, F. D. (1975a) ^{99}Tc^m methylene diphosphonate—a superior agent for skeletal imaging: comparison with other technetium complexes. *Journal of Nuclear Medicine*, 16, 744–755

SUBRAMANIAN, G., MCAFEE, J. G., BLAIR, R. J. and THOMAS, F. D. (1975b) An evaluation of ^{99m}Tc labelled phosphate compounds as bone imaging agents. In: *Radiopharmaceuticals*, G. Subramanian, B. Rhodes and J. F. Cooper (eds.), New York: Society of Nuclear Medicine, pp. 319–328

SY, W. M., WESTRING, D. W. and WEINBURGER, G. (1975) 'Cold' lesions on bone imaging. *Journal of Nuclear Medicine*, 16, 1013–1016

7 Protocols of procedures

D. L. Hastings and M. C. Prescott

The details of the procedures described in this book vary between departments and institutions according to logistical considerations and the availability of radio-pharmaceuticals and instrumentation. The protocols presented here are based on those used at present at Manchester Royal Infirmary and represent examples which may be used as a general guide.

It should be noted that no special preparation of the patient is necessary for any of the tests; for renography a state of dehydration should be avoided.

The question of blocking the thyroid gland is often raised in connection with the use of agents containing radioisotopes of iodine and technetium. In the majority of cases the purity of modern radiopharmaceuticals, their effective half-life and the quantity of activity administered should be such that this is unnecessary. However, if indicated, it may be done by the oral administration of 3–6 mg/kg body weight of potassium perchlorate at 30–60 minutes prior to the test. This has been recommended, for example, when 400 MBq ^{99m}Tc-pertechnetate is used for dynamic perfusion studies.

Renography

Gamma camera renography

Clinical procedure

1. Select the radiopharmaceutical and prepare the appropriate dose for injection (*see* *Table 7.1*). In some circumstances (e.g. study of reflux in duplex systems) it may be appropriate to increase the dose.
2. Set up the gamma camera for the gamma ray energy of the radionuclide, and select the appropriate collimator (*Table 7.1*). Set up for sequential analogue images of, for example, 5-minute duration.
3. Set up the computer for a dynamic acquisition of 20-second frames for 40 minutes.
4. Ensure that the patient is adequately hydrated; in hot weather give a 500-ml drink.
5. Send the patient to empty his bladder, and then position the patient for a posterior view, in the sitting position. The kidneys should be just above the centre of the field of view with the bladder at the bottom of the picture (for pelvic or horseshoe kidneys an anterior view is preferable).
6. Inject the radiopharmaceutical into a vein in the antecubital fossa. In the case of neonates, or patients in whom a vein is difficult to find, it may be necessary to use an indwelling butterfly needle, and flush the dose through with saline immediately after injection.
7. At the time of injection start the computer and analogue acquisitions.
8. If diuresis is not required, acquisition may be terminated at 20 minutes.
9. If diuresis is considered, judgement on whether to give frusemide should be made at approximately 20 minutes, and the time of administration of diuretic should be noted. Image acquisitions should then be continued until significant elimination is seen, or until 10–15 minutes after the diuretic (*see* p. 17).
10. Develop the analogue films.
11. If the patient has a pelvic kidney which is hidden by the bladder at the end of the study, a further 5-minute image of the kidney should be obtained after the patient has emptied the bladder. Similarly, if a urostomy bag interferes with a renal image a further 5-minute image should be taken after the bag has been drained.
12. Carry out the computer analysis as described below.

Computer analysis

In gamma camera renography it is desirable to represent counts in the computer-derived renogram as a percentage of the injected dose. This is achieved by advance

TABLE 7.1. Dosage and settings for gamma camera renography

Study and radiopharmaceutical	Adult dose		Child dose				Camera settings	
	(MBq)	(µCi)	Dose/kg body wt.		Minimum dose		Energy (keV)	Collimator
			(MBq)	(µCi)	(MBq)	(µCi)		
Standard renography								
^{99m}Tc-DTPA	75	2000	1.0	27	4	100	140	Low energy
^{123}I-OIH	12	300	0.2	5.4	3	80	159	Low energy
^{131}I-OIH	4	100	0.06	1.6	2	50	364	High energy
Transplant renography								
^{123}I-OIH	3	80	0.05	1.3	2	50	159	Low energy
^{131}I-OIH	3	80	0.05	1.3	2	50	364	High energy

determination of the sensitivity of the gamma camera to a given radionuclide contained in a phantom simulating a kidney within the torso. The sensitivity, or calibration, factor in cps/MBq is obtained for each radionuclide, gamma camera and collimator combination. The resulting set of calibration factors is stored in the computer and a user-written program selects the appropriate factor when analysing a renogram.

1. View the images using a dynamic display. Check for patient movement and validity of data.
2. Sum the first 10–20 frames and several frames near the end of the study so that the kidneys and bladder can be seen clearly.
3. Delineate regions of interest for the left kidney, right kidney, bladder and a background region between the upper parts of—and extending to just above—the kidneys (see Figure 2.3). If indicated, also delineate segmental regions of interest and regions for separate moieties.
4. Generate curves corresponding to the regions.
5. Correct the curves for background and convert the counts to percentage dose using the stored calibration factor for the radionuclide used.
6. Determine the relative function of the left and right kidney (see p. 15) and the relative function of other renal regions if required.
7. Produce a hard copy of the results by plotting the analysed curves as percentage dose against time with appropriate labels and tabulating the values of relative function. (User programs may be written to carry out steps 5, 6 and 7.)

Deconvolution analysis

1. View the images using dynamic display. Check for patient movement and validity of data.
2. Sum the first 10–20 frames so that the kidneys can be seen clearly.
3. Delineate regions of interest for each kidney, and a blood region in a vascular area above the left kidney over the lower borders of the heart.
4. Display the whole kidney regions of interest on a later image in which the renal pelvis is visualized clearly. Delineate, for each kidney, a parenchymal region within the original whole kidney region but excluding the pelvic area.
5. Generate curves corresponding to the regions.
6. Run the computer program to carry out deconvolution analysis, which generates impulse retention functions for each kidney and parenchyma and calculates the mean transit time for each region.
7. Produce a hard copy of the results by plotting the count rate curves and the impulse retention functions and by tabulating the mean transit times.

Probe renography

1. Draw up a dose of ^{131}I-OIH in a syringe—1 MBq (27 μCi) for the normal adult (for children approximately 0.015 MBq/kg, but not less than 0.2 MBq (5 μCi)).
2. Position all detectors looking at the dose. Adjust each pulse height analyser and high voltage unit to give the peak count rate.
3. Set the ratemeter time constant to 3 seconds. Set the ratemeter scales to 300 cps for detectors 1 and 2 (chest and bladder), and 1000 cps for detectors 3 and 4 (right and left kidney).
4. Adjust the chart recorder pen position to zero and check its function.
5. Ensure the patient is adequately hydrated; in hot weather give him a 500-ml drink.
6. Send the patient to empty his bladder and then position him in a chair with detectors

3 and 4 over the kidneys, detector 1 over the infraclavicular region and detector 2 over the bladder.

7. Inject the OIH and acquire data for at least 20 minutes.
8. If an obstruction is suspected, and one or both renograms remain flat or continue rising, consider diuresis (*see* the procedure below).
9. Switch off the chart recorder and label the tracings.

Diuresis renography (using gamma camera or probes)

Diuresis from start of test

1. Ensure that the patient is in a good state of hydration and that there is no clinical reason why diuresis should not be induced.
2. Ask the patient to empty his or her bladder.
3. Ask the patient to drink one or two cups of water (approximately 300 ml).
4. Insert a butterfly needle into a suitable vein. Inject frusemide at a dose of 0.5 mg/kg body weight. Wait 15 minutes before starting step 5.
5. Inject the radiopharmaceutical as for a routine renogram.
6. Continue the renogram as normal. If the patient needs to pass urine in the middle of the test, leave the system running and reposition after the patient returns. Continue the renogram until 20 minutes after the OIH injection. Measure the volume of the urine voided.
7. Warn the patient that the diuretic effect will last for a couple of hours.

Diuresis at 20 minutes

1. Ensure that the patient is in a good state of hydration and that there is no clinical reason why diuresis should not be induced.
2. Perform the standard renography procedure.
3. Give the patient a drink of water (approximately 300 ml).
4. At 20 minutes inject frusemide at a dose of 0.5 mg/kg body weight. Note the time. Continue with renography until significant elimination occurs, or until 10–15 minutes after the diuretic was administered (*see* p. 17).
5. Measure the volume of urine at the end of the test.
6. Warn the patient that the effect of diuresis will last for a couple of hours.

Repeat with diuresis immediately after standard renogram

This method may only be used if most of the activity has been excreted from the kidney by the end of the routine renogram.

1. Check that the patient is in a good state of hydration and that there is no clinical reason why diuresis should not be induced.
2. Let the routine renogram continue to at least 20 minutes, until most activity has been excreted from the kidney.
3. Ask the patient to drink one or two cups of water (approximately 300 ml).
4. Inject frusemide at a dose of 0.5 mg/kg body weight. Wait 15 minutes before beginning step 5.
5. Inject a further dose of the radiopharmaceutical. A second dose equal to the initial dose should be sufficient.
6. Continue as from step 6 of the first method (*see* p. 17).

Renal imaging

Renal imaging with first circulation: gluconate or DTPA

1. Prepare a dose of 400 MBq ^{99m}Tc-calcium gluconate or ^{99m}Tc-DTPA. Draw up 10 ml normal saline into a separate syringe.
2. Set up the gamma camera for ^{99m}Tc with a low-energy parallel hole collimator. Set the multi-formatter for 12 analogue images of 5 seconds' duration.
3. Set up the computer for a dynamic acquisition of 60 frames, each of 1 second's duration, followed by 5 frames each of 2 minutes' duration.
4. Position the patient, seated if possible, for a posterior view of the kidneys.
5. Take an intermittent infusion needle (butterfly cannula with a rubber diaphragm) and insert the needle into a vein in the antecubital fossa. Take both saline and radiopharmaceutical syringes, complete with needles, and insert them together into the rubber diaphragm of the cannula. Establish a flow of saline and then inject the radiopharmaceutical as a bolus, maintaining pressure on the saline plunger to prevent backflow. Flush with more saline.
6. At the time of injection start the computer and analogue acquisitions.
7. When the sequence of 12 images showing the perfusion is complete, change to a new film cassette.
8. For the parenchymal study at 2 minutes after injection, acquire an image of the same size as the first 12 images, and of 40 seconds' duration, onto position 1 of the multi-formatter.
9. Without changing the film cassette, set the multi-formatter to a 2 × 2 format to begin acquisition at the second position. Starting at 5 minutes after injection acquire two further images in sequence, each of 2 minutes' duration.
10. For the fourth and final position of the multi-formatter, reposition the patient for an anterior view of the kidneys and acquire a 2-minute image.
11. Develop the two analogue films.

Renal imaging using ^{99m}Tc-DMSA

1. Prepare the required dose of ^{99m}Tc-DMSA: 1 MBq/kg body weight.
2. Two hours prior to imaging inject the DMSA into a vein in the antecubital fossa.
3. Set up the gamma camera for ^{99m}Tc with a low-energy parallel hole collimator. Set a preset count limit of 400 000 counts and a zoom factor of 2.
4. Set up the computer for the static acquisition of 5-minute images.
5. Acquire both analogue and computer images for each of the following views: anterior, posterior, left posterior oblique and right posterior oblique.
6. On the computer images of both posterior and anterior views delineate regions of interest for each kidney and a background area between the kidneys.
7. Normalize the counts in each region for region size and correct the kidney counts by subtracting the background. For each kidney calculate the geometric mean of the corrected counts by taking the square root of the product of counts from the anterior and posterior views. If these figures are L for the left kidney and R for the right kidney then the relative function of each kidney is given by:

$$\frac{L}{L + R} \times 100\% \quad \text{and} \quad \frac{R}{L + R} \times 100\% \tag{1}$$

Gallium imaging

1. Prepare a dose of 80 MBq ^{67}Ga-citrate, and inject it intravenously.
2. Take images as below after 24, 48 and 72 hours (or as appropriate).

3. Set up the gamma camera for ^{67}Ga with a high-energy, high-sensitivity parallel collimator. If possible set three windows for the three ^{67}Ga photopeaks at 93, 185 and 300 keV and sum the three outputs. If only one window setting is possible, the 185 keV photopeak is preferable.
4. Position the patient supine for anterior and posterior views as required. If the test is for the investigation of pyrexia of unknown origin, then anterior and posterior views of the whole body may be required. However, if there is a more specific problem, for example a possible renal abscess, then anterior and posterior views of the kidney area may be sufficient.
5. If excess gut activity is a problem at 72 hours, the images may be repeated 24 hours later, when the distribution of activity in the gut will probably have changed, or an enema may be administered to the patient.

Transplant studies

Renal transplant renography

Clinical procedure

1. Select the radiopharmaceutical and prepare the dose for injection (*see Table 7.1*).
2. Set up the gamma camera for the gamma ray energy of the radionuclide and select the appropriate collimator. Set up for sequential analogue images of 5 minutes' duration.
3. Set up the computer for a 60-second image.
4. Position the patient with the camera over the iliac fossa containing the transplanted kidney. If possible the bladder and some of the contralateral iliac fossa should also be in the field of view.
5. Obtain a 60-second background image on the computer.
6. Reset the computer for a dynamic acquisition of 90 × 20-second frames.
7. Inject the dose intravenously and start the computer and analogue acquisitions.
8. Measure the remaining activity in the dose syringe and calculate the net dose injected.
9. Obtain 6 × 5-minute analogue images throughout the 30-minute study.
10. At 30 minutes obtain the following computer images:
    (a) 60-second repositioned bladder image if the bladder is not completely within the field of view on the dynamic images;
    (b) 60-second catheter image if a catheter is present. The catheter should be imaged through at least 2-cm thick tissue-equivalent rubber;
    (c) 60-second injection site image if any residual activity remains in the area;
    (d) 60-second drainage bag image if any drainage bags contain fluid.
11. Carry out the computer analysis as described below.

Computer analysis of renal transplant renography

1. View the images using a dynamic display. Check for patient movement and validity of data.
2. Sum all the frames of the dynamic study.
3. Delineate regions of interest for the transplanted kidney, bladder and background region, if possible, in the contralateral iliac fossa. In addition delineate regions for the areas of interest in any images acquired in step 10 of the clinical procedure above.
4. Generate curves for the kidney, bladder and background.
5. Correct the curves for background, smooth them, and convert the counts to percentage dose using the stored calibration factor (as described above, p. 79) for

the radionuclide used. If necessary make a correction for any residual activity at the injection site as seen on image (c) in step 10 above.

6. Determine the time at which the renogram attains its peak value and the total activity (as percentage of dose) in kidney, bladder and catheter at 30 minutes (called 'total removal', *see* p. 131).

7. Produce a hard copy of the results by plotting the analysed curves as percentage dose against time with appropriate labels, time of renogram peak, and total removal amount. (User programs may be written to carry out steps 5, 6 and 7.)

Renal transplant perfusion studies

These are performed as for renal imaging using ^{99m}Tc-DTPA described above (p. 81) with the following exception.

Position the patient with the camera over the iliac fossa containing the kidney. If possible some of the lower aorta and distal iliac artery should be included in the field of view. The position should remain unchanged throughout the study.

Clearance studies

Glomerular filtration rate

1. Select the radiopharmaceutical and prepare the appropriate dose. For ^{51}Cr-EDTA use 3 MBq (80 μCi). For ^{99m}Tc-DTPA, if the GFR is to be determined concurrently with renography or a first circulation study, then the dose will be the same as for that study, i.e. 75 MBq (2 mCi) for renography or 400 MBq (10 mCi) for first circulation. Otherwise 20 MBq (0.5 mCi) ^{99m}Tc-DTPA is sufficient. This lower activity may also be used if the GFR is to be determined concurrently with a ^{131}I-OIH transplant scan.

2. Prepare a further aliquot of the radiopharmaceutical for use as a standard.

3. Calibrate the dose and standard and dilute the standard to 1 litre using one of the calibration methods on p. 85.

4. Take a 10 ml heparinized blood sample from the patient for use as a background.

5. Inject the patient using an antecubital vein and note the time. Retain the syringe if using calibration method (1) or (3).

6. Take four 10 ml heparinized blood samples at 90, 150, 210, 270 minutes post injection. Take the blood samples from a different site from that used for injection and note the exact collection times.

7. Centrifuge the blood samples and, from each, dispense 2 ml of plasma into appropriately labelled sample tubes. Into another sample tube dispense 2 ml from the standard flask.

8. Count the samples, the standard and a room background for the same times, using a scintillation well counter set up for the radionuclide. Correct all plasma counts for background by subtracting the background plasma sample count, and correct the standard counts by subtracting the room background.

9. Using log-linear graph paper plot the plasma count (log scale) against time.

10. Find the best straight line fit and determine the intercept at time zero (time of injection) and the half time of clearance ($t_{1/2}$) in minutes.

11. Calculate the volume of dilution and the GFR from the following formulae:

$$\text{Volume of dilution, } V = \frac{(\text{Standard counts}) \times (\text{dose/standard ratio})}{\text{Intercept}} \text{ litres} \qquad (2)$$

$$\text{GFR} = \frac{V \times 0.693}{t_{1/2}} \times 1000 \text{ ml/minute} \qquad (3)$$

Effective renal plasma flow

The labelled OIH used for ERPF measurement should be of high radiochemical purity: it should not contain more than 0.5% free iodide.

Multiple blood sample method

1. Prepare the dose and a standard syringe containing 2 MBq and 0.75 MBq respectively of ^{125}I-OIH. The test may be done concurrently with renography using ^{123}I-OIH or ^{131}I-OIH, in which case the renogram dose may be exploited for both tests, and only an additional standard is needed.
2. Calibrate the dose and standard. Dilute the standard to 1 litre using one of the calibration methods on p. 85.
3. Place an intermittent infusion needle (butterfly) in a suitable vein and withdraw a 10 ml blood sample into a heparinized vial for use as a background.
4. Inject the dose through the butterfly needle. Flush the butterfly with saline. Retain the syringe if using calibration methods (1) or (3).
5. Insert a butterfly needle into a vein of the arm opposite to that used for injection. Take 5 ml heparinized blood samples at 10-minute intervals up to an hour after injection, noting the time of each sample. Before taking each sample, first withdraw and discard approximately 1 ml of fluid to empty the cannula. Keep the cannula open between samplings using saline.
6. Centrifuge all the blood samples.
7. Dispense 2 ml samples of plasma and diluted standard into labelled sample tubes.
8. Count all the samples, the standard and a room background in a scintillation well counter.
9. Correct the count rates by subtracting the background count rate.
10. Using log-linear graph paper plot the corrected plasma count rate (log scale) against time. Fit an exponential by finding the best straight line through the later part of the curve. Read off the intercept (C_2) and measure the half-time in minutes. Calculate the slope (λ_2). Peel off this fitted exponential from the observed plasma curve (by subtracting values at appropriate intervals) and fit the best straight line to the subtracted values to give the first exponential component. Read the intercept (C_1) and measure the slope (λ_1) as above.
11. Calculate the ERPF from the formula:

$$ \text{ERPF} = \frac{\lambda_1 \lambda_2}{C_1 \lambda_2 + C_2 \lambda_1} \cdot C_s \cdot \text{R} \cdot 1000 \, \text{ml/min} \tag{4} $$

where C_s is the corrected count rate from the diluted standard and R is the dose/standard ratio.

Single sample method

1. Prepare dose and standard syringes containing 2 MBq (50 μCi) and 0.75 MBq (20 μCi) respectively of ^{125}I-OIH. The test may be done concurrently with renography using ^{123}I-OIH or ^{131}I-OIH, in which case the renogram dose may be exploited for both tests, and only an additional standard is needed.
2. Calibrate the dose and standard, and dilute the standard using one of the calibration methods on p. 85.
3. Place an intermittent infusion needle (butterfly) in a suitable vein and withdraw a 10 ml blood sample into a heparinized vial for use as a background.
4. Inject the dose through the butterfly needle. Flush the butterfly with saline. Retain the syringe if using calibration methods (1) or (3).

5. If the test is being carried out concurrently with a ^{99m}Tc-DTPA renogram the DTPA may be injected at this stage using the same butterfly.
6. The patient should be kept resting until the next blood sample.
7. At 44 minutes after injection (42–46 minutes is acceptable) take a 10 ml heparinized blood sample from the opposite arm to that used for the injection.
8. Centrifuge the two blood samples.
9. Dispense 2 ml of plasma from each sample and 2 ml from the diluted standard into labelled samples tubes.
10. Count the plasma samples, the standard and a room background in a scintillation well counter. If the patient had a concurrent ^{99m}Tc study the samples must be kept for 3 days before counting to allow the ^{99m}Tc to decay.
11. Correct the 44-minute plasma count by subtracting the background plasma sample count, and correct the standard count by subtracting the room background.
12. Calculate the volume of dilution and the ERPF from the following formulae:

$$V = \frac{(\text{Standard counts}) \times (\text{dose/standard ratio})}{(\text{44-minute plasma counts})} \text{ litres} \qquad (5)$$

$$\text{ERPF} = 5.5 \times V \text{ ml/min}$$

Calibration of dose and standard for clearance studies

Three methods are described here for calibration of dose and standard in clearance studies. Use method (1) for ^{99m}Tc. Use method (2) for ^{125}I, ^{131}I or ^{51}Cr in situations when all of the dose can be injected with certainty (i.e. blood can be withdrawn into syringe after injection, and reinjected to remove residue of dose). Otherwise method (3) is a useful back-up technique which corrects for residue in syringe.

Method (1): isotope calibrator

Measure the activity contained in both dose and standard syringes in the isotope calibrator (ionization chamber). After injection, re-measure the used dose syringe and subtract the residual activity to give the net dose activity. Expel the contents of standard syringe into a 1-litre volumetric flask and make up to 1 litre with water. Re-measure the used standard syringe and subtract the residual activity to give the net standard activity. Calculate the ratio, R, of net dose activity to net standard activity.

Method (2): weighing

Weigh accurately two empty syringes, each fitted with needle and needle guard, one marked 'dose' and the other marked 'standard'. Draw up the required volumes of radiopharmaceutical solution into each syringe and re-weigh them. Calculate the net weights of dose and standard, and derive the ratio, R, of dose to standard. When injecting the dose, be sure to use all of it by withdrawing blood back into the used syringe and re-injecting the residue of radioactivity. Similarly, when making up the standard dilution to 1 litre in a volumetric flask, be sure to wash out all the radioactivity into the flask.

Method (3): scintillation counter jig

This method requires a jig, or support, for the syringes so that they may be positioned reproducibly in front of a scintillation detector (e.g. a well counter) in such a way that the sensitivity of the detector to activity in the syringes is reduced to eliminate dead-time effects, and that the sensitivity of the detector is reasonably independent of volume of solution in the syringe. Measure the count rate from both dose and standard syringes. Inject the dose, preserving the syringe for a residue measurement in the jig. Subtract the result of the residue measurement from the original dose count rate to obtain the net dose count rate. Expel the contents of the standard syringe into a 1-litre volumetric flask and make up to exactly 1 litre. Measure the residue in the syringe as above and obtain the net standard count rate. Derive the ratio, R, of net dose count rate to net standard count rate.

Indirect micturating cystography

1. This test will normally follow ^{123}I-OIH gamma camera renography, but if carried out by itself, a dose of 40 MBq (1 mCi) of ^{123}I-OIH should be administered intravenously (for children, 0.5 MBq (15 μCi)/kg body weight). Following renography a suitable delay is advisable to ensure that little or no residual activity remains in the kidneys. The patient should not be allowed to go to the toilet between the renography and this test. If possible no diuretic should be given with the preceding renogram.
2. Set up the gamma camera for ^{123}I with a low-energy parallel collimator.
3. Set up the computer for a dynamic acquisition of 60 frames each of 5 seconds' duration.
4. When the patient is ready to micturate, position him/her in front of the camera for a posterior view to include the bladder and both kidneys. It may be convenient to use a commode.
5. When the patient feels ready to void start the computer acquisition and acquire a few frames before allowing the patient to micturate. If possible the patient should first strain without voiding.
6. After the patient has voided allow the computer to acquire a few more frames before terminating acquisition.
7. Measure the volume of urine passed.
8. On the computer delineate regions of interest over each kidney and the bladder and generate count vs. time curves for each region.
9. Plot the curves.
10. Obtain hard copy images from the computer of any reflux seen.

Direct micturating cystography

1. Insert a catheter into the bladder via the urethra (or by suprapubic stab) under the usual aseptic conditions.
2. Connect the catheter to an infusion set for bladder irrigation—normal saline should be connected.
3. Set up the camera for ^{99m}Tc with a low-energy parallel collimator (for a small field of view camera a diverging collimator may be necessary).
4. Set up the computer for a 20-minute dynamic acquisition of 20-second frames.
5. Position the patient in front of the camera for a posterior image with the bladder at the bottom of the field of view and the kidney area in the middle or upper part.
6. Infuse 100 ml (approximately) of normal saline into the bladder.
7. Inject 37 MBq (1 mCi) ^{99m}Tc-pertechnetate into the catheter. Direct needle puncture of a rubber catheter is usually adequate. If preferred it can be administered via an infusion set from a small-volume infusion bottle.

8. Start the computer.
9. Continue to infuse normal saline at approximately 50–100 ml/min until the bladder is well distended and the patient complains of discomfort and an urgent desire to micturate.
10   Discontinue the infusion.
11. Stop the computer and reset for a 10-minute dynamic acquisition of 5-second frames.
12. Restart the computer.
13. Deflate the urethral catheter retaining balloon.
14. Disconnect the infusion set and either remove the catheter or ensure it will fall into the commode when the patient micturates.
15. Ask the patient to strain without voiding.
16. Ask the patient to micturate.
17. After the patient has voided acquire a few more frames before terminating the acquisition.
18. Measure the voided volume.
19. For each dynamic study delineate regions of interest over each kidney and bladder and generate count-versus-time curves.
20. Plot the curves.
21. Obtain hard copy images from the computer of any reflux seen.

It is the practice of some urologists to give antibiotic cover when a urinary catheter has been inserted.

Residual bladder volume

1. This test will follow either ^{123}I-OIH or ^{99m}Tc-DTPA gamma camera renography and no additional dose is required.
2. Set up the gamma camera for ^{123}I or ^{99m}Tc with a low-energy parallel collimator.
3. Set up the computer to acquire static images of 1 minute's duration.
4. When the patient's bladder is reasonably full, as indicated by the amount of activity it contains following renography, position the patient for an anterior view of the bladder.
5. Acquire a 1-minute image on the computer.
6. Send the patient to the toilet to collect all urine passed. Measure the volume of urine (V ml).
7. Reposition the patient for another anterior view of the bladder.
8. Acquire a 1-minute image on the computer.
9. For each of the two computer images delineate two regions of interest, one for the bladder and one for an area of background above the bladder.
10. Normalize the background count to the same area as the bladder region on each image and subtract from the bladder count to give a background corrected bladder count: A for pre- and B for post-micturition images.
11. Calculate the initial bladder volume and the residual bladder volume:

$$\text{Initial bladder volume} = \frac{A}{A - B} \times V \, \text{ml} \tag{6}$$

$$\text{Residual bladder volume} = \frac{B}{A - B} \times V \, \text{ml} \tag{7}$$

Bone scanning

1. Prepare a dose of 550 MBq (15 mCi) ^{99m}Tc-MDP.
2. Inject the dose intravenously. Advise the patient to drink plenty of fluid and to empty the bladder frequently.
3. Wait 3 hours.
4. Set up the gamma camera for ^{99m}Tc with a low-energy parallel collimator and for 3-minute analogue images.
5. Ask the patient to empty bladder.
6. Obtain the following views:

   (a) posterior pelvis
   (b) posterior femurs and hips
   (c) posterior lumbar spine
   (d) posterior thoracic spine
   (e) posterior shoulders and skull
   (f) anterior thorax

   If specifically indicated, obtain additional views:

   (g) arms
   (h) hands
   (i) legs
   (j) feet

   Further anterior and lateral images of any views may be taken if necessary for clarification.

Part 2

Clinical applications

8 Obstructive uropathy

P. H. O'Reilly and E. W. Lupton

Obstructive uropathy in its various forms accounts for a large proportion of the workload of urology and nephrology departments. In the past, biochemical tests and intravenous or retrograde urography were the only investigations used for its assessment. Now nuclear medicine, ultrasound, CT scanning, antegrade pyelography and pressure flow studies are also available. This chapter examines the specific role of nuclear medicine in the investigation of urinary obstruction and its relationship to the other tests in current use.

The pathophysiology of obstructive uropathy is complex. Obstruction may be acute or chronic, complete or incomplete, persistent or intermittent. Impedance to flow, urinary tract dilatation, reduction in urine flow rates, variations in intrarenal pressures and impairment of function are all involved. The individual role each of these plays in producing renal damage is not fully understood. Intrarenal pressures undoubtedly rise temporarily in acute obstruction but measurements in chronic obstructive states are often normal (Underwood, 1937; Kiil, 1957; Djurhuus et al., 1976a). In experimental partial ureteric occlusion studies, intrapelvic pressures have been demonstrated to remain normal while dilatation persists or even progresses (Boyarsky and Martinez, 1964; Weaver, 1968; Schweitzer, 1973; Djurhuus et al., 1976b; Weiss, 1980). An assessment of obstructive uropathy based solely on the measurement of pressure is incomplete. The guidelines for investigation must embrace broader concepts. It is more logical that emphasis be placed on urine flow. This immediately renders static anatomical means of assessment such as the IVU unhelpful except for structural considerations. More dynamic data are required. Dilatation and obstruction can be independent entities; the appreciation that they may be mutually exclusive has radically changed the approach to the evaluation of urodynamics in obstruction. Alternatively, investigation can concentrate on the ultimate rationale for the treatment of the obstructed urinary tract, the preservation of renal function. Quantification of the contribution of the individual kidney to the overall renal function becomes essential.

Consideration of such pathophysiological criteria underlines the clinicians' role in obstructive uropathy—to diagnose and remove the obstruction, to preserve renal function and to reverse any damage which may have occurred. In acute cases it may be possible to achieve all these aims. In the chronic situation, selection for and timing of surgery are far from straightforward. They may be complicated by decisions regarding which kidney to operate on first in bilateral disease and by doubts about the persisting effects of previous obstructive episodes or surgery in recurrent disease. There is also the

TABLE 8.1

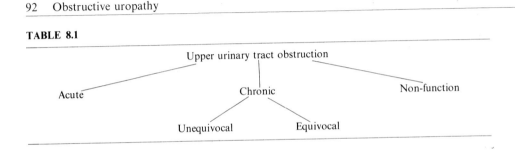

need to distinguish between patients with true obstruction and those with similar urographic appearances from non-obstructive dilatation or ureteric reflux.

The place of nuclear medicine in the investigation of obstructive uropathy is unique. This specialty alone can offer simultaneous quantification of individual renal function and dynamic analysis of individual urine flow rates—the two parameters of most importance in obstruction. To examine these in more detail it is useful to divide the all-embracing term 'obstructive uropathy' into the various sub-groups shown in *Table 8.1* and to consider them individually.

Acute obstruction

Acute obstruction is frequently encountered in clinical practice. Stone disease is the most common cause, and this alone is responsible for 7% of urgent admissions to general hospitals. In acute obstruction the plain abdominal X-ray and intravenous urogram are of great clinical value. The maintenance of renal blood flow and glomerular filtration combined with slow (obstructed) intratubular transit of urine mean that renal input exceeds output, and a diagnostic dense nephrogram is produced (*Figure 8.1a*). Delayed pictures will usually show a dilated pelvicalyceal system or ureter down to the level of the obstructing lesion (*Figure 8.1b*). If ureteric visualization fails to occur, retrograde ureterography will delineate the anatomy and site of obstruction. Ultrasound, CT scanning and antegrade studies are unlikely to be needed. Gamma camera renography is useful, however, to establish an objective baseline of divided renal function and to monitor the functional and urodynamic response to conservative or surgical management. Inspection of the gamma camera images may give some indication of the extent and site of obstruction which is of considerable value with a plain abdominal radiograph in patients allergic to contrast media.

Unequivocal chronic obstruction

Stones, ureteroceles, retroperitoneal fibrosis, ureteric and bladder tumours and extrinsic malignancies such as those involving the colon and pelvic organs are examples of situations where the urinary tract may be chronically but unequivocally obstructed by a demonstrable organic lesion. In the majority of these conditions, examination by intravenous urography, retrograde ureterography, ultrasound, CT scanning or contrast studies will make a definite diagnosis, and surgical intervention will be forthcoming. While diagnosis of the underlying cause may be relatively straightforward, one further piece of information is essential to management—the underlying divided renal function and its implications regarding the management of the patient. Routine biochemical evaluations such as blood urea or blood urea nitrogen, serum creatinine, creatinine clearance or maximum urinary concentrating ability determine

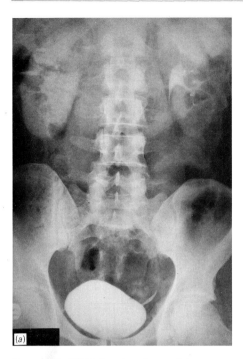

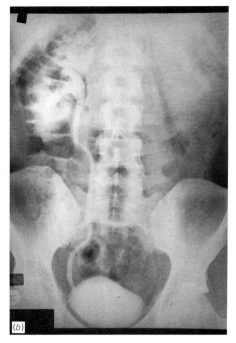

Figure 8.1a IVU showing dense right nephrogram in case of acute obstruction

Figure 8.1b Delayed film (19 hours) demonstrating dilatation down to juxta-vesical ureter

total renal capability. Conventional divided clearances or concentrating ability require selective ureteric catheterization which is invasive and carries the likelihood of failure to pass the obstruction or the introduction of infection into an already compromised urinary tract with potentially disastrous consequences. Gamma camera renography using ^{123}I-OIH or ^{99m}Tc-DTPA will objectively analyse the accumulation, transit and elimination of tracer activity by each kidney to produce the renogram curves described in Chapter 2. The simple and non-invasive nature of the procedure is an added advantage, and it is at last becoming widely used in urological practice, in both its routine and its more sophisticated forms (Piepz *et al.*, 1978; Raynaud, 1978; Holten and Storm, 1979; Buck, MacLeod and Blacklock, 1980; Dubovsky *et al.*, 1980).

This development has in no small way been the result of a growing appreciation of the unreliability of the intravenous urogram as an indicator of the functional status of the kidneys. The anatomical size of the kidneys means little. It is possible to have a hugely dilated pelvicalyceal system with an apparently thin but merely attenuated and potentially normal rim of functioning parenchyma on its periphery. The physiological determinants of urographic contrast visualization and the lack of standardization of dose on a volume-for-weight basis combine to obscure grossly reductions in function (Banner and Pollack, 1980). This is compounded by misleadingly excellent collecting system visualization and by the subjective 'eyeballing' nature of urogram interpretation with its large observer bias. The radionuclide methods are free from these disadvantages. They are objective, quantitative and dynamic and accurately complement the anatomical urogram data.

If renal function is affected by obstruction the slope of the second phase of the renogram curve will be depressed to various degrees according to the duration and extent of the obstruction. This will be reflected in the computer-derived analysis of

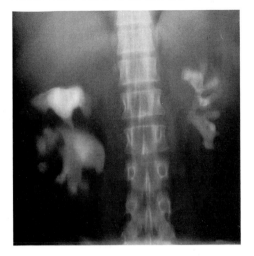

Figure 8.2A IVU showing large staghorn calculus in right kidney with smaller stones in left kidney

divided renal function. The earliest effect on the third phase will be flattening of the usual upper concavity of the curve. This is always a suspicious sign, and, even if underlying divided function is equal, such patients should be observed with care. In more severe or chronic cases the curve will show increasingly pronounced degrees of obstruction until the third phase is completely absent (*Figure 8.2*). In long-standing obstruction analysis of the third phase will be less easy since uptake will be compromised and renal activity will be insufficient to make meaningful comment on excretion patterns. Ultimately uptake will be absent and the appearances will be those of a non-functioning kidney. These findings will be the same whatever the cause of the obstruction. Renography does not always ascertain aetiology—this is the task of the other available imaging procedures.

Gamma camera renography is invaluable in unequivocal chronic obstruction. Vital decisions regarding renal conservation or nephrectomy should not be taken without such studies, although consideration of all the available imaging and radiographic data is often necessary. It must be remembered that dehydration, poor radionuclide injection technique and undue movements during the examination will affect renogram data. If any doubt exists about the result a second study will clarify the situation in the majority of cases. Decisions to sacrifice a kidney should not be taken solely on the result of an isolated radionuclide investigation.

Unfortunately no convincing method exists at present to predict preoperatively recovery of renal function that would occur following relief of chronic unequivocal obstruction. The nearest approach lies in percutaneous puncture of the renal pelvis, using modern pig-tail catheters, which will allow antegrade pyelography to determine the site of obstruction and subsequent decompression of the system. If decompression results in recovery of function, conservation may be recommended (*Figure 8.3*). This remains the only practical prognosticator at present and can be of considerable value in selected cases. Its invasive nature should stimulate efforts to replace it by a non-invasive alternative.

Equivocal chronic obstruction

Urinary tract dilatation without a demonstrable organic lesion to account for it is a common urological problem. It may occur in idiopathic hydronephrosis, primary megaureter and vesico-ureteric reflux, or after operations such as pyeloplasty,

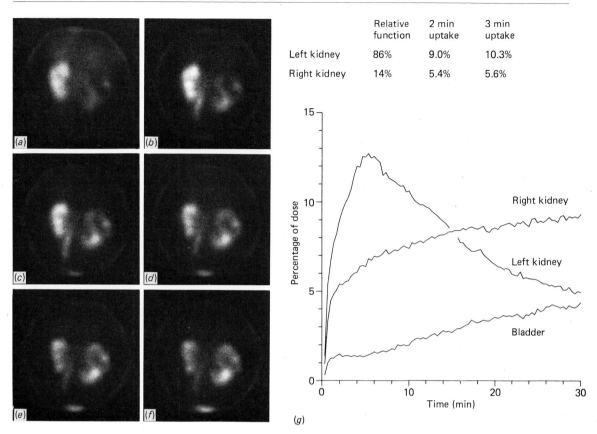

	Relative function	2 min uptake	3 min uptake
Left kidney	86%	9.0%	10.3%
Right kidney	14%	5.4%	5.6%

Figure 8.2B Renogram showing an obstructive pattern on the right side: (*a*) to (*f*) analogue images at 0–5, 5–10, 10–15, 15–20, 20–25 and 25–30 minutes; (*g*) derived renogram curves

pyelolithotomy, ureterolithotomy, ureteric re-implantation and urinary diversions. Such dilatation immediately raises the question: is obstruction present? It is indefensible to operate on a dilated urinary tract without objective evidence that it is obstructed, and equally dangerous not to operate where obstruction exists. This dilemma has resulted in the development of two specific nuclear medicine methods to clarify such cases: diuresis renography and radionuclide parenchymal transit time estimations.

Diuresis renography

The principle behind this procedure is that, in a genuinely obstructed upper urinary tract, obstruction will be present at low and high urine flow rates. In a dilated, non-obstructed system, an obstructed renogram curve caused by stasis will be 'unmasked' by diuresis, and washout of radionuclide will occur from the upper tract. The technique requires a standard ^{123}I-OIH gamma camera renogram to be performed. One of three modifications is then employed.

1. If the standard renogram is normal, it is repeated 15 minutes after an intravenous injection of frusemide 0.5 mg/kg;
2. If the standard renogram is obstructed with no elimination at 20 minutes, the frusemide is given at this stage while the study continues uninterrupted;

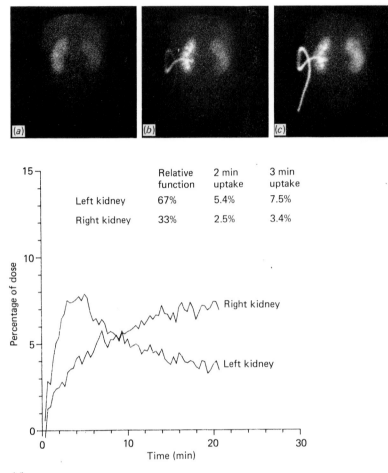

(d)

Figure 8.3 Renogram in patient with bilateral obstruction showing indwelling antegrade pigtail catheter inserted for the relief of obstruction: (*a*) to (*c*) analogue images at $0-2\frac{1}{2}$, $2\frac{1}{2}-5$ and 5–10 minutes; (*d*) derived renogram curves

3. If the renogram shows spontaneous but slow elimination, the frusemide is given while the study continues, but the renogram is repeated giving the diuretic from the start if there is any difficulty in interpretation.

Four responses may occur as summarized in *Figure 8.4.*

1. Both renograms are normal, excluding obstruction (response I);
2. An initially obstructive curve remains obstructive, confirming genuine obstruction (response II) (*Figure 8.5*);
3. An initially obstructive curve is converted to 'normal' with rapid, complete elimination of tracer, indicating a dilated but non-obstructed system (response IIIa) (*Figure 8.6*);
4. An obstructive curve shows a partial response only to diuresis, indicating a sub-total degree of obstruction or a kidney functioning too poorly to respond to the diuretic (response IIIb) (*Figure 8.7*).

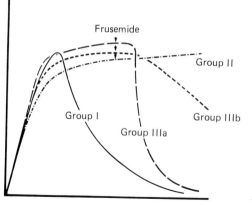

Figure 8.4 Diuresis renogram responses

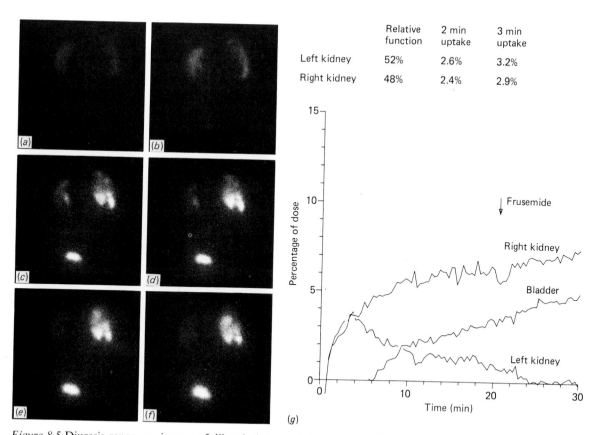

	Relative function	2 min uptake	3 min uptake
Left kidney	52%	2.6%	3.2%
Right kidney	48%	2.4%	2.9%

Figure 8.5 Diuresis renogram in case of dilated obstructed right upper urinary tract; frusemide injected 20 minutes after radiopharmaceutical: (*a*) to (*f*) analogue images at 0–2½, 2½–5, 5–10, 15–20, 20–25 and 25–30 minutes; (*g*) derived renogram curves. Note persistent retention of tracer in right renal pelvis on images and lack of response to frusemide in derived curves

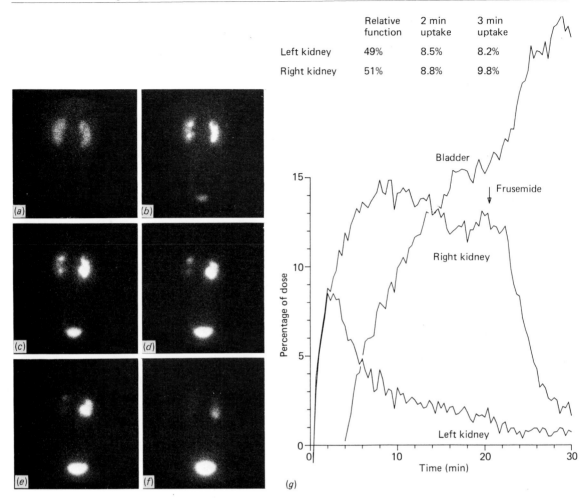

	Relative function	2 min uptake	3 min uptake
Left kidney	49%	8.5%	8.2%
Right kidney	51%	8.8%	9.8%

Figure 8.6 Diuresis renogram in case of dilated non-obstructed right upper urinary tract; frusemide injected 20 minutes after radiopharmaceutical: (*a*) to (*f*) analogue images at $0-2\frac{1}{2}$, $2\frac{1}{2}-5$, 5–10, 15–20, 20–25 and 25–30 minutes; (*g*) derived renogram curves. Note rapid washout of tracer from right kidney images and rapid response to frusemide in derived curves

The diuresis renogram gives simultaneous evaluation of function and urodynamics under normal and high flow states. Reports from several centres have confirmed its value (O'Reilly *et al.*, 1978; Koff, Thrall and Keyes, 1979; O'Reilly *et al.*, 1979; Kreuger *et al.*, 1980; O'Reilly *et al.*, 1981; Stage and Lewis, 1981; O'Reilly and Gosling, 1982). It requires adequate renal function if information on urodynamic behaviour is to be obtained. A good response to the diuretic can be expected down to clearances of 15–20 ml/min. Below this level, the effect of small doses of intravenous frusemide is less predictable; below 10 ml/min the technique is of doubtful value because of the combination of poor tracer uptake and poor diuretic response. Increasing the administered dosage of frusemide may achieve an increased total diuresis in damaged kidneys, but it will not increase the initial (i.e. 3–10 minutes) response upon which interpretation of the diuresis renogram is based.

For this reason, equivocal responses to diuresis renography must be viewed with care. If the underlying renal function is good, even minor degrees of curve abnormality

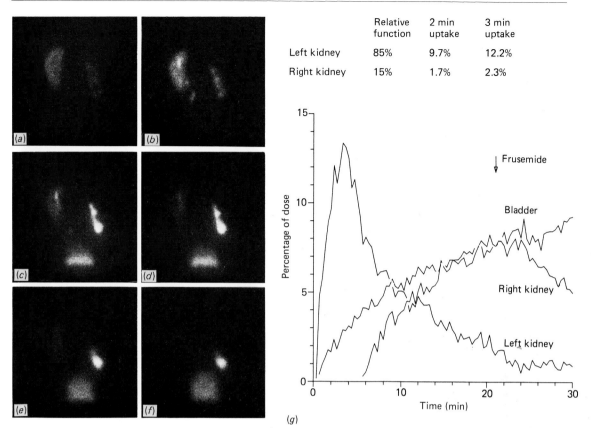

	Relative function	2 min uptake	3 min uptake
Left kidney	85%	9.7%	12.2%
Right kidney	15%	1.7%	2.3%

Figure 8.7 Diuresis renogram in case of dilated right upper urinary tract showing partial response to diuresis; frusemide injected 20 minutes after radiopharmaceutical: (*a*) to (*f*) analogue images at $0-2\frac{1}{2}$, $2\frac{1}{2}-5$, 5–10, 15–20, 20–25 and 25–30 minutes; (*g*) derived renogram curves

are significant. If renal function is poor, it must be established whether poor washout is due to a good diuretic response occurring against a genuinely impeded outlet, or a poor diuretic response through a normal, non-obstructed outlet. Other studies such as parenchymal transit times or perfusion pressure flow studies may be of some help for classification. English (1983) has investigated further the problem of equivocal cases. In a series of 35 patients with idiopathic hydronephrosis who showed preserved underlying function but equivocal tracer washouts the renogram was repeated giving the diuretic 15 minutes before the radiopharmaceutical instead of the classic 3 minutes. In some cases, a previously equivocal response became normal, in others a hypotonic pattern became obstructed (*Figure 8.8*) or reverted to normal (*Figure 8.9*). It is suggested that, at 15 minutes, the urinary flow rate after frusemide will be at its maximum and possibly greater than that after 3–5 minutes. This will stress the outflow tract still more, akin to increasing the perfusion rates during pressure flow studies, and may help to clarify the small number of cases which are equivocal.

It has been suggested that, in some patients, good tracer washout indicating a non-obstructive diuresis renogram pattern might be achieved only at the expense of a high (and by implication damaging) proximal pressure rise due to incipient obstruction. Mininberg at Cornell University, New York, has looked into this problem by

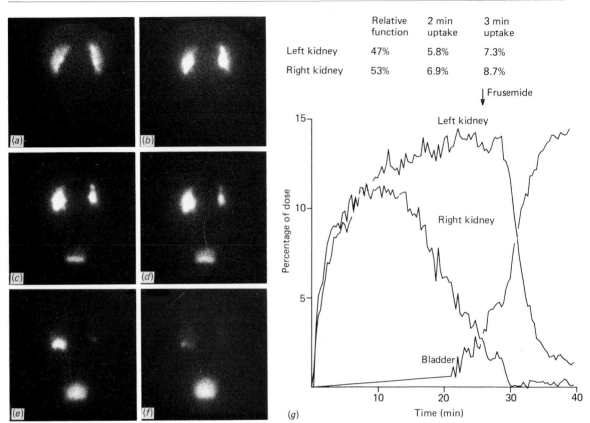

	Relative function	2 min uptake	3 min uptake
Left kidney	47%	5.8%	7.3%
Right kidney	53%	6.9%	8.7%

Figure 8.8A Diuresis renogram in case of bilateral upper tract dilatation; frusemide injected 20 minutes after radiopharmaceutical: (*a*) to (*f*) analogue images at 0–5, 5–10, 20–25, 25–30, 30–35 and 35–40 minutes; (*g*) derived renogram curves. Note fast response to diuresis on left

comparing the curve changes during diuresis renography with actual renal intrapelvic pressures measured directly through nephrostomy tubes in 15 patients. Three sub-groups were defined. Seven patients had prompt washout of tracer under diuresis and renal pelvic pressures remained normal. All these patients were unobstructed. Two patients showed obstructive diuresis renograms with simultaneous rising pressures. Six patients had slower than normal (equivocal) washout after diuresis accompanied by only a moderate increase in intrapelvic pressure. These studies showed good agreement between intrapelvic pressures and diuresis renogram responses 'reconfirming its effectiveness in evaluating obstructive uropathy' (D. Mininberg, personal communication, 1983).

However, some workers have encountered one or two cases where there *was* a pressure rise during a good diuresis-induced washout. If a number of such cases do come to light, it will need to be determined if the pressure elevations are damagingly high, or if this represents a physiological response similar to the pressure rises found in normal kidneys subjected to diuresis.

Parenchymal transit time estimation

This technique, using ^{99m}Tc-DTPA or ^{123}I-OIH, relies on the ability to separate the renal parenchyma from the collecting system while replaying images from data

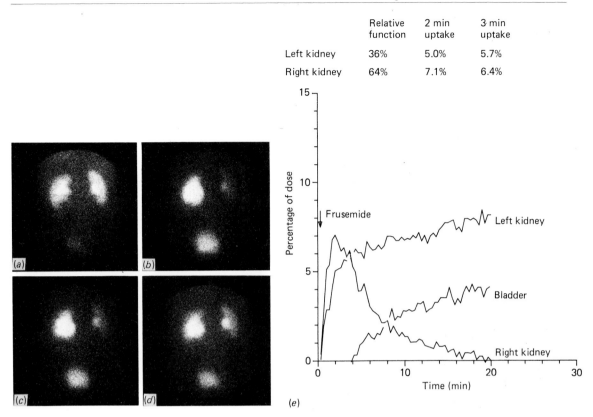

	Relative function	2 min uptake	3 min uptake
Left kidney	36%	5.0%	5.7%
Right kidney	64%	7.1%	6.4%

Figure 8.8B Diuresis renogram in same case; frusemide injected 15 minutes *before* radiopharmaceutical: (*a*) to (*d*) analogue images at 0–5, 5–10, 10–15 and 15–20 minutes; (*e*) derived renogram curves. Note obstructive pattern on left

acquired during gamma camera renography. This distinction can be made by subjective assessment during visual display of sequential images. Alternatively the areas can be separated by displaying the renogram data as a functional image of the distribution of mean times, thereby improving the accuracy of pelvicalyceal definition (Whitfield *et al.*, 1978). Areas of interest are flagged over the whole kidney, the renal parenchyma and a vascular region. Activity–time curves are derived for each area. The process of deconvolution is then applied to both the whole kidney and parenchymal renograms (*see* Chapter 15), and retention functions are obtained. From these it is possible to calculate the transit times for the radionuclide across both the whole kidney and the parenchyma alone. With significant obstruction both the whole kidney and parenchymal transit times are prolonged (*Figure 8.10*). In the dilated, non-obstructed system, whole-kidney transit time may be prolonged but parenchymal transit is not (*Figure 8.11*).

Parenchymal transit time estimation is therefore another non-invasive method of assessing dilated upper urinary tracts. It gives quantitative information relating to the effects of obstruction on parenchymal function. Possible disadvantages are the necessity of complex computer programs and difficulties in separating parenchyma and pelvis, especially where there is a thin cortical layer. Recent reports have claimed that this technique can diagnose obstruction even in the presence of very poor renal function (Nawaz *et al.*, 1983). However, the time of onset of delayed parenchymal transit and the ability to distinguish obstructive from other forms of nephropathy

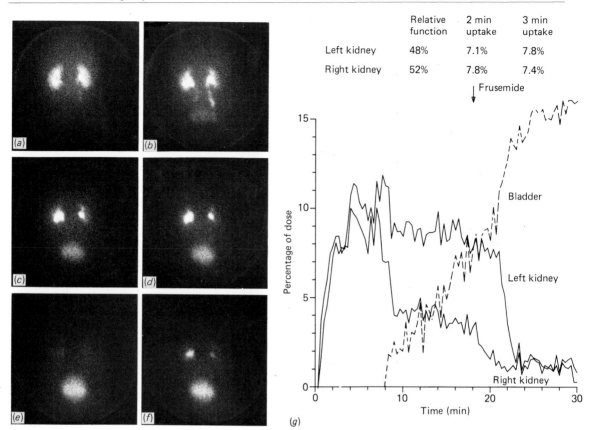

	Relative function	2 min uptake	3 min uptake
Left kidney	48%	7.1%	7.8%
Right kidney	52%	7.8%	7.4%

Figure 8.9A Diuresis renogram in case of left dilated upper tract; frusemide injected 20 minutes after radiopharmaceutical: (*a*) to (*f*) analogue images at 0–5, 5–10, 10–15, 15–20, 20–25 and 25–30 minutes; (*g*) derived renogram curves. Note left dilated non-obstructive pattern

remain uncertain. Lupton *et al.* (1979a) have shown agreement between the results of diuresis renography and parenchymal transit times in 80% of 46 cases of renal pelvic dilatation. The discrepancies occurred mainly in patients with atypical hydronephrosis, possibly due to chronic pyelonephritis or reflux.

Perfusion pressure-flow studies

A further method to investigate the dilated upper urinary tract involves the percutaneous antegrade puncture of the renal pelvis or ureter proximal to the site of suspected obstruction and perfusion of saline or contrast medium at a fixed rate of 10 ml/minute—the so-called Whitaker test. If the pressure rises above 22 cmH$_2$O during perfusion, obstruction is said to be diagnosed. A rise of less than 15 cmH$_2$O excludes obstruction while the intervening range is equivocal. Such perfusion pressure-flow studies are a more direct approach to assess the ability of the renal collecting system to transport fluid (Pfister and Newhouse, 1979; Whitaker, 1979). They assume the premise that, if the ureter will not transmit perfusate at 10 ml/minute without a significant pressure rise, surgical intervention is necessary to relieve obstruction. They are invasive, unsuitable for repeat studies and give no information on renal function although they do not require renal function to be performed. Comparisons of diuresis

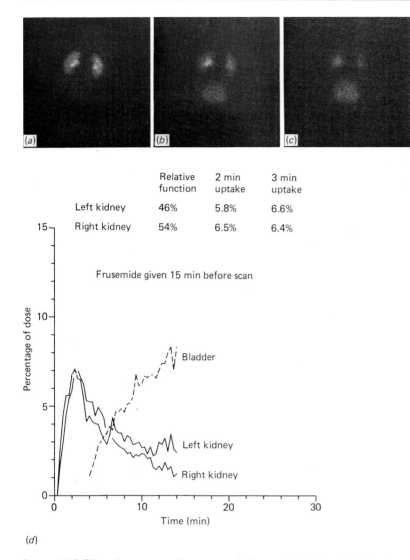

	Relative function	2 min uptake	3 min uptake
Left kidney	46%	5.8%	6.6%
Right kidney	54%	6.5%	6.4%

Frusemide given 15 min before scan

(d)

Figure 8.9B Diuresis renogram in same case; frusemide injected 15 minutes *before* radiopharmaceutical: (a) to (c) analogue images at 0–5, 5–10 and 10–15 minutes; (d) derived renogram curves. Note normal pattern

renography with the Whitaker test have shown agreement between the results in 70–90% of cases (Koff, 1982; Lupton, 1985). Parenchymal transit times also showed good correlation with pressure-flow studies in 90% of the small number of cases reported by Whitfield *et al.* (1977).

All these techniques are now accepted in clinical practice and are undergoing continuing evaluation (Lupton *et al.*, 1979b, 1980; Nawaz *et al.*, 1983). They are an impressive and considerable advance in accurately assessing over 80% of patients who, before their availability, presented a huge clinical problem. Their individual and combined application to equivocal obstruction has been a considerable help to the clinician faced with making the correct management decision in this difficult situation.

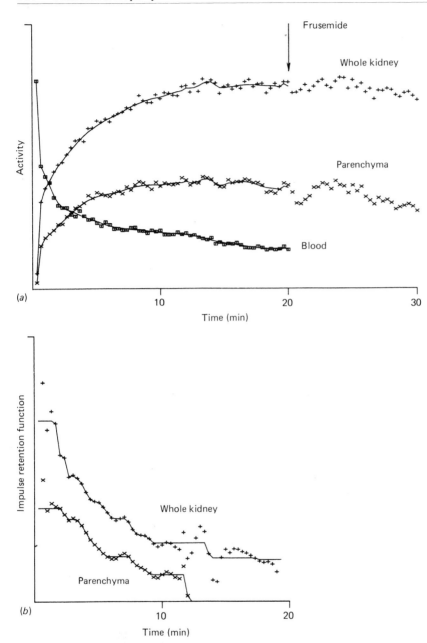

Figure 8.10 Deconvolution applied to an obstructed kidney. Both the whole kidney mean transit time (> 8.4 minutes) and the parenchyma mean transit time (6.8 minutes) are prolonged. Deconvolution is only valid up to the time at which frusemide is administered. (*a*) Standard activity–time curves. The points indicate the raw data and the solid lines the smoothed curves used for deconvolution. (*b*) Impulse retention functions. The first point in each curve, which includes the background contribution, is off the top of the scale. Points beyond the time at which the curve reaches zero have been suppressed for clarity. The solid line indicates the retention function after it has been trimmed to remove background and constrained to be a monotonically decreasing function

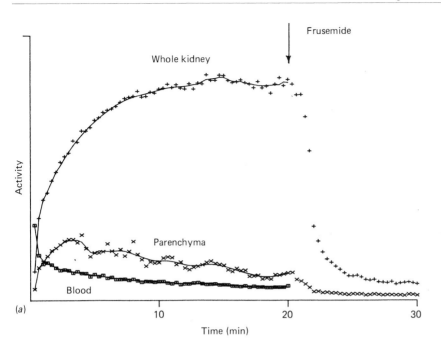

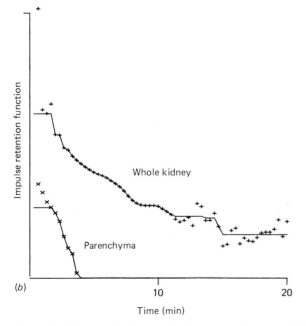

Figure 8.11 Deconvolution applied to a non-obstructed kidney. Although the whole kidney mean transit time is prolonged (>9.9 minutes) the parenchyma mean transit time is normal (2.7 minutes): (*a*) standard activity–time curves— same format as *Figure 8.10a*; (*b*) impulse retention functions—same format as *Figure 8.10b*

The non-functioning kidney

The finding of a urographic non-functioning kidney raises a number of questions. Is the kidney present? If so, is non-opacification due to irreversible parenchymal disease or reversible obstruction? If the latter, how long has it been present and what is the likelihood of functional improvement if the condition is operated upon? In this situation, ultrasound is the investigation of choice. Its simple, non-invasive nature promotes it above retrograde ureteropyelography (which is invasive and carries the risk of introducing infection into an already compromised urinary tract), radionuclide studies and CT scanning. Its value is two-edged. In most cases it should be possible to ascertain if the kidney is present, and if so whether the ureter, pelvis or calyces are dilated (suggesting an obstructive aetiology) or not. Agenesis may ultimately require cystoscopy to demonstrate an absent hemitrigone, while radionuclide or CT scanning will help to locate ectopic renal tissue if this is suspected as a cause of non-opacification in the normal anatomical position (*see* also Chapters 3 and 9). Two reports have suggested that vascular isotope scanning and delayed ^{131}I-OIH camera scanning may be of further value in complementing the anatomical information available from ultrasound (Lome, Persky and Levy, 1979; Sherman and Blaufox, 1980). The former assesses renal blood-flow in non-functioning kidneys while the latter will show some kidneys which are not visible urographically. It should be added that, with modern high-dose urogram techniques and nephrotomography, the vast majority of kidneys will be visible urographically. Such studies are not always performed *de novo*, however, and the standard urogram which demonstrates a non-functioning kidney is better followed up by ultrasound and radionuclide studies than by bringing the patient back for further urograms.

In the standard uronephrological practice, upper urinary tract obstruction will comprise a large proportion of day-to-day clinical work. Ultrasound and CT scanning have now been added to intravenous and retrograde urography, and sophisticated nephrotomography and antegrade pyelography have become more widely used. These procedures, however, do not give detailed simultaneous information on the two parameters of most importance in obstructive uropathy, i.e. divided renal function and upper tract urodynamics. This deficiency has been corrected by the development of urological nuclear medicine. Consequently the establishment of quantitative divided renal function, the ability to monitor upper tract urodynamics, the means to evaluate changes with respect to therapy and the distinction between genuine obstruction and other conditions which may mimic it are now within the realms of clinical possibility.

Without these developments dynamic functional assessments in obstructive uropathy could not be made with any degree of objective confidence. Reliance would be placed instead on anatomical criteria such as contrast opacification, pelvicalyceal and ureteric dilatation or kidney size. Patients would run the risk of inaccurate or incomplete assessment, or inappropriate surgery without any objective means to justify such decisions. Fortunately, the combination of specialized nuclear medicine with the various available radiological imaging procedures has allowed the urologist to assess obstructive uropathy with reference to the physiological criteria discussed earlier, providing considerable benefit to patient care.

References

BANNER, M. P. and POLLACK, H. M. (1980) Evaluation of renal function by excretory urography. *Journal of Urology*, **124**, 437–443

BOYARSKY, S. and MARTINEZ, S. (1964) Pathophysiology of the ureter; partial ligation of the ureter in dogs. *Investigative Urology*, **2**, 173–176

BUCK, C., MACLEOD, M. A. and BLACKLOCK, N. J. (1980) The advantages of ^{99m}Tc-DTPA in dynamic renal scintigraphy and measurement of renal function. *British Journal of Urology*, **52**, 174–183

DJURHUUS, J. C., NERSTROM, B., IVERSON-HANSEN, R. and RASK-ANDERSON, H. (1976a) Incomplete ureteral duplication. *Scandinavian Journal of Urology and Nephrology*, **10**, 111

DJURHUUS, J. C., NERSTROM, B., GYRD-HANSEN, N. and RASK-ANDERSON, H. (1976b) Experimental hydronephrosis. *Acta chirurgica Scandinavica*, Suppl., **427**, 17

DUBOVSKY, E. V., BUESHEN, A. J., TOBIN, M., SCOTT, J. W. and TAUXE, W. N. (1980) A comprehensive computer assisted renal function study: a routine procedure in clinical practice. In: *Radionuclides in Nephrology*, N. K. Hollenberg and S. Lange (eds.), Stuttgart, New York: Georg Thieme, pp. 52–58.

ENGLISH, P. J., TESTA, H. J., LAWSON, R. S., CARROLL, R. N. P. and CHARLTON-EDWARDS, E. (1983) Modified diuresis renography in the assessment of equivocal pelvi-ureteric junction obstruction. *Nuclear Medicine Communications*, **4**, 136 (abstract)

HOLTEN, I. and STORM, H. H. (1979) Kidney scintigraphy with ^{99m}Tc-DMSA and ^{131}I-hippuran. *Scandinavian Journal of Urology and Nephrology*, **13**, 275

KIIL, F. (1957) *The Function of the Renal Pelvis and Ureter*, Oslo: University Press.

KOFF, S. A., THRALL, J. H. and KEYES, J. W. J. R. (1979) Diuretic radionuclide urography. *Journal of Urology*, **122**, 451–454

KOFF, S. A. (1982) Experimental validation of diagnostic methods in idiopathic hydronephrosis. In: *Idiopathic Hydronephrosis*, P. H. O'Reilly and J. A. Gosling (eds.), Berlin, Heidelberg and New York: Springer Verlag

KREUGER, R. P., ASH, J. M., SILVER, M. M., KASS, E. J., GILMOUR, R. F., ALTON, D. J., GILDAY, D. J. and CHURCHILL, B. M. (1980) Primary hydronephrosis. *Urologic Clinics of North America*, **7**, 231

LOME, L., PERSKY, S. and LEVY, L. (1979) Dynamic renal scanning in the non-visualised kidney. *Journal of Urology*, **121**, 148–153

LUPTON, E. W., LAWSON, R. S., SHIELDS, R. A., TESTA, H. J. and HERMAN, K. J. (1979a) Presentation to the British Nuclear Medicine Society Annual Meeting, London, April 1979

LUPTON, E. W., O'REILLY, P. H., TESTA, H. J. *et al.* (1979b) Diuresis renography and morphology in urinary tract obstruction. *British Journal of Urology*, **51**, 10

LUPTON, E. W., TESTA, H. J., LAWSON, R. S., CHARLTON EDWARDS, E., CARROLL, R. N. P. and BARNARD, R. J. (1980) Diuresis renography and the results of surgery for idiopathic hydronephrosis. *British Journal of Urology*, **51**, 449–453

LUPTON, E. W., RICKARDS, P., TESTA, H. J., GILPIN, S. A., GOSLING, J. A. and BARNARD, R. J. (1985) A comparison of diuresis renography, the Whitaker test and renal pelvic morphology in idiopathic hydronephrosis. *British Journal of Urology*, **57**, 119–123

NAWAZ, M. K., BRITTON, K. E., NIMMON, C. C. *et al.* (1983) Parenchymal transit time index (PTTI) and frusemide diuresis (FD): a comparison in obstructive nephropathy. *Nuclear Medicine Communications*, **4**, 138 (abstract)

O'REILLY, P. H., TESTA, H. J., LAWSON, R. S., FARRAR, D. J. and CHARLTON EDWARDS, E. (1978) Diuresis renography in equivocal urinary tract obstruction. *British Journal of Urology*, **50**, 76–80

O'REILLY, P. H., LAWSON, R. S., SHIELDS, R. A. and TESTA, H. J. (1979) Idiopathic hydronephrosis. *Journal of Urology*, **121**, 153–155

O'REILLY, P. H., LUPTON, E. W., TESTA, H. J., SHIELDS, R. A., CARROLL, R. N. P. and CHARLTON EDWARDS, E. (1981) The dilated non-obstructed renal pelvis. *British Journal of Urology*, **53**, 205–210

O'REILLY, P. H. and GOSLING, J. A. (eds.) (1982) *Idiopathic Hydronephrosis*, Berlin, Heidelberg and New York: Springer Verlag

PFISTER, R. C. and NEWHOUSE, J. H. (1979) Antegrade pyelography and ureteral perfusion. *Radiologic Clinics of North America*, **17**, 341–350

PIEPZ, A., DENIS, R., HAM, H. R., DOBBELAIR, A. and SCHULMAN, C. (1978) A simple method for measuring separate GFR using a single injection of ^{99m}Tc-DTPA and the scintillation camera. *Journal of Pediatrics*, **93**, 769–774

RAYNAUD, E. C. (1978) *The Renal Uptake of Radioactive Mercury*, Springfield, Illinois: Thomas

SCHWEITZER, F. A. W. (1973) Intra pelvic pressure and renal function studies in experimental chronic partial ureteric obstruction. *British Journal of Urology*, **45**, 2–8

SHERMAN, R. A. and BLAUFOX, M. D. (1980) Clinical significance of non-visualisation with ^{131}I-hippuran renal scan. In: *Radionuclides in Nephrology*, N. K. Hollenberg and S. Lange (eds.), Stuttgart and New York: Georg Thieme

STAGE, K. H. and LEWIS, S. (1981) Use of the radionuclide washout test in evaluation of suspected upper urinary tract obstruction. *Journal of Urology*, **125**, 379–386

UNDERWOOD, W. E. (1937) Recent observations on the pathology of hydronephrosis. *Proceedings of the Royal Society of Medicine*, **30**, 817–819

WEAVER, R. G. (1968) Reabsorptive patterns and pressures in hydronephrosis with a clinical application. *Journal of Urology*, **100**, 112–116

WEISS, R. M. (1980) Ureteral obstruction. *Dialogues in Paediatric Urology*, **3**, 12

WHITAKER, R. H. (1979) The Whitaker test. *Urologic Clinics of North America*, **6**, 529–539

WHITFIELD, H. N., BRITTON, K. E., FRY, I. K., NIMMON, C. C., TRAVERS, P. and WICKHAM, J. E. A. (1978) The obstructed kidney: Correlation between renal function and urodynamic assessment. *British Journal of Urology*, **49**, 615–619

9   Urological tumours

P. H. O'Reilly, H. J. Testa and M. C. Prescott

Radionuclide studies can play an important role in the investigation of urological malignancies, particularly renal carcinoma, adrenal and testicular tumours and metastatic disease. Furthermore bone scanning is essential for accurate staging in carcinoma of the prostate.

Renal carcinoma

Carcinoma of the kidney is thirteenth in frequency of all carcinomas and represents 2.8% of the total (Bennington and Kradjian, 1967). If the nephroblastoma, which occurs in children and rarely presents diagnostic problems, is excluded, the growths comprise adenocarcinoma (hypernephroma, clear cell carcinoma), transitional cell carcinoma (urothelial carcinoma) and squamous cell carcinoma. Hypernephroma accounts for 83% of such renal tumours in all age groups and 90% in adults (Lucke and Schlumberger, 1957). It is the commonest renal tumour likely to be referred to radiological and nuclear medicine departments for identification.

In most cases, the possibility of a hypernephroma is first detected as a space-occupying lesion on intravenous urography. Subsequent investigation is dominated by the need to determine if the lesion is a renal neoplasm or a benign condition such as cyst, abscess, carbuncle, pseudotumour, xanthogranuloma, angiomyolipoma, arteriovenous malformation or infarct. Within this pathological range, the two commonest conditions will be tumour and cyst, making this distinction the primary clinical demand. The intravenous urogram with nephrotomography will often distinguish between tumour and cyst. The classic simple cyst is radiolucent and non-calcified with a thin, well-defined margin (Figure 9.1), while a carcinoma is usually at least as dense as normal parenchyma, has an irregular wall with poorly defined margins and sometimes shows calyceal amputation and calcification (Figure 9.2) (Chynn and Evans, 1960; Evans, 1968; Peterson, Jackson and Moore, 1968; Clayman, Williams and Fraley, 1979). In practice, however, surgical decisions can be made with confidence following the IVU in less than 75% of cases. Where urogram and histological diagnoses have been compared, a 10% false negative rate (cancer misdiagnosed as benign) has been reported (Clayman, Williams and Fraley, 1979). In current urological practice, it is usually judged necessary to have confirmatory evidence of malignancy before proceeding to nephrectomy.

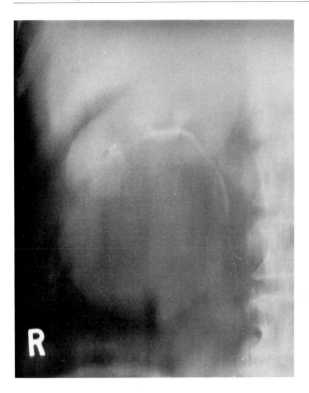

Figure 9.1 IVU in patient with renal cyst

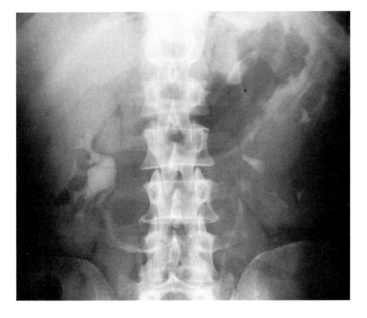

Figure 9.2 IVU in patient with left hypernephroma

In recent years a formidable choice of options has become available for this purpose. As well as radionuclide studies, these include ultrasound, computed tomography, arteriography, cyst puncture, digital angiography and magnetic resonance imaging. There is no generally agreed protocol for their use. Until the advent of such tests, surgical exploration was the traditional approach to the problem (Kropp *et al.*, 1967). The magnitude of this procedure was justified by the assurance of histological confirmation (Ambrose *et al.*, 1977). The introduction of modern imaging procedures has challenged this approach in the expectation that, in the majority of cases, diagnosis should be possible without surgical invasion. Selective renal angiography was the first and most widely used procedure to achieve this. Using arteriography, the renal blood vessels are seen to be stretched around the margin of the avascular cystic lesion, and to constrict in response to an intravenous injection of adrenaline. In tumours, multiple abnormal blood vessels are seen with vascular pooling and the classic hypervascular blush of a tumour circulation within and around the lesion (*Figure 9.3*). The abnormal vessels are unresponsive to adrenaline. Unfortunately 10% of hypernephromas are hypovascular or avascular and will mimic cysts, while abscesses, angiomyolipomata and xanthogranulomatous pyelonephritis in particular can resemble malignancy. The procedure has a false negative rate of 3.6% and false positive rate of 2.9% (Lang, 1963; Meaney, 1969; Watson, Fleming and Evans, 1968). It is invasive, and serious complications can be expected in 0.71% of cases; minor complications affect 2.9% of cases (Lang, 1963; Halpern, 1964).

In recent years radionuclide scanning, ultrasound and CT scanning have emerged as non-invasive alternatives to arteriography. The purpose of radionuclide scanning in renal space-occupying disease is to determine if the lesion is vascular or avascular. The study, as described in Chapter 3, involves the visualization of the passage of the agent through aorta, renal arteries and individual kidneys and the production of subsequent parenchymal images. The vascular and parenchymal phases are then compared to

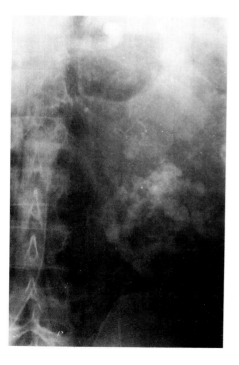

Figure 9.3 Renal arteriogram in patient with hypernephroma arising in lower pole of left kidney

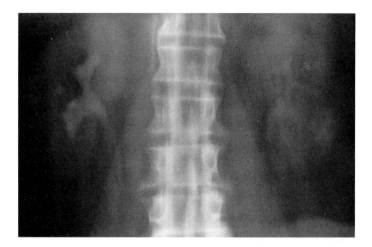

Figure 9.4A IVU in patient with right renal cyst and multiple left renal cysts

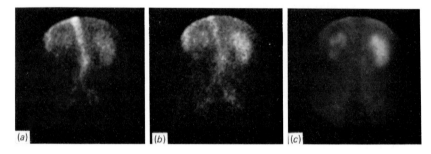

Figure 9.4B Gamma camera study using ^{99m}Tc-gluconate in same patient: (*a*) and (*b*) 5-second images of first circulation; (*c*) 2-minute image of parenchymal uptake. Note non-vascular areas in both kidneys and lack of uptake in corresponding areas on parenchymal image

assess the nature of any abnormality found. In renal cysts, the area on the vascular study corresponding to the site of the lesion on the parenchymal study will be avascular or 'cold' (*Figure 9.4*). In tumours, the area will be hypervascular or 'hot' (*Figure 9.5*).

Ultrasound imaging depends on the reflection or impedance of projected sound-waves directed at a suspect lesion. The patient usually lies prone and arachis oil is used to ensure good acoustic coupling. Multiple transverse and longitudinal sections are examined and Polaroid films can be obtained for reporting if desired. The fluid contents of a cyst are transonic and the distal border will be easily delineated sonographically (*Figure 9.6A*). In contrast, a neoplasm has poorly defined margins and a heterogenous composition creating complex internal echoes and poor beam transmission (*Figure 9.6B*).

CT scanning assesses the morphological structure of tissues by producing transverse cross-sectional images of X-ray absorption. The kidneys are usually scanned at 1-cm intervals with a spatial thickness of 13 mm and scan speeds of about 20 seconds. The examination is complemented by computer tomographic angiography and contrast enhancement (*Figure 9.7*).

For most clinicians ultrasound is the most readily available of these procedures. The best figures for its use are those of Sherwood, who reported an accuracy rate of 98% for renal cysts and 86% for tumours (Sherwood, 1975). However, it is highly operator-dependent. Problems may arise from renal movement during scanning, changing

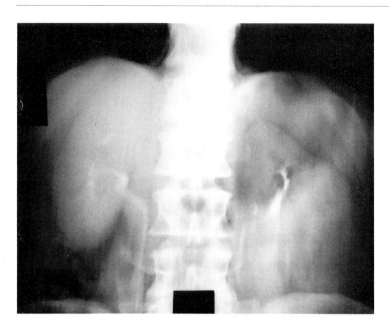

Figure 9.5A IVU in patient with
left hypernephroma

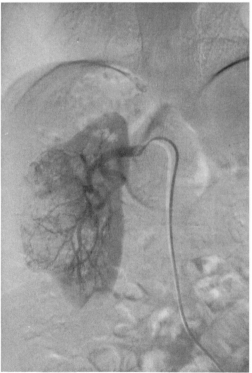

Figure 9.5B Renal arteriogram in same patient

positions of overlying bowel, and bony interference with high or low-lying kidneys.
Necrotic tumours sometimes appear transonic. Nevertheless the technique is simple,
quick, non-invasive, does not require renal function for visualization and does not use
ionizing radiation. With the expansion of nuclear medicine facilities the use of the

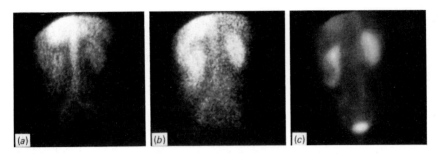

Figure 9.5C Gamma camera study using ^{99m}Tc-gluconate in same patient: (*a*) and (*b*) 5-second images of first circulation; (*c*) 2-minute image of parenchymal uptake. Note tumour circulation in left kidney and lack of uptake in corresponding area on parenchymal images

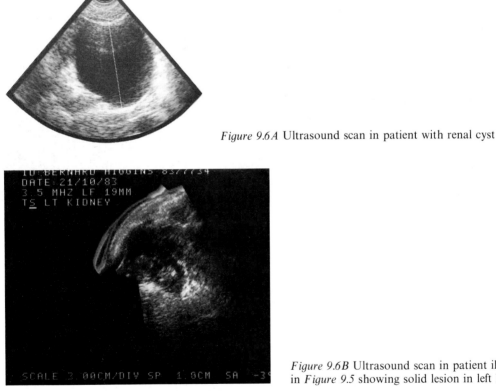

Figure 9.6A Ultrasound scan in patient with renal cyst

Figure 9.6B Ultrasound scan in patient illustrated in *Figure 9.5* showing solid lesion in left kidney

radionuclide method has also become widely available. Using this technique, O'Reilly *et al.* (1979) reported an accuracy of 96% for cysts and 81% for hypernephroma. The technique requires an intravenous injection but, like ultrasound, is simple, easy and quick to perform. The radiation dose is small, about 17 mSv (1.7 rad) to the kidneys and 0.9 mSv (0.09 rad) to the whole body. However, it has a resolution of the order of 1 cm and some renal function is a prerequisite for its success.

Several papers and textbooks, when describing radionuclide studies in renal imaging, deal only with static parenchymal techniques using such agents as ^{197}HgCl,

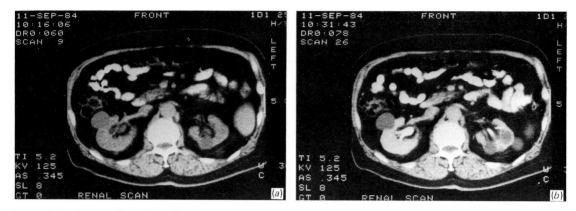

Figure 9.7A CT scan in patient illustrated in *Figure 9.4* showing cyst in right kidney and multiple cysts in left kidney: (*a*) before contrast; (*b*) after contrast

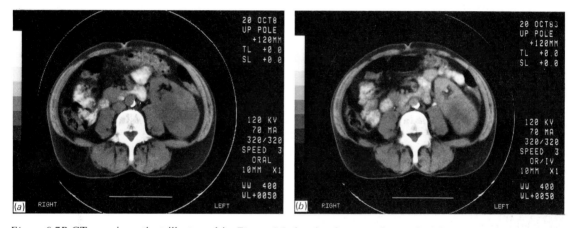

Figure 9.7B CT scan in patient illustrated in *Figure 9.5* showing hypernephroma in left kidney: (*a*) before contrast; (*b*) after contrast

but attempts to distinguish between a tumour and a cyst *cannot* be made on the basis of a parenchymal scan alone. It will be misleading to draw conclusions solely on the basis of criteria such as the contours of the margins of the lesion or its apparent cortical invasion. Until the vascular scan is seen, no firm statements on the nature of the lesion are valid. In a recent prospective study comparing ultrasound with radionuclide studies (O'Reilly *et al.*, 1981) the accuracy figures for ultrasound were 86% for cysts and 90% for tumours, and for radionuclide studies 100% for cysts and 80% for tumours (*Table 9.1*). Perhaps the most important point in this study was the fact that, in those cases where the two procedures agreed, there were no false results. Their combination assesses both the internal structure and the vascular characteristics of the suspected lesion.

Computed tomography gives detailed anatomical information on the kidney and its immediate relationships. The radiation dose is about the same as arteriography. The maximum entry dose for a 20-second single section is 15 mSv (1.5 rad), while seven adjacent sections at 13-mm spacing result in 29 mSv (2.9 rad) (Isherwood, Pullan and Ritchings, 1978). The results of a comparison between radionuclide scanning, ultrasound and CT scanning are summarized in *Table 9.2* (O'Reilly *et al.*, 1981). The CT scan is highly accurate but inappropriate for routine use after urography in all renal

TABLE 9.1. Results of combined use of radionuclide and ultrasound scanning in the investigation of renal space-occupying lesions

Final diagnosis	No. of cases	Radionuclide scan		Ultrasound scan	
		Diagnosis	No.	Diagnosis	No.
Renal cyst	14	Avascular	14	Cystic	12
				Not visualized	2
Renal adenocarcinoma	10	Vascular	8	Solid	9
		Avascular	2	Cystic	1
Pseudotumour	2	Normal	2	Normal	2
Xanthogranulomatous pyelonephritis	1	Vascular	1	Solid	1

space-occupying lesions. It is best reserved for cases remaining equivocal after ultrasound and radionuclide studies.

Many radiologists are now adept at cyst puncture. Where a suspected lesion on ultrasound appears to be cystic it is possible to carry out immediate puncture and aspiration. A non-invasive procedure is thereby converted into an invasive one in the interests of decompressing the lesion, obtaining fluid for cytology and confirming the diagnosis. With experience, success should be possible in up to 96% of cases (Jeans, Penry and Roylance, 1972; Thornbury, 1972; Pollack, Goldberg and Bagash, 1974). No deaths have been reported, although there is a risk of abscess formation, pneumothorax and retroperitoneal haemorrhage. Inadvertent puncture of a carcinoma has not resulted in seeding and this possibility should not be a discouragement (Dean, 1939; Schreeb *et al.*, 1967).

Some enthusiasts believe that if ultrasound is accompanied by cyst puncture, CT scanning should never be required; it will only duplicate the relevant information (Abrams and McNeil, 1978). Where a local expert in cyst puncture is not available, however, difficult cases are best served by CT scanning. *Figure 9.8* shows a logical protocol for the use of these procedures. In practice, the use of these various tests will depend on local availability and clinical preferences. In many cases it may be possible to make clinical decisions after urography alone, or after urography and one of the other tests. Some cases will require all the investigations. Even with all the available tests, 5–8% of renal mass lesions will defy preoperative diagnosis (Murphy and Marshall, 1980).

The hypernephroma is suitable for investigation by radionuclide studies due to its hypervascularity. This is not so for the less common tumours such as transitional cell carcinoma, which does not have the same degree of neovascularization. Arteriography, for example, will demonstrate an abnormal circulation in only 10% of cases (Wright and Walker, 1975). Accurate preoperative diagnosis is more likely by ultrasound or CT scanning.

No renal tumour-specific radiopharmaceutical is yet known. [67]Ga, which has been used for the detection of lymphomas, melanoma and bronchogenic carcinoma, has occasionally shown positive uptake in renal carcinoma (Validya *et al.*, 1970; Antoniades *et al.*, 1973; Sauerbrunn, Andrews and Hubner, 1978; Adler, Greweldinger and Conradi, 1981). However, Frankel *et al.* (1975) reviewed 20 cases in which the ^{67}Ga scan showed increased renal uptake. Tissue diagnoses included leukaemia, lymphoma and metastatic melanoma but there was no case of primary renal tumour. The main role of this isotope in renal studies would appear to be in inflammatory conditions (Hopkins, Hey and Meade, 1976; Hurwitz *et al.*, 1976; *see* Chapter 14). Focal renal uptake of ^{99m}Tc-polyphosphate, used in bone scanning, has been claimed to be specific

TABLE 9.2. Results using radionuclide, ultrasound and computed tomographic scanning in the investigation of renal space-occupying lesions

Final diagnosis	No. of cases	Radionuclide scan		Ultrasound scan		Computed tomographic scan	
		Result	No.	Result	No.	Result	No.
Renal adenocarcinoma	12	Vascular	9	Solid	12	Neoplasm	12
		Avascular	2				
		Equivocal	1				
Renal cyst	7	Avascular	5	Cystic	4	Cystic	6
		No lesion	2	Solid	3	Haemorrhagic cyst/neoplasm	1
Transitional cell tumour of renal pelvis	1	Non-functioning kidney	1	Solid lesion in renal pelvis	1	Neoplasm	1
Bilateral metastatic tumours	1	Avascular space-occupying lesion	1	Solid tumour	1	Bilateral neoplasms	1
		Normal	1	Normal	1		
Xanthogranulomatous pyelonephritis	1	Avascular lesion of kidney	1	?Tumour ?Pyonephrosis	1	Hypernephroma	1
Parapelvic cyst	1	Enlarged renal pelvis	1	Normal	1	Parapelvic cyst	1

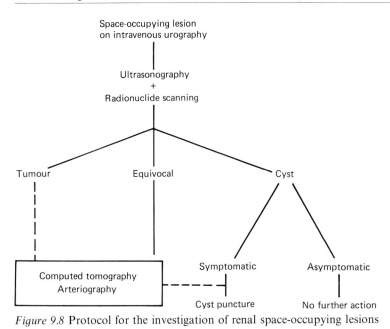

Figure 9.8 Protocol for the investigation of renal space-occupying lesions

for metastatic renal squamous cell carcinoma (Pitzer, 1975), but doubt has been cast on this hypothesis (Harbert, 1976; Vieras and Boyd, 1976; Winter, 1976). All these examples constitute individual case reports, but they reflect the widespread interest which exists in finding a tumour-specific agent.

Benign lesions

The accurate exclusion of renal tumour in space-occupying disease is as important as its confirmation. In this respect, the identification of benign conditions is mandatory if unnecessary laparotomies and nephrectomies are to be avoided. *Cysts* will show the classic 'cold' areas in both vascular and parenchymal studies. False positive results suggesting malignancy are rare, but can occur if the cyst is surrounded by large cortical vessels (Quinn, 1968). *Abscesses* may also give a double cold result, and in this respect the vascular study can be of great importance in differentiating an abscess from focal pyelonephritis. In the former the vascular study shows a cold central area sometimes surrounded by a hypervascular rim, while in focal pyelonephritis a localized blush is normally seen (Rosenthall and Reed, 1968). Another inflammatory condition where radionuclide studies are valuable is *renal carbuncle* (O'Reilly *et al.*, 1980). This is essentially a parenchymal disease. Intravenous urography is non-specific, showing a lumbar scoliosis concave to the affected side, loss of the psoas shadow and a possible soft tissue mass. Radionuclide scans usually show a large, avascular intrarenal lesion expanding the affected kidney, indicative of either a cyst or an abscess. Taken in the context of the patient's symptoms, the differential diagnosis should include renal carbuncle. Arteriography is seldom diagnostic, while ultrasound can show either transonic or complex echoes. Blatt, Hayt and Freeman (1974) have demonstrated the value of radionuclide studies in patients with *tuberous sclerosis*. Eighty per cent of these cases suffer from angiomyolipomatous malformations in both kidneys, a benign condition indistinguishable from polycystic disease on excretion urography. In this condition the perfusion study will show vascularization of the lesions, contrasting sharply with the appearances in polycystic disease. This technique may thus preclude the need for arteriography. While this is true for the distinction between cyst and vascular malformation, these patients also have a high incidence of bilateral hypernephroma, and the scan will not distinguish between these and angiomyolipomata, for both will be vascular. CT scanning or arteriography are recommended in this situation.

Radionuclide imaging can be very useful in the identification of cortical bulges due to *pseudotumours*—localized lobulation or unfolding and hypertrophy of the renal columns of Bertin into the renal sinus. Such bulges frequently mimic tumours on urography and their clarification is vital. Since the tissue is composed of normal parenchyma rather than a foreign space-occupying tissue, the area will not only show normal perfusion, but will also take up radiopharmaceutical in the same way as parenchyma (Williams and Parker, 1982).

Prostatic cancer

There are approximately 5700 new cases of cancer of the prostate in the UK (Tate *et al.*, 1979) and 42 000 in the USA (Klein, 1979) annually, and the incidence is increasing. Treatment depends on tumour stage, cell grade, and the age and general condition of the patient. No matter what other criteria for evaluation—such as serum hormone changes, tumour markers, cytology, histology and prostatic ultrasound—are used, assessment is incomplete without radionuclide bone scanning. Twenty per cent of patients presenting with cancer of the prostate and normal skeletal surveys will have positive bone scans (Chisholm, 1980), and the procedure holds a central place in the management of such patients. The technique is described in detail in Chapter 6.

Tumours of the testis

Paterson, Peckham and McCready (1976) have reported consistent tumour localization using ^{67}Ga in patients with seminoma of the testis. In this series, 13 out of 15 scans performed in patients with disseminated disease in relapse gave good imaging of all the disease areas. It was found to be useful, both for initial staging and for subsequent routine follow-up. The technique is simple and consists of the intravenous injection of 75 MBq (2 mCi) of the radiopharmaceutical followed by 48-hour bowel preparation to eliminate gastrointestinal activity. Scanning is performed at 48 hours and again 24 hours later if necessary. An example of the resulting images is shown in *Figure 9.9*. The procedure is of little use in teratoma. In nine cases reported by Paterson and colleagues (1976) the scan was negative in seven and showed only a faint image in two. However, they indicated that a positive scan which subsequently reverted to negative might be suggestive of transition from seminoma to teratomatous change.

Liver metastases

Liver scanning is occasionally required in urological practice to investigate the possibility of metastatic disease. Its primary purpose is to save the incurably ill patient either surgical laparotomy to confirm the presence of such metastases, or definitive treatment to a primary tumour when the presence of secondary deposits makes such treatment pointless. The usual approach to such scanning is based on phagocytosis of radioactive colloid particles by the Kupffer cells of the liver. These are reticulo-

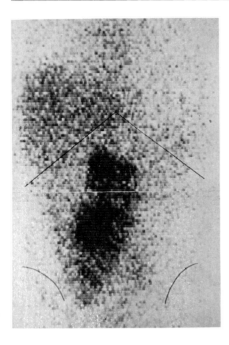

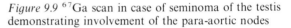

Figure 9.9 ^{67}Ga scan in case of seminoma of the testis demonstrating involvement of the para-aortic nodes

endothelial cells, and over 90% of the RE elements in the body are located in the liver, allowing excellent static scanning following intravenous injection of such particles; 75 MBq (2 mCi) of ^{99m}Tc-tin colloid is injected intravenously. Ten minutes after injection the scan is performed using a gamma camera. Anterior, posterior and right lateral views are taken. The finding of multiple focal defects is non-specific, but in the presence of a known primary tumour is highly suggestive of metastases. Examples of the normal liver scan and a scan demonstrating multiple metastases are shown in *Figure 9.10.*

False negative results are found in a small proportion of patients, and it has been suggested that ultrasound and CT scanning have rather better specificity (Finlay, Meek and Gray, 1982). In practice there is little to choose between radionuclide scanning and ultrasound; the choice is usually dictated by local availability and preferences. CT scanning is rarely the first investigation of choice for the detection of liver metastases, although it is of undoubted value in equivocal cases.

Adrenal scintigraphy

The major application of adrenal scintigraphy is in the localization of sites of hypersecretion of hormones in Cushing's syndrome, Conn's syndrome and phaeochromocytoma. The use of adrenal scintigraphy in determining the nature of an unexplained mass in the renal area is limited. In those patients with a 'functioning' tumour the signs and symptoms of excessive hormone production will direct attention to the adrenal gland. A mass will only occasionally be found in the absence of any signs of excess hormone production. In non-functioning tumours, however, a large mass may develop before the patient complains of any symptoms. The nature of such an abdominal mass may be difficult to determine on physical examination. A radionuclide liver or renal scan can help distinguish a large liver or spleen from a large kidney and

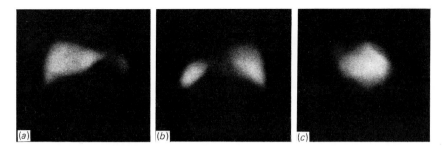

Figure 9.10A Normal liver scan: (*a*) anterior view; (*b*) posterior view; (*c*) right lateral view

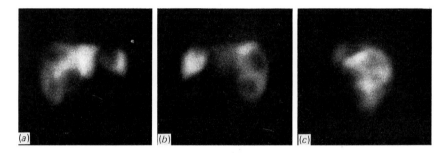

Figure 9.10B Liver scan in metastatic disease: (*a*) anterior view; (*b*) posterior view; (*c*) right lateral view. Note multiple widespread focal defects corresponding to metastatic deposits

vice versa. If the studies are performed together, an adrenal lesion may be inferred if there is a cold area separating the kidney from the liver; normally the two images should be contiguous. However, a space-occupying lesion on the inferior border of the liver or the upper pole of the kidney may produce a similar image, as could a retroperitoneal tumour extending anteriorly.

The traditional methods of adrenal phlebography or arteriography with venous sampling have been useful and reasonably accurate but they are highly invasive. Infarction, haematoma, false aneurysms and pressor crises have all been reported (Gold *et al.*, 1972; Melby, 1972). Non-invasive alternatives such as ultrasound and computed tomography (CT) are now used initially, and they will usually identify the site of the tumour. CT scanning is an accurate imaging procedure in adrenal tumours (Dunnick *et al.*, 1982; Snell *et al.*, 1983). It is reported to be superior to ultrasound. In a prospective study CT scanning gave a 90% success rate compared with a figure of 70% for ultrasound (Abrams *et al.*, 1982). However, if excess hormone production is present, or widespread metastatic disease is a possibility (especially in the case of phaeo-chromocytoma), then radionuclide scanning may be the initial investigation, with CT reserved for more detailed anatomical images of areas of abnormality on the scintiscan (Francis *et al.*, 1983).

Many compounds have been investigated for the imaging of adrenal glands (Beierwaltes *et al.*, 1976, 1978; Knapp, Ambrose and Callahan, 1980). Iodine-labelled cholesterols were used initially (Blair *et al.*, 1971; Lieberman *et al.*, 1971; Thrall, Freitas and Beierwaltes, 1978) with ^{131}I-6β-iodomethyl-19-norcholesterol being one of the most effective (Sarkar *et al.*, 1977). More recently ^{75}Se-19-

selenomethylcholesterol has become available. It has better adrenal concentration than [131]I-19-iodocholesterol, and it is more stable *in vitro*, allowing it to be stored at room temperature. Moreover the thyroid gland does not require blocking. Its use, therefore, is becoming more widespread. Although it has been reported that there is concentration in the adrenal medulla of dogs (Sarkar *et al.*, 1976), its main application is in the localization of cortical hormone-producing tumours. Imaging is performed 7 and 14 days after an intravenous injection of 7.5 MBq (200 μCi) ^{75}Se-selenocholesterol. The percentage of dose uptake in each adrenal area is quantified, making any depth corrections necessary. The normal range is 0.07–0.3% of the administered dose (Britton, 1983). The pattern of uptake depends on the lesion present. In adrenal carcinoma the picture is variable, some large tumours producing corticosteroids may not be visualized as uptake per gram of tissue is too low, but the normal adrenal is not visualized either as it is suppressed by the excess hormone. However, if the tumour secretes insufficient cortisol or aldosterone or androgens, the contralateral adrenal will not be suppressed and hence it is visualized. Other combinations of uptake occur in different endocrine conditions and dexamethasone suppression may be used to evaluate further the abnormalities seen (Conn *et al.*, 1972; Hogan *et al.*, 1976; Seabold *et al.*, 1976; Thrall, Freitas and Beierwaltes, 1978; Britton, 1983). It has been reported that metastatic lesions can sometimes be detected using radiocholesterol (Forman *et al.*, 1974; Watanabe *et al.*, 1976; Drane, Graham and Nelp, 1983).

Phaeochromocytoma, a tumour of the adrenal medulla, is visualized by metaiodobenzylguanidine (MIBG). The patient's thyroid must be blocked before injection and for at least 4 days after the test if ^{131}I is used. Imaging is performed daily for 2–3 days starting the day after a slow intravenous injection of 18.5 MBq ^{131}I-MIBG. Some later images may be required (Sisson *et al.*, 1981; Valk *et al.*, 1981; Winterberg, Fischer and Vetter, 1982). Higher doses of ^{123}I-MIBG may be used, but then the normal adrenal may be visualized (Lynn *et al.*, 1984). Usually a normal adrenal is not seen or only faintly visualized (Nakajo *et al.*, 1983). The body is imaged from the skull to the pelvis, as these lesions may be multiple or metastatic and any areas of abnormal uptake may be investigated in more detail by the administration of a bone, renal or liver imaging agent as appropriate at the end of the test (Sutton *et al.*, 1982; Francis *et al.*, 1983; Troncone *et al.*, 1984). MIBG is taken up in both benign and malignant phaeochromocytomas, and it has been used to treat metastatic malignant lesions. Large doses are required—at least 3700 MBq (100 mCi) at a time, and this may need to be repeated. The results have been mixed. This is partly due to the relatively poor uptake by these tumours. Despite being clearly visualized on the images, the amount of the dose in each lesion may only be 1 or 2%, although a few may take up more (Nakajo *et al.*, 1983; McDougall, 1984). Metaiodobenzylguanidine has also been shown to concentrate in neuroblastomas (Kimmig *et al.*, 1984), and can be used in the localization of these tumours in a manner similar to the localization of phaeochromocytomas.

In summary, two radiopharmaceuticals are currently in use for the direct visualization of the adrenal glands: radioiodocholesterol for adrenal cortical lesions and iodine-labelled metaiodobenzylguanidine for phaeochromocytomas and neuroblastomas. They should be used in conjunction with CT scanning, and their main value is in assessing the adrenal lesions associated with endocrine disorders and in the detection of metastatic lesions, especially in phaeochromocytoma.

Phantom kidneys

It is not uncommon, on a perfusion study performed postoperatively on patients after nephrectomy, to see an apparent image of a vascularized kidney on the side operated on, without a corresponding parenchymal image. This may be of some relevance after nephrectomy for carcinoma, where such an abnormal perfusion might suggest recurrent vascular tumour or malignant glands. The phenomenon also occurs after nephrectomy for benign reasons and in renal agenesis. Sometimes it may be confused with splenic or hepatic circulation, but the majority of these occurrences can be demonstrated as separate from the renal areas, the splenic circulation usually being seen on the early frames of the vascular study above and lateral to the renal area, and the hepatic image occurring later, being a reflection of the slower, portal circulation.

The phenomenon has been explained by Holmes and his colleagues (1977) as being due to perfusion in a malpositioned jejunum and colon lying in the space normally occupied by the kidneys. It is apparent because of the lack of attenuation of renal tissue and the proximity of the bowel, lying in the renal fossa, to the posteriorly placed gamma camera. This is in keeping with similar reports on angiography in renal agenesis and ectopia (Meyers, Whalen and Evans, 1973). It provides a nice explanation for the phantom. We have not yet demonstrated the cause to be other than this even in patients after malignant nephrectomy. It is unlikely that secondary deposits would be sufficiently vascular to appear on the radionuclide perfusion study. Appreciation of this phenomenon is important if difficulties in interpretation are to be avoided.

References

ABRAMS, H. L. and MCNEIL, B. J. (1978) Medical implications of computed tomography (CAT scanning). *New England Journal of Medicine*, **298**, 255–261, 310–318

ABRAMS, H. L., SIEGELMAN, S. S., ADAMS, D. F. *et al.* (1982) Computed tomography versus ultrasound of the adrenal gland: A prospective study. *Radiology*, **143**, 121–128

ADLER, J., GREWELDINGER, J. and CONRADI, H. (1981) Gallium-67 scans in renal tumours. *Urological Radiology*, **3**, 27–29

AMBROSE, S. S., LEWIS, E. L., O'BRIEN, D. P., WALTON, I. V. and ROSS, J. R. (1977) Unsuspected renal tumours associated with renal cysts. *Journal of Urology*, **117**, 704–708

ANTONIADES, J., HONDA, T., CROLL, M. N. and BRADY, L. W. (1973) Gallium-67 scan in renal cell carcinoma. *Journal of Urology*, **109**, 564

BEIERWALTES, W. H., WIELAND, D. M., ICE, R. D. *et al.* (1976) Localisation of radiolabeled enzyme inhibitors in the adrenal gland. *Journal of Nuclear Medicine*, **17**, 998–1002

BEIERWALTES, W. H., WIELAND, D. M., YU, T., SWANSON, D. P. and MOSLEY, S. T. (1978) Adrenal imaging agents: rationale, synthesis, formulation and metabolism. *Seminars in Nuclear Medicine*, **VIII**, 1, 5–22

BENNINGTON, J. L. and KRADJIAN, R. M. (1967) *Renal Carcinoma*, Philadelphia: Saunders

BLAIR, R. J., BEIERWALTES, W. H., LIEBERMAN, L. M. *et al.* (1971) Radiolabeled cholesterol as an adrenal scanning agent. *Journal of Nuclear Medicine*, **12**, 176–182

BLATT, C. J., HAYT, D. B. and FREEMAN, L. M. (1974) Radionuclide imaging of the kidneys in tuberous sclerosis. *Journal of Nuclear Medicine*, **15**, 699

BRITTON, K. E. (1983) Adrenal imaging. In: *Clinical Nuclear Medicine*, M. N. Maisey, K. E. Britton and D. L. Gilday (eds.), London: Chapman and Hall, pp. 249–257.

CHISHOLM, G. D. (1980) Urological malignancy: Prostate. In: *Tutorials in Post-graduate Medicine: Urology*, G. D. Chisholm (ed.), London: Heinemann Medical, pp. 223–246

CHYNN, K. Y. and EVANS, J. A. (1960) Nephrotomography in the differentiation of renal cyst from neoplasm: a review of 500 cases. *Journal of Urology*, **83**, 21–24

CLAYMAN, R. V., WILLIAMS, R. D. and FRALEY, E. E. (1979) Current concept in cancer. The pursuit of the renal mass. *New England Journal of Medicine*, **300**, 72–74

CONN, C. J., MORITA, R., COHEN, E. C. *et al.* (1972) Primary aldosteronism—photoscanning of tumours after administration of [131]I-19-iodocholesterol. *Archives of Internal Medicine*, **129**, 417–425

DEAN, A. L. (1939) Treatment of solitary cyst of the kidney by aspiration. *Transactions of the American Association of Genito-Urinary Surgeons*, **32**, 91–95

DRANE, W. E., GRAHAM, M. M. and NELP, W. B. (1983) Imaging of an adrenal cortical carcinoma and its skeletal metastasis. *Journal of Nuclear Medicine*, **24**, 710–712

DUNNICK, N. R., DOPPMAN, J. L., GILL, J. R., STROTT, C. A., KEISER, H. R. and BRENNAN, M. F. (1982) Localisation of functional adrenal tumours by computed tomography and venous sampling. *Radiology*, **142**, 429–433

ELL, P. J., DEACON, J. M., DUCASSON, D. and BRENDEL, A. (1980) Emission and transmission brain tomography. *British Medical Journal*, **280**, 422–438

EVANS, J. A. (1968) The accuracy of diagnostic radiology: Arteriography and nephrotomography. *Journal of the American Medical Association*, **204**, 223–226

FINLAY, I. G., MEEK, D. R., GRAY, H. W., DUNCAN, J. G. and McARDLE, C. B. (1982) Incidence and detection of occult hepatic metastases in colorectal cancer. *British Medical Journal*, **284**, 803–805

FORMAN, B. H., ANTAR, M. A., TOULOUKIAN, R. J., MULROW, P. J. and GENEL, M. (1974) Localisation of metastatic adrenal carcinoma using ^{131}I-19-iodocholesterol. *Journal of Nuclear Medicine*, **15**, 332–334

FRANCIS, I. R., GLAZER, G. M., SHAPIRO, B., SISSON, J. C. and GROSS, B. H. (1983) Complementary roles of CT and ^{131}I-MIBG scintigraphy in diagnosing pheochromocytoma. *American Journal of Roentgenology, Radium Therapy and Nuclear Medicine*, **141**, 719–725

FRANKEL, R. S., ROCHMAN, S. D., LEVENSON, S. M. and JOHNSTON, G. S. (1975) Renal localisation of ^{67}gallium citrate. *Radiology*, **114**, 393

GOLD, R. E., WISINGER, B. M., GERACI, A. R. and HEINZ, L. M. (1972) Hypertensive crisis as a result of adrenal venography in a patient with phaeochromocytoma. *Radiology*, **102**, 579–580

HALPERN, M. (1964) Percutaneous transfemoral arteriography. An analysis of the complications in 1,000 consecutive cases. *American Journal of Roentgenology, Radium Therapy and Nuclear Medicine*, **92**, 918–934

HARBERT, J. C. (1976) Focal renal activity in bone scans. *Journal of Nuclear Medicine*, **17**, 426 (letter)

HOGAN, M. J., McRAE, J., SCHAMBELAN, M. and BIGLIERI, E. G. (1976) Location of aldosterone producing adenomas with ^{131}I-19-iodocholesterol. *New England Journal of Medicine*, **294**, 410–414

HOLMES, E. R., KLINGENSMITH, W. C., KIRSCHNER, P. T. and WAGNER, H. N. (1977) Phantom kidney in ^{99m}Tc DTPA studies of renal blood flow. *Journal of Nuclear Medicine*, **18**, 702–705

HOPKINS, C. B., HEY, R. L. and MEADE, C. (1976) ^{67}Ga scintigraphy for the diagnosis and localisation of perinephric abscesses. *Journal of Urology*, **109**, 564

HURWITZ, S. R., KESSLER, E. O., ALAZAKU, P. and ASHBURN, W. K. (1976) ^{67}Ga imaging to localise urinary tract infection. *British Journal of Radiology*, **49**, 156–160

ISHERWOOD, I., PULLAN, B. R. and RITCHINGS, R. T. (1978) Radiation dose in neuroradiology procedures. *Neuroradiology*, **16**, 478–481

JEANS, W. D., PENRY, J. B. and ROYLANCE, J. (1972) Renal puncture. *Clinical Radiology*, **23**, 298–311

KIMMIG, B., BRANDEIS, W. E., EISENHUT, M., BUBECK, B., HERMANN, H. J. and ZUM WINKEL, K. (1984) Scintigraphy of a neuroblastoma with ^{131}metaiodobenzylguanidine. *Journal of Nuclear Medicine*, **25**, 773–775

KLEIN, L. A. (1979) Prostatic carcinoma. *New England Journal of Medicine*, **300**, 824–833

KNAPP, F. F. Jr., AMBROSE, K. R. and CALLAHAN, A. P. (1980) Tellurium-123m labeled 23-(isopropyl telluro)-24nor-5α-cholan-3βol: A new potential adrenal imaging agent. *Journal of Nuclear Medicine*, **21**, 251–257

KROPP, K. A., FRAYHACK, J. T. and WENDEL, R. M. (1967) Morbidity and mortality of renal exploration for cyst. *Surgery, Gynecology and Obstetrics*, **125**, 803–806

LANG, E. K. (1963) Complications of retrograde percutaneous arteriography. *Journal of Urology*, **90**, 604–610

LIEBERMAN, L. M., BEIERWALTES, W. H., CONN, J. W., ANSARI, A. N. and NISHIYAMA, H. (1971) Diagnosis of adrenal disease by visualization of the human adrenal glands with ^{131}I-19-iodocholesterol. *New England Journal of Medicine*, **285**, 1387–1393

LUCKE, B. and SCHLUMBERGER, H. I. (1957) Tumors of the kidney renal pelvis and ureter. In: *Atlas of Tumor Pathology*, Washington DC: Armed Forces Institute of Pathology

LYNN, M. D., SHAPIRO, B., SISSON, J. C. *et al.* (1984) Portrayal of pheochromocytoma and normal human adrenal medulla by m^{123}I-iodobenzylguanidine. *Journal of Nuclear Medicine*, **25**, 436–440

McDOUGALL, I. R. (1984) Malignant pheochromocytoma treated by I-131-MIBG. *Journal of Nuclear Medicine*, **25**, 249–250

MEANEY, T. F. (1969) Errors in angiographic diagnosis of renal masses. *Radiology*, **93**, 361–366

MELBY, J. C. and MARSHALL, F. F. (1980) Renal cyst versus tumour: a continuing dilemma. *Journal of Urology*, **127**, 566–570

MEYERS, M. A., WHALEN, J. P. and EVANS, J. A. (1973) Malposition and displacement of the bowel in renal agenesis and ectopia: New observations. *American Journal of Roentgenology, Radium Therapy and Nuclear Medicine*, **117**, 323–333

MURPHY, J. B. and MARSHALL, F. F. (1980) Renal cyst versus tumour: a continuing dilemma. *Journal of Urology*, **127**, 566–570

NAKAJO, M., SHAPIRO, B., COPP, J. *et al.* (1983) The normal and abnormal distribution of the adrenomedullary imaging agent m[I-13] iodobenzylguanidine (I^{131}MIBG) in man: Evaluation by scintigraphy. *Journal of Nuclear Medicine*, **24**, 672–682

O'REILLY, P. H., SHIELDS, R. A. and TESTA, H. J. (1979) *Nuclear Medicine in Urology and Nephrology*, London: Butterworths

O'REILLY, P. H., LUPTON, E. W., TESTA, H. J. and CHARLTON EDWARDS, E. C. (1980) A case of renal carbuncle—the role of radionuclides. *British Journal of Radiology*, **53**, 504–506

O'REILLY, P. H., OSBORN, D. E., TESTA, H. J., ASBURY, D. L., BEST, J. J. K. and BARNARD, R. J. (1981) Renal imaging. A comparison of radionuclide ultrasound and CT scanning in investigation of renal space occupying lesions. *British Medical Journal*, **282**, 943–945

PATERSON, A. H. G., PECKHAM, M. J. and McCREADY, V. R. (1976) Value of gallium scanning in seminoma of the testis. *British Medical Journal*, **1**, 1118–1121

PETERSON, C. C. Jr., JACKSON, J. H. Jr. and MOORE, J. G. (1968) A re-evaluation of nephrotomography stressing limitations of the procedure. *Journal of Urology*, **98**, 721–727

PITZER, P. M. (1975) Renal imaging in ^{99m}Tc polyphosphate bone scanning. Focal increased renal uptake in metastatic carcinoma of the lung. *Journal of Nuclear Medicine*, **16**, 602

POLLACK, H. M., GOLDBERG, B. B. and BAGASH, M. (1974) Changing concepts in the diagnosis and management of renal cysts. *Journal of Urology*, **111**, 326–329

QUINN, J. C. (1968) Editorial comment. In: *Year Book of Nuclear Medicine*, Vol. 3, Chicago: Year Book Medical Publishers, p. 251

ROSENTHALL, L. and REED, E. C. (1968) Radionuclide distinction of vascular and non-vascular lesions of the kidney. *Canadian Medical Association Journal*, **98**, 65

SARKAR, S. D., ICE, R. D., BEIERWALTES, W. H., GILL, S. P., BALACHANDRAN, S. and BASMADJIAN, G. P. (1976) Selenium 75-19-selenocholesterol. A new adrenal scanning agent with high concentration in the adrenal medulla. *Journal of Nuclear Medicine*, **17**, 212–217

SARKAR, S. D., COHEN, E. L., BEIERWALTES, W. H., ICE, R. D., COOPER, R. and GOLD, E. N. (1977) A new and superior adrenal imaging agent ^{131}I-6β-iodomethyl-19-nor-cholesterol (NP59). Evaluation in humans. *Journal of Clinical Endocrinology and Metabolism*, **45**, 353–362

SAUERBRUNN, B. J., ANDREWS, G. A. and HUBNER, K. F. (1978) ^{67}Gallium citrate imaging in tumours of the genitourinary tract: report of co-operative study. *Journal of Nuclear Medicine*, **19**, 470–475

VON SCHREEB, T., ARNER, O., SKORSTED, G. et al. (1967) Renal adenocarcinoma. Is there a risk of spreading tumour cells in diagnostic puncture. *Scandinavian Journal of Urology and Nephrology*, **1**, 270–276

SEABOLD, J. E., COHEN, E. L., BEIERWALTES, W. H. et al. (1976) Adrenal imaging with ^{131}I-19-iodocholesterol in the diagnostic evaluation of patients with aldosteronism. *Journal of Clinical Endocrinology and Metabolism*, **42**, 41–51

SHERWOOD, T. (1975) Renal masses and ultrasound. *British Medical Journal*, **4**, 682–685

SISSON, J. C., FRAGER, M. S., VALK, T. W. et al. (1981) Scintigraphic localization of pheochromocytoma. *New England Journal of Medicine*, **305**, 12–17

SNELL, M. E., LAWRENCE, R., SUTTON, D., SEVER, P. S. and PEART, W. S. (1983) Advances in the techniques of localisation of adrenal tumours and their influence on the surgical approach to the tumour. *British Journal of Urology*, **55**, 617–621

SUTTON, H., WYETH, P., ALLEN, A. P. et al. (1982) Disseminated malignant phaeochromocytoma: localisation with iodine-131-labelled metaiodobenzylguanidine. *British Medical Journal*, **285**, 1153–1154

TATE, H. C., RAWLINSON, J. B. and FREEDMAN, L. S. (1979) Randomised comparative studies in the treatment of cancer in the UK: room for improvement? *Lancet*, **2**, 623–625

THORNBURY, J. R. (1972) Needle aspiration of avascular renal lesions: Correlation contrast medium injection with cytologic and arteriographic diagnosis. *Radiology*, **105**, 299–302

THRALL, J. H., FREITAS, J. E. and BEIERWALTES, W. H. (1978) Adrenal scintigraphy. *Seminars in Nuclear Medicine*, **8**, 1, 23–41

TRONCONE, L., MAINI, C. L., DE ROSA, G. et al. (1984) Scintigraphic localisation of a disseminated malignant phaeochromocytoma with the use of ^{131}I meta-iodobenzylguanidine. *European Journal of Nuclear Medicine*, **9**, 429–432

VALIDYA, S. G., CHAUDRI, M. A., MORRISON, R. and WHAIT, D. (1970) Localisation of ^{67}Ga in malignant neoplasm. *Lancet*, **2**, 94

VALK, T. W., FRAGER, M. S., GROSS, M. D. et al. (1981) Spectrum of pheochromocytoma in multiple endocrine neoplasia. *Annals of Internal Medicine*, **94**, 762–767

VIERAS, P. and BOYD, C. M. (1976) Focal renal activity in bone scans. *Journal of Nuclear Medicine*, **17**, 429 (letter)

WATANABE, K., KAMOI, I., NAKAYAMA, C., KOGA, I. and MATSUURA, K. (1976) Scintigraphic detection of hepatic metastases with ^{131}I labelled steroid in recurrent adrenal carcinoma: Case report. *Journal of Nuclear Medicine*, **17**, 904–906

WATSON, R. C., FLEMING, R. J. and EVANS, J. A. (1968) Arteriography in the diagnosis of renal carcinoma: A review of 100 cases. *Radiology*, **91**, 888–897

WILLIAMS, E. D. and PARKER, C. (1982) Kidney pseudotumour diagnosed by emission computer tomography. *British Medical Journal*, **285**, 1379–1380

WINTER, P. F. (1976) Focal renal activity in bone scans. *Journal of Nuclear Medicine*, **17**, 429 (letter)

WINTERBERG, B., FISCHER, M. and VETTER, H. (1982) Scintigraphy in phaeochromocytoma. *Klinische Wochenschrift*, **60**, 631–633

WRIGHT, F. W. and WALKER, M. M. (1975) Radiological diagnosis in avascular renal tumours. *British Journal of Urology*, **47**, 253

10 Renal transplantation

M. C. Prescott and R. W. G. Johnson

Renal failure is a major clinical problem. In the United Kingdom there are 40 new cases of end-stage renal failure per million of the population per year. For many of these patients the treatment of choice is renal transplantation.

The technique of renal transplantation has been established for many years. The use of a cadaver kidney in the treatment of renal failure was first described in 1945 by Hufnagel, working in Boston. Since then there have been great advances in surgical technique, kidney preservation, tissue typing and immunosuppression, making renal transplantation a very effective and established treatment. However, despite the improved selection of compatible kidneys there are still problems with rejection. During recent years there has been an increasing awareness of the dangers of prolonged treatment with high-dose immunosuppression, and a more sparing use of high-dose steroids has actually improved the patient's prognosis (Johnson *et al.*, 1977). The desire to avoid unnecessary immunosuppressive therapy has led to a continuing search for improved diagnostic methods for the detection of rejection and its distinction from other complications such as acute tubular necrosis, vascular thrombosis, ureteric obstruction and urinary extravasation.

If the new kidney works well from the day it is transplanted, the serum biochemistry and urine volume can be used to monitor its progress. However, cadaver kidneys do not always work well immediately, as they may have suffered some ischaemic damage and show signs of acute tubular necrosis. The degree of impairment is very variable, ranging from the polyuric phase of acute renal failure to anuria. In the latter case the patient requires supportive dialysis, sometimes for several weeks, before sufficient renal function returns. During this time the serum biochemistry cannot be used to monitor the kidney as it is altered by dialysis. Furthermore, clinical signs of rejection, for example pyrexia and kidney tenderness, can be caused by other complications. Therefore other methods are needed to monitor kidney function, to assist in the diagnosis of surgical complications and, if possible, to make a positive diagnosis of rejection.

The definitive test for kidney rejection is the renal biopsy. The histological picture is characteristic and distinct in acute and chronic rejection. However, biopsy carries a small risk of renal damage due to haemorrhage, and it is not a test that can be repeated frequently. Instead, several radiological and nuclear medicine procedures have been put forward as alternatives for routine use.

The need to monitor renal function when the patient is undergoing dialysis has led to the increasing use of nuclear medicine studies in these patients' routine management. The radionuclide investigations that have been developed for the measurement of renal function in non-transplanted kidneys have been adapted and used to monitor the progress of renal grafts. They have the advantages of being non-invasive and may be repeated frequently—important in a situation where the clinical condition may change rapidly. In addition, several radionuclide techniques have been developed specifically for the identification of rejection. The fact that there are several different methods used to follow the kidney's progress suggests that there is not one which is ideal, but the most commonly adopted procedures are perfusion studies, using a bolus of ^{99m}Tc, and renography and clearance studies using ^{131}I-OIH or ^{99m}Tc-DTPA.

Renal perfusion and blood flow measurement

Perfusion may be evaluated by gamma camera imaging following an injection of ^{99m}Tc-DTPA.

During rejection episodes renal blood flow is reduced (Jackson and Mannick, 1964; Hollenberg et al., 1968, 1972), and this means that renal perfusion studies can be used to indicate rejection. Perfusion studies are usually performed with 400–600 MBq ^{99m}Tc-DTPA given as a rapid bolus.

The gamma camera is positioned over the iliac fossa containing the kidney. The lower aorta and distal iliac artery should be in the field of view. One-second images are stored on the computer and appropriate analogue images taken at the same time (see Chapters 3 and 7). The vein chosen for administration of the bolus should be as large as possible. Those in the antecubital fossa are usually suitable. However, in some of these patients a smaller vein may have to be accepted as those in the antecubital fossa may have been damaged by repeated use. This is especially so where only one arm is available for injections or venepunctures as the other is used for dialysis access only.

First-pass activity–time curves are derived from the data for the kidney and lower aorta. The ratio of the slopes for renal and aortic curves constitutes the kidney-to-aortic blood flow or K/A ratio (Kirchner et al., 1978). There is considerable overlap of values between groups of patients, and the ratio is best used in serial studies to show a change in blood-flow, a decrease often indicating rejection.

Another method of quantifying perfusion is to use the iliac artery distal to the kidney to compare with the kidney. Normalized activity–time curves are generated from these regions of interest, and then the area under each curve up to the peak of the arterial curve is calculated. The ratio of the arterial area to the kidney area is used as a perfusion index. As blood-flow falls this index increases, so rejection and renal artery stenosis both cause an increase in this index (Hilson et al., 1978). Again the absolute value of this perfusion index shows overlap between the groups, and its value is in determining the change between studies. Both these methods require good bolus injections; as veins may be poor in some of the renal transplant patients some studies will not be suitable for quantification.

Even if blood-flow indices are not calculated, the flow study can be used qualitatively to assess perfusion compared with the iliac vessels and the upper and lower poles in relation to each other, especially important if more than one renal artery was present. Areas of renal infarction can be seen (*Figure 10.1*), as can delayed perfusion to one pole (*Figure 10.2*). Patchy distribution of the tracer in the images taken 5–10 minutes after the perfusion study can indicate rejection. The role of qualitative assessment of the perfusion study will be discussed further in relation to its use with gamma camera renography.

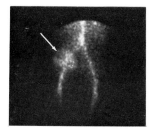

Figure 10.1 A perfusion study. One 5-second frame showing an area of infarction (arrow) at the upper pole of the transplanted kidney

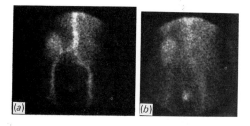

Figure 10.2 A perfusion study in a transplanted kidney with two renal arteries. Delayed flow to the lower pole. There is a 30-second interval between (*a*) and (*b*)

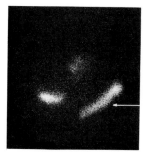

Figure 10.3 An image 30 minutes after injection of ^{123}I-OIH. Most of the activity has left the kidney and is in the bladder. The linear area of activity on the right (arrow) corresponds to the wound dressing and indicates urine leakage from the wound

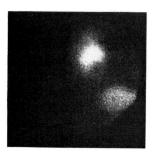

Figure 10.4 A transplanted kidney showing a dilated renal pelvis

Gamma camera renography

Gamma camera renography is one of the more commonly used investigations for monitoring a renal graft and the one most used by the authors. The method is adapted from that used for 'normal' kidneys: many different parameters of the renogram have been quantified and used by many different authors. They include: time to peak of the renogram, half time of the elimination phase, blood clearance curve, ratio of bladder

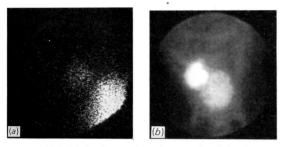

Figure 10.5 (*a*) An image 30 minutes after injection of ^{131}I-OIH showing part of a large bladder area (bottom right)
(*b*) An image 10 minutes after injection of ^{99m}Tc-DTPA showing the large bladder. In this instance a blockage of the urinary catheter was causing urine retention

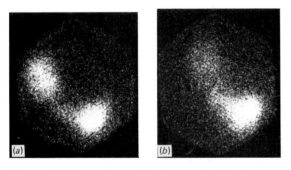

Figure 10.6 (*a*) An image 25 minutes after injection of ^{131}I-OIH. The bladder is visualized despite a catheter *in situ*
(*b*) An image 18 hours after the same injection. Despite a patent bladder catheter the bladder is still seen. There is increased activity between the bladder and kidney. The 'bladder' activity was extravasated urine collecting in the pelvis

and kidney curve heights, bladder appearance time, kidney-to-background ratio (Rosenthall *et al.*, 1974), and bladder-to-kidney ratios (Hayes and Moore, 1971, 1972; Hayes, Moore and Taplin, 1972; Hong-Yoe *et al.*, 1976). An accumulation ratio can also be calculated which is an integral of kidney counts in the first 2 minutes as a fraction of the dose count: a fall in this ratio indicates rejection (Hong-Yoe *et al.*, 1976). An excretion index can be calculated by expressing bladder activity at 20 minutes as a percentage of the predicted value calculated from the effective renal plasma flow (Dubovsky *et al.*, 1975, 1980, 1982).

The method of gamma camera renography is described in detail in Chapter 7. The radiopharmaceutical used is OIH labelled with ^{131}I, or ^{123}I when it is available. Following the intravenous administration of the OIH, computer and analogue dynamic images are obtained for 30 minutes. At the end of the study any catheter or wound drainage bags present are imaged for 60 seconds each. Interpretation of the results is both qualitative and quantitative.

The images are studied to look for evidence of urinary extravasation (*Figure 10.3*) or a dilated pelvis which may indicate obstruction (*Figure 10.4*). If a large bladder image is seen with a 'free draining' catheter *in situ*, two possibilities should be considered: either the catheter is not draining the bladder effectively or urine is leaking into the pelvic space and mimicking a bladder image (*Figures 10.5* and *10.6*).

After the patency of the catheter has been checked a repeat delayed image is taken. If there is no change in the image, with considerable activity in the bladder area, or the outline of the activity is irregular, then extravasation of urine is the most likely diagnosis (*Figure 10.6b*). Areas with relatively decreased uptake of OIH or slow uptake may indicate ischaemic areas. This is most likely to be seen where there was more than one renal artery with separate anastomoses.

The derived renogram curve is plotted as a percentage of the injected dose. The dose syringe is calibrated both before and after injection and the injection site is also imaged for any retention of the dose. The final dose used to derive the renogram is that obtained after correction both for retained activity in the syringe and retained activity at the injection site. The latter correction is needed only infrequently, usually when the doctor injecting is aware of a problem. However, many of these patients have difficult venous access and just occasionally some of the dose is retained at the venepuncture site. As the percentage uptake by the kidney is used to monitor its function it is important to get as accurate an assessment as possible of the dose available to the kidney.

The 'normal' renogram described in Chapter 2 is not often seen even in a 'good graft'. It is seen most frequently in live donor transplants where the ischaemic time of the kidney is minimal (*Figure 10.7*). The usual renogram curve in a 'normal' transplanted kidney shows a slightly prolonged excretion phase (*Figure 10.8*). The qualitative assessment of the curve (the nearer to the 'normal' shape the better) is combined with the quantitative measurements. As has been mentioned, many parameters can be calculated from the renogram. The time of the renogram peak, and the total activity in the kidney, bladder and any catheter drainage bags present at the end of the test (total removal), have been found to be a good indication of renal function. Any significant activity in the wound drainage bag, while contributing to total removal when calculating the kidney's function, is indicative of a urine leak and is diagnostic of such even if the source of the leakage is not visible on the renogram images.

Using the method of acquisition and analysis described and repeating the study at regular intervals, it has been shown that a prolongation of the renogram peak by more than 5 minutes and a decrease in the 'total removal' of more than 5% of the injected dose gives a predictive value for rejection of 74%. An improvement in either parameter correctly indicates improvement in the patient's condition in 90% of tests. If a OIH clearance study is performed simultaneously, then a change of more than 50 ml/min appears significant. If there is a deterioration in all three measurements the predictive value for definite rejection is 83% (Prescott, 1982).

There are two exceptions to the use of a 5% reduction in total removal as being indicative of a fall in renal function. One is when the kidney is working well, and there is good OIH uptake by the kidney and excellent elimination into the bladder and catheter. Usually at an early stage the patient has a free draining urinary catheter *in situ*, and most of the activity is in the catheter bag by 30 minutes. This activity must be counted to add to the 'total removal'. The catheter should always be counted over tissue-equivalent rubber, to simulate the absorption that would have occurred if the activity had been in the bladder, as the figure is to be used for subsequent comparison when the activity will be in the bladder. Despite this, however, there is a tendency to 'overestimate' the activity in the catheter. Where this is a considerable amount, a 10%-of-the-dose fall in total removal is usually taken before a significant fall is reported on the subsequent renogram.

The second exception is when the initial renogram after transplantation shows more

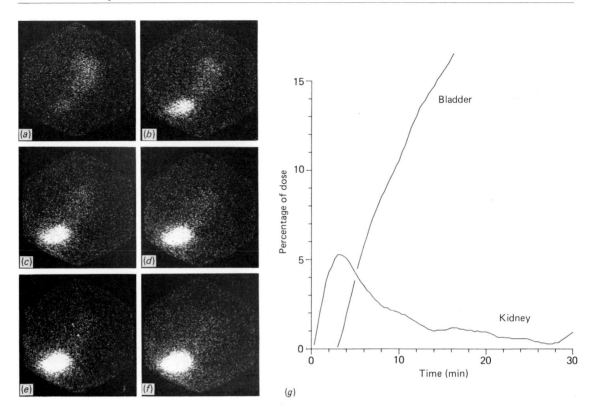

Figure 10.7 A normal study. Six 5-minute images following an intravenous injection of 3 MBq ^{131}I-OIH, and the renogram derived from the 90 20-second frames acquired in the computer

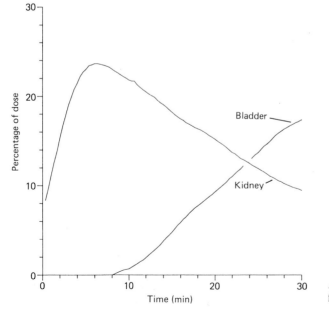

Figure 10.8 The 'usual' renogram obtained from a well functioning renal transplant

than 50% of the dose cleared in 30 minutes. This is most likely to show a decline without any evidence of rejection. A repeat renogram in 48 hours is advisable to give a more realistic baseline.

If the renogram is to be used in the monitoring of renal function, serial studies should be performed. Apart from its use in detecting surgical complications, a single isolated renogram is of little value: it is the change in uptake from one renogram to another that is important. Many centres rightly suggest that a first renogram is performed 24 hours after the operation. It should also be accompanied by a qualitative perfusion study for future comparison. We would suggest that patients with well functioning grafts should have a renogram routinely at least every 4 days, including one following catheter removal and one when stable function has been achieved.

Of course, more frequent scans may be performed when there is a clinical problem. Patients with acute tubular necrosis should have studies on alternate days. The value of this is illustrated diagrammatically in *Figure 10.9*. The initial study shows moderate uptake, this improves on day 3 and again on day 5 although the kidney is still not excreting the OIH and the patient is still requiring haemodialysis. On day 7 the kidney rejects and the renogram uptake falls to that seen on day 1. This is sufficient to suggest rejection. However, if only the first and last renogram were compared a report of no change would be given. Initially the patient may have few clinical symptoms of rejection, as the serum biochemistry and urine volume are of no help in a patient on haemodialysis, and the diagnosis may be missed until a further renogram shows a continuing decrease in function.

A repeat study should always be performed following anti-rejection therapy—and during therapy if there is any doubt about the response to treatment.

On any single study it is not always possible to make a differential diagnosis between

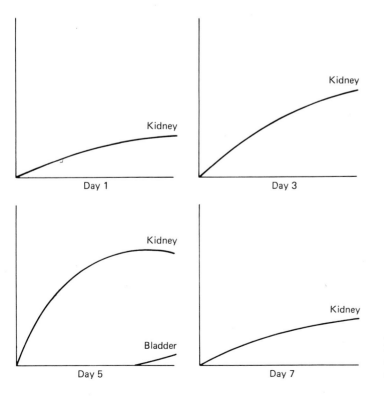

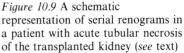

Figure 10.9 A schematic representation of serial renograms in a patient with acute tubular necrosis of the transplanted kidney (*see* text)

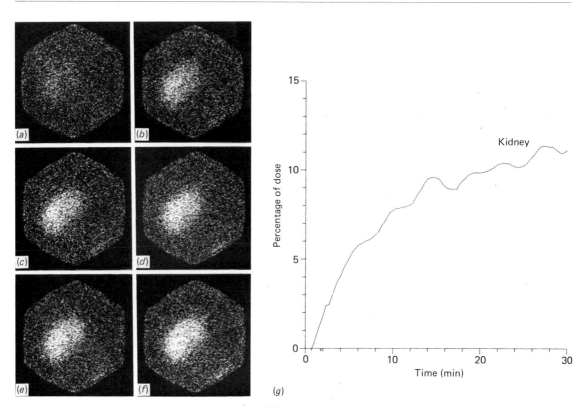

Figure 10.10A The images and renogram from an ^{131}I-OIH study in a patient with acute tubular necrosis of the transplanted kidney

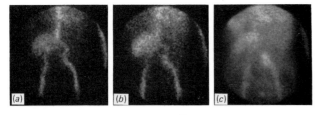

Figure 10.10B The images from a ^{99m}Tc-DTPA perfusion study in the same patient as *10.10A*: (a) and (b) two 5-second frames of the circulation showing good perfusion of the transplanted kidney. An image 1 minute later showing uniform distribution of the activity

acute tubular necrosis (ATN), rejection and obstruction. They may all give a constantly rising renogram curve. However, on day 1 the cause is most likely to be acute tubular necrosis especially if no dilated collecting systems are seen. If the renogram is studied in conjunction with a perfusion study it may help to distinguish ATN from rejection, as classically ATN has good OIH uptake but no elimination and a good circulation and blood pool image (*Figure 10.10*). Rejection may have a similar OIH appearance but rather less perfusion and a patchy blood pool image. We have found this to be true as a rule, although on qualitative assessment of the images a mild rejection may seem to have quite satisfactory perfusion. Conversely poor perfusion may be demonstrated initially in some kidneys with acute tubular necrosis—especially those much travelled and hence severely affected by ischaemia. If a change occurs from a normal to a rising curve—provided no hypotensive episode has occurred—then it is more likely to be due to rejection or obstruction than to ATN.

Obstruction of the ureter causes a rising renogram and sometimes a prominent pelvis on the images. A prominent pelvis of itself does not indicate obstruction (*Figure 10.11*), but the appearance of the pelvis when it was not previously seen, together with a change from a normal to a rising renogram, is strongly suggestive of obstruction.

The use of a diuresis renogram has been disappointing in our experience. The response of a transplanted kidney to a given amount of diuretic is variable and usually slower than normal, and so it is difficult to quantify. More than the standard 0.5 mg/kg of frusemide (*see* Chapter 2) may be required to produce any diuresis. It is not usually needed in a graft with good function to distinguish obstruction from a dilated non-obstructed system, but it may be used occasionally when there is a slight fall in function, to be certain that there is no obstruction.

While it has been said that there is only a significant deterioration in function if there is a fall in the total removal of more than 5% of the injected dose between one study and

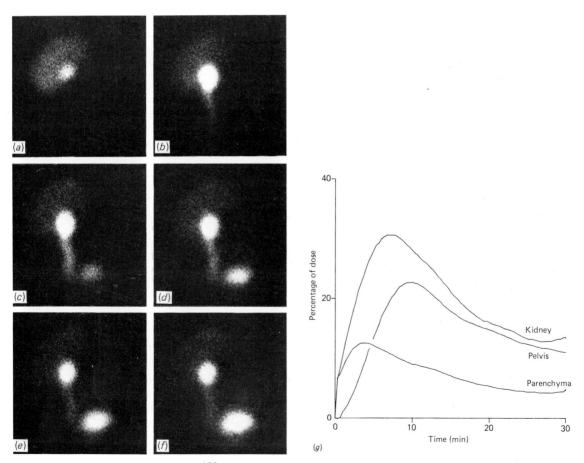

Figure 10.11 A transplant study using ^{123}I-OIH showing a prominent renal pelvis. The renogram demonstrates good drainage from the kidney

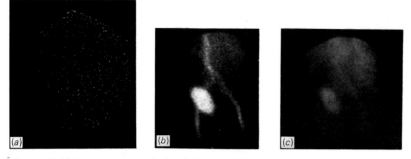

Figure 10.12 A renogram and circulation study in a patient with severe acute tubular necrosis in the transplanted kidney: (*a*) absent OIH uptake; (*b*) good perfusion of the renal transplant; (*c*) good blood pool in the kidney. This patient's kidney eventually achieved satisfactory function

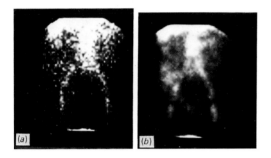

Figure 10.13 A ^{99m}Tc-DTPA circulation study in severe rejection: (*a*) poor perfusion; (*b*) poor blood pool in the kidney on the 4-minute image. The iliac arteries have as much activity as the kidney

the next, it is important to review all the patient's renograms, for it is possible that a more insidious form of rejection is occurring, unlike the usual acute episodes normally seen in the early stage. In this case each renogram may drop by 3% or so. Over a period of a week there may be a significant fall in function without any dramatic change from one renogram to the next.

There is sometimes a complete absence of OIH uptake in the kidney, and there are three possible causes for this (once technical problems, such as incorrect positioning of the camera, have been excluded!). These are: severe rejection, severe acute tubular necrosis and vascular thrombosis. A perfusion study should help distinguish these. As has been mentioned, acute tubular necrosis should have good perfusion and blood pool images. Severe rejection should have poor perfusion and patchy blood pool images while vascular thrombosis shows no perfusion (*Figures 10.12–14*). Occasionally rejection may be so severe as to show no perfusion. In this case it is not possible to distinguish it from an arterial thrombosis, but regrettably the treatment is usually the same—transplant nephrectomy. If a ring of hyperaemia is seen around a photon-deficient kidney area the kidney is certainly beyond rescue (*Figure 10.15*).

Exceptionally, it has been reported that a kidney with apparently absent perfusion does recover some function following treatment of rejection but some surgeons are prepared to explore the kidney on the evidence of the perfusion study alone, especially if it is similar on two successive occasions. However, before absent perfusion is reported, every other explanation for the poor perfusion must be eliminated. *Figure 10.16* shows the images from a patient with an abdominal hernia causing the intestines to overlie the kidney area. When perfusion was severely reduced it was impossible to see the kidney against the general background. On this occasion a report of absent perfusion was given with reservations because of the background. Arteriograms showed a poorly perfused kidney.

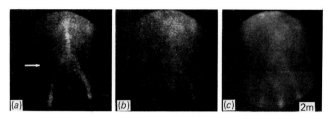

Figure 10.14 A ^{99m}Tc-DTPA circulation study showing absent perfusion and blood pool: (*a*) and (*b*) 5-second images; (*c*) image at 2 minutes post injection. The position of the transplanted kidney is arrowed

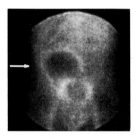

Figure 10.15 A 40-second image 2 minutes post injection of ^{99m}Tc-DTPA for a perfusion study. The ring of hyperaemia is seen around a necrotic kidney (arrow)

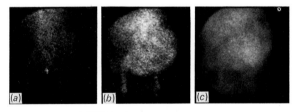

Figure 10.16 A ^{99m}Tc-DTPA perfusion study. Anterior views: (*a*) and (*b*) 5-second frames during the circulation phase; (*c*) an image at 2 minutes. The transplanted kidney was lying in the left iliac fossa

Renal artery stenosis is a surgical complication which is seen less frequently when a Carrel patch is used rather than an end-to-end anastomosis. Its effect on the renogram depends on its severity, but it tends to cause slow uptake and excretion. On the perfusion study there tends to be slow flow into the kidney; once activity reaches the kidney it is well visualized. It is not possible to diagnose renal artery stenosis positively with current nuclear medicine techniques, but if the diagnosis is suspected then renal arteriograms or a DIVA study should be performed.

Renography may be performed with DTPA instead of OIH, and some centres perform a renogram and a perfusion study together. In well functioning grafts there is little difference in the results produced by the two compounds (OIH and DTPA), although the figures for uptake as a percentage of dose and changes in total removal will not, of course, hold. We have found that, in the presence of poor function, it is even more difficult to obtain an accurate renogram with DTPA than with OIH. Because of the high background levels, the percentage uptake by the kidney depends critically on where the background region is taken. The images may also be misleading as a blood pool image can be obtained with DTPA due to the higher activity given, even when there is no function (*see Figures 10.12* and *10.13*). Provided a correct background region is taken, the renogram should show no uptake in such cases, but in the iliac fossae and pelvic regions it is not always possible to obtain a suitable background region so the renogram may show a falsely high uptake.

Probe renography

Probe renography is still useful for qualitative assessment of renal function where a gamma camera is not readily available. The procedure described in Chapters 2 and 7 may be modified to investigate the transplanted kidney, the probe being placed over the kidney in the iliac fossa. Additional information can be obtained by placing further probes over the right upper thorax, contralateral iliac fossa (to measure background activity) and bladder. As the kidney and bladder are in close proximity it is important that the probes are collimated adequately. Even then it is not always possible to distinguish kidney activity from that in the bladder. A dose of 1 MBq ^{131}I-OIH is administered intravenously and the activity from each detector fed to a chart recorder for the following 30 minutes. This is mainly a qualitative assessment, although methods of quantification have been described (Magnusson *et al.*, 1967; Staab *et al.*, 1969). The blood clearance curves obtained at the time of renography can be used to calculate half-time ($t_{1/2}$) (Joekes, Constable and Hyne, 1974). A prolongation of blood clearance $t_{1/2}$, delayed uptake and delayed elimination (provided there is no bladder interference) all indicate deteriorating function and are consistent with rejection.

Isotope clearance studies

The clearance studies described in Chapter 5 can also be used to monitor the progress of the transplanted kidney. Variations of these methods have been described, including the use of a single blood sample and external monitoring (Rossing, Bojsen and Frederiksen, 1978; Kristiansen, Frederiksen and Jeppesen, 1982) to give an estimation of glomerular filtration rate, or the use of external monitoring alone to give a $t_{1/2}$ for clearance (Sampson, Macleod and Warren, 1981). It must be remembered that these patients may have been subjected to many investigations for years, and their venous access may be poor; techniques requiring only one blood sample—for example, the single sample technique for effective renal plasma flow (Tauxe, Maher and Taylor, 1971; Tauxe *et al.*, 1982) and glomerular filtration rate (Constable *et al.*, 1980)—may be preferable to those needing multiple samples. However, if only a single sample at a specified time is to be relied on, it is advisable to ensure venous access well in advance of the time required: otherwise the time taken in obtaining the sample may invalidate the test.

A method of measuring glomerular filtration rate in the renal transplant recipient without blood sampling has been reported by Hutchings (Hutchings *et al.*, 1984). He studied 25 patients using ^{99m}Tc-DTPA and correlated the total kidney and bladder activity at 22 minutes after injection, with a standard determination of GFR using ^{51}Cr-EDTA. As a result he suggests that the 22-minute uptake value can be used to predict GFR in patients whose creatinine clearance is in the range 14–120 ml/min.

The usual detector for external monitoring of clearance is a sodium iodide detector. However, several groups have validated the use of a cadmium telluride (CdTe) detector (Kristiansen, Frederiksen and Jeppesen, 1982; Macleod and Sampson, 1982). This can be much smaller than the corresponding sodium iodide detector and may be attached to a patient and linked to a portable recorder for long periods of monitoring. The patient is free to move about if required, and yet the clearance can be calculated at varying times for up to 24 hours following a single injection of ^{99m}Tc-DTPA. A fall in the clearance may indicate rejection.

Influences of drugs on the renogram

Many commonly prescribed drugs may interfere with renal function. Some (e.g. diuretics) increase urine flow, while others may impair renal function. In a patient with a good creatinine clearance a mild reduction in function for a short while will cause no clinical problems. In a patient with function that is already compromised a further insult will lead to a rise in serum creatinine and urea, and this may be confused with a rejection episode. Renal transplant recipients often have many concurrent clinical problems and may receive many drugs during the postoperative course. Beta-adrenergic blocking agents, antibiotics, diuretics, corticosteroids and cyclosporin A (CyA) are among the commonest used that may alter renal function and hence affect the renogram.

Some β-adrenergic blocking agents are known to reduce renal plasma flow (Falch, Norman and Ødegaard, 1978). When given to patients with chronic renal failure and hypertension they can produce further deterioration in function (Warren, Swainson and Wright, 1974). Some reports suggest that the fall in function may only be transitory (Kincaid-Smith and Hua, 1974; Thompson and Joekes, 1974); others suggest that the renal plasma flow may remain constantly depressed (Falch, Ødegaard and Norman, 1979). Most patients given β-blockers have been taking them constantly prior to transplantation for hypertension control so their effect on the renogram, if any, is present from day 1 and should be constant. However, the person reporting should be aware of any changes in therapy as this may cause a temporary change in OIH clearance by the kidney. Antibiotics are a different case. They are usually given in short courses and may interfere with OIH uptake. Although non-nephrotoxic agents are usually prescribed, agents such as gentamicin are occasionally required and can impair renal uptake of OIH (Milman and Dahlger, 1980). Decreased uptake on the renogram in this situation may not indicate rejection.

Cyclosporin A is a relatively new immunosuppressive agent, and it appears to be very effective in reducing rejection. It does have some nephrotoxic effects (Calne *et al.*, 1978; Klintmalm, Iwatsuki and Starzel, 1981); these are a potential source of confusion in renal transplant recipients (Klintmalm, Iwatsuki and Starzel, 1981). There is a tendency for serum creatinine and urea to be slightly higher than normal (but stable) in patients taking this drug, but in acute toxicity the serum creatinine may rise quite steeply, raising the question of rejection. Unfortunately the renogram is often of no help in distinguishing these conditions. A fall in uptake and a delay in the renogram peak may occur in both states (Prescott *et al.*, 1982). A perfusion study may not help either. There have been reports of studies in patients with nephrotoxicity from the use of CyA in liver transplantation showing an ATN type picture and also ones mimicking rejection (Klintmalm, Iwatsuki and Starzel, 1981; Klintmalm *et al.*, 1981).

Diuretics can cause both increased uptake and increased urine flow (Clorius *et al.*, 1979). It is important therefore for serial studies to be done in roughly the same time relation to any maintenance diuretic on successive occasions, and if a large bolus is to be given it should be given after, rather than before, the renogram if at all possible. The same applies to corticosteroids which may of themselves improve renal clearance (Hayes and Moore, 1972).

Techniques for positive identification of rejection

During acute rejection, fibrin thrombi form in the glomerular and peritubular vessels of the kidney, and radioiodinated fibrinogen has been used to detect this (Salaman, 1970, 1972a, b). Following intravenous injection of ^{125}I, fibrinogen counts are obtained over the heart and kidney. The measurements are repeated over several days and an increased kidney-to-heart ratio indicates rejection. False positives occur, however, in the presence of wound and perirenal haematomas, renal vein thrombosis and urinary extravasation (Salaman, 1972b; Yeboah et al., 1973). Urinary obstruction may also cause false positive results, as fibrinogen fragments are known to be excreted in the urine during the first 2 weeks following transplantation (Braun and Merrill, 1968). Free iodide resulting from the breakdown of the compound is also excreted in the urine, hence urine obstruction will give a positive uptake. If ^{123}I is used to label the fibrinogen, then gamma camera images can be performed. This helps to distinguish perirenal haematoma from renal uptake (Swanson, Chatterjee and Denardo, 1979). However, the limited availability of ^{123}I prevents this from being used routinely.

^{99m}Tc-sulphur colloid is another radiopharmaceutical that has been advocated for the diagnosis of acute rejection. Following intravenous administration kidney uptake is compared with bone marrow uptake. Uptake equal to or greater than bone marrow is considered to indicate rejection. This method appears to have mixed results. Some have found it accurate with no false positives (Leonard et al., 1980), but others have found it more helpful in chronic rejection with little or no uptake in acute rejection (George et al., 1975). As colloid uptake has been reported in non-transplanted kidneys where patients have congestive cardiac failure (CCF) (Higgins et al., 1974; Klingensmith, Datu and Burdick, 1978), it is not surprising that false positive results have been reported in transplant patients with CCF (Kim et al., 1977). Kim reported that positive uptake was also seen in association with sepsis, and this, together with a report of positive studies in acute tubular necrosis (Frick et al., 1976), makes this technique of doubtful value in the diagnosis of rejection.

^{67}Ga-gallium citrate has also been suggested for the diagnosis of acute rejection. However, its urinary excretion means that imaging must be delayed for at least 24 hours, and false positives can still occur if there is little urine output, as in obstruction or acute tubular necrosis. Gallium may be taken up by the kidney for 4–5 weeks after the operation without any evidence of rejection, even though this is the time when most acute rejection episodes occur (Fawwaz and Johnson, 1979). This, and its known association with sepsis and acute tubular necrosis (Kumar and Coleman, 1976), have caused it to be discarded.

More recently, labelling of platelets, lymphocytes and leucocytes have all been suggested as possible methods for the diagnosis of rejection. Labelled leucocytes are taken up by the kidney in acute and chronic rejection (Frick et al., 1979). A delay of at least 24 hours is required between injection of autologous labelled white cells and imaging, and occasionally, in severely neutropenic patients, it is difficult to obtain sufficient white cells for labelling. This method will give false positive results in the presence of infection.

Labelled platelets have been suggested as platelet aggregation is known to occur in glomerular and peritubular capillaries in acute rejection. Platelet injections are given early in the postoperative period and images are obtained every day. Top-up injections are given weekly (Leithner et al., 1982a). The results of these studies are mixed. Some reports say that positive uptake occurs only in acute rejection (Heyns et al., 1982). Others report that both acute and chronic rejection show positive uptake in the kidney although acute rejection has more marked uptake (Leithner et al., 1980). Chandler and colleagues (1983) have attributed some prognostic significance to the platelet uptake. They correlated the degree of platelet uptake, especially after anti-rejection therapy, with the kidney status 2 years later. Those with low uptakes still had good function while those with high uptake either had had a nephrectomy because of rejection or had chronic rejection. Other workers, however, have not found platelet uptake to be so useful (Hilson *et al.*, 1982). False positive results have been reported in renal vein thrombosis (Chandler *et al.*, 1983) and haemolytic uraemic syndrome (Leithner *et al.*, 1982b). Contamination of the platelet preparation with plasma will mean labelling of transferrin (Hawker, Hawker and Wilkinson, 1978). A blood pool image will be obtained as a result, and contamination with white cells will mean a false positive scan in infection.

All the methods described above will give false negative results when rejection is accompanied by severely impaired blood-flow. Moreover their true value needs to be assessed more fully.

Other diagnostic techniques

The intravenous urogram (IVU) gives good anatomical information and may be useful in demonstrating surgical complications. However, at low levels of function it becomes less satisfactory, and it is not suitable for frequent studies. Renal arteriography gives excellent information about the vessels of the kidney and is most helpful in detecting renal artery stenosis for which it has been the investigation of choice. Changes do occur in rejection and include prolonged circulation time and stretching and narrowing of the interlobar and arcuate arteries, but these changes may not be seen in early rejection (Laasonen and Kock, 1978). Arteriography is invasive; it may be technically difficult; and it is certainly not suitable for multiple repeat studies. It has been reported that the contrast media used in arteriography may induce complement activation and so precipitate rejection (Heideman, Claes and Nilson, 1976), and that high doses of contrast media may of themselves make renal failure worse (Braun *et al.*, 1984; Mudge, 1980). Intravenous digital angiography, which is relatively non-invasive, has proved helpful in the diagnosis of renal artery stenosis, but it still has the drawback of requiring high-dose contrast media.

X-ray computed tomography (CT) is also used to investigate renal transplant recipients. It gives little information about function: its main use is in the diagnosis of complications such as abscesses, lymphoceles and haematomas. Antegrade pyelography is most helpful in identifying the site of ureteric obstruction in a poorly functioning graft, but it plays no part in the diagnosis of rejection.

Ultrasound is non-invasive and does not disturb the patient. It involves no dose of ionizing radiation, and, although no information on renal function can be obtained, it has been suggested that an increase in kidney size, together with decreased echogenicity of renal pyramids and patchy sonolucent areas in the cortex, may indicate rejection (Singh and Cohen, 1980; Frick *et al.*, 1981). This is less helpful with the non-oedematous rejection seen in patients taking CyA. The great advantage of ultrasound is the ability to detect a dilated renal pelvis and fluid collections in the renal area—for example, lymphoceles and urinomas which may be producing ureteric obstruction.

Methods of immunological surveillance are being developed and hold promise for the future, but are not yet suitable for routine use.

This chapter has concentrated on the use of radiopharmaceuticals in the monitoring of renal function and the diagnosis of postoperative complications directly related to the kidney. It should also be remembered that these patients are subject to an increased risk

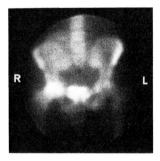

Figure 10.17 A bone scan. Anterior view showing increased uptake in the right hip. The patient was complaining of pain in the hip and had been on long-term corticosteroid therapy. The final diagnosis was avascular necrosis of the femoral head

of thromboembolism, as in any surgical procedure, and an increased risk of malignancy, related in part to the immunosuppression. The standard nuclear medicine procedures of isotope venography, lung, liver and bone imaging may be useful to help diagnose these complications, as for any other patient. Bone scintigraphy may also be used in the diagnosis of avascular necrosis of the femoral head, which occurs in some patients following long-term steroid therapy. Abnormalities may be seen in the affected hip before there are significant radiological changes (*Figure 10.17*).

No single, non-invasive test has yet emerged as the investigation of choice in the follow-up care of transplant recipients. A combination of radiology, nuclear medicine and ultrasound should be used. Renography reflects the change in function of the kidney consequent on rejection; it does not positively diagnose rejection. Labelled platelets are more rejection-specific, although there are some problems with false negative results when the rejection episode severely impairs the blood supply to the kidney. Ultrasound's main advantage is in the diagnosis of ureteric dilatation and perirenal fluid collections.

Which tests are used will depend in part on the expertise and equipment available in any given centre, but if some of the techniques described in this chapter are used to complement each other, in combinations appropriate to the suspected clinical diagnosis, they should provide a highly accurate diagnostic service.

References

BRAUN, W. E. and MERRILL, J. P. (1968) Urine fibrinogen fragments in human renal allografts. A possible mechanism of renal injury. *New England Journal of Medicine*, **278**(25), 1366–1371

BRAUN, W. E., PHILLIPS, D. F., VIDT, D. G. *et al.* (1984) Coronary artery disease in 100 diabetics with end stage renal failure. *Transplantation Proceedings XVI*, **3**, 603–607

CALNE, R. Y., THIRU, S., MCMASTER, P. *et al.* (1978) Cyclosporin A in patients receiving renal allografts from cadaver donors. *Lancet*, **2**, 1323–1327.

CHANDLER, S. T., BUCKELS, J., HAWKER, R. J., SMITH, N., BARNES, A. D. and MCCOLLUM, C. N. (1983) Indium labeled platelet uptake in rejecting renal transplants. *Surgery, Gynecology and Obstetrics*, **157**(3), 246–248

CLORIUS, J. H., DREIKHORN, K., ZELT, J., RAPTON, E., WEBER, D., RUBINSTEIN, K., DAHM, D. and GEORGI, P. (1979) Renal graft evaluation with pertechnetate and ^{131}I-hippuran. A comparative clinical study. *Journal of Nuclear Medicine*, **20**, 1029–1037

CONSTABLE, A. R., HUSSEIN, M. M., ALBRECHT, M. P. and JOEKES, A. M. (1980) Renal clearance determined from single plasma samples. *Proceedings IVth International Symposium of Radionuclides in Nephrology*, Boston, Basel: S. Karger, pp. 62–66

DUBOVSKY, E. V., LOGIC, J. R., DIETHELM, A. G., BALCH, C. M. and TAUXE, W. N. (1975) Comprehensive evaluation of renal function in the transplanted kidney. *Journal of Nuclear Medicine*, **16**(12), 1115–1120

DUBOVSKY, E. V., TAUXE, W. N., DIETHELM, A. G. and WHELCHEL, J. D. (1980) Quantitative functional evaluation of kidney transplants: Dynamic patterns of various complications based on 1950 studies in 436 patients. *Journal of Nuclear Medicine*, **21**(6), P39

DUBOVSKY, E. V., TAUXE, W. N., DIETHELM, A. G., WHELCHEL, J. D., RIVERA, R. and YESTER, M. (1982) Dynamic patterns of kidney transplant complications using quantitative functional evaluation. In: *Radionuclides in Nephrology*, A. M. Joekes, A. R. Constable, N. J. G. Brown and W. N. Tauxe (eds.), London: Academic Press, pp. 257–262

FALCH, D. K., NORMAN, M. and ØDEGAARD, A. E. (1978) Renal plasma flow and cardiac output during hydralazine and propranolol treatment in essential hypertension. *Scandinavian Journal of Clinical and Laboratory Investigation*, **38**, 143

FALCH, D. K., ØDEGAARD, A. E. and NORMAN, N. (1979) Decreased renal plasma flow during propranolol treatment in essential hypertension. *Acta medica Scandinavica*, **205**, 91–95

FAWWAZ, R. A. and JOHNSON, P. M. (1979) Localisation of gallium 67 in the normally functioning allografted kidney. *Journal of Nuclear Medicine*, **20**(3), 207–209

FRICK, M. P., LOKEN, M. K., GOLDBERG, M. E. and SIMMONS, R. L. (1976) Use of ^{99m}Tc S. colloid in evaluation of renal transplant complications. *Journal of Nuclear Medicine*, **17**(3), 181–183

FRICK, M. P., HENKE, C. E., FORSTROM, L. A., SIMMONS, R. A., McCULLOUGH, J. and LOKEN, M. K. (1979) Use of ^{111}In labelled leucocytes in evaluation of renal transplant rejection. A preliminary report. *Clinical Nuclear Medicine*, **4**(1), 24–25

FRICK, M. P., FEINBERG, S. B., SIBLEY, R. and IDSTROM, M. E. (1981) Ultrasound in acute renal transplant rejection. *Radiology*, **138**, 657–660

GEORGE, E. A., CODD, J. E., NEWTON, W. T., HENRY, R. and DONATI, R. M. (1975) Further evaluation of ^{99m}Tc sulfur colloid accumulation in rejecting renal transplant in man and a canine model. *Radiology*, **116**, 121–126

HAWKER, R. J., HAWKER, L. M. and WILKINSON, A. R. (1978) Use of indium-111 oxine to label human platelets. *Lancet*, **2**, 481

HAYES, M. and MOORE, T. C. (1971) Early detection and classification of renal transplant rejection by B/K scan ratio and blood isotope clearance data. *Transplantation*, **12**(2), 139–141

HAYES, M. and MOORE, T. C. (1972) Early detection of canine renal allograft rejection by reduction in the scan bladder/kidney isotope ratio. *Surgery*, **71**(1), 60–65

HAYES, M., MOORE, T. C. and TAPLIN, G. V. (1972) Radionuclide procedures in predicting early renal transplant rejection. *Radiology*, **103**(3), 627–631

HEIDEMAN, M., CLAES, G. and NILSON, A. E. (1976) The risk of renal allograft rejection following angiography. *Transplantation*, **21**(4), 289–293

HEYNS, A. du.P., LOTTER, M. G., PIETERS, H., PAUW, F. H., BADENHORST, P. N., WESSELS, P. and MINNAAR, P. C. (1982) A quantitative study of indium III-oxine platelet kinetics in acute and chronic transplant rejection. *Clinical Nephrology*, **18**(4), 174–182

HIGGINS, C. B., TAKETA, R. M., TAYLOR, A., HALPERN, S. E. and ASHBURN, W. L. (1974) Renal uptake of ^{99m}Tc S colloid. *Journal of Nuclear Medicine*, **15**(7), 565–567

HILSON, A. J. W., MAISEY, M. N., BROWN, C. B., OGG, C. S. and BEWICK, M. S. (1978) Dynamic renal transplant imaging with ^{99m}Tc DTPA (Sn). Supplemented by a transplant perfusion index in the management of renal transplants. *Journal of Nuclear Medicine*, **19**(9), 994–1000

HILSON, A. J. W., LAZARUS, C., PARBTANI, A., CAMERON, J. S. and MAISEY, M. N. (1982) In^{111} Platelets in early detection of kidney graft rejection. In: *Radionuclides in Nephrology*, A. M. Joekes, A. R. Constable, N. J. G. Brown and W. N. Tauxe (eds.), London: Academic Press, pp. 295–298

HOLLENBERG, N. K., RETIK, A. B., ROSEN, S. M., MURRAY, J. E. and MERRILL, J. P. (1968) The role of vasoconstriction in the ischaemia of renal allograft rejection. *Transplantation*, **6**(1), 59

HOLLENBERG, N. K., BIRTCH, A., RASHID, A., MANGEL, R., BRIGGS, W., EPSTEIN, M., MURRAY, J. E. and MERRILL, J. P. (1972) Relationships between intrarenal perfusion and function: Serial haemodynamic studies in the transplanted human kidney. *Medicine*, **51**(2), 95–106

HONG-YOE, O., EPHRAIM, K. H., JESSURUN, R. F. M., NIEUWENHUIS, M. G. and STUYVENBERG, A. (1976) Quantitative assessment of renal transplant function on renogram performed with computer assisted gamma camera. *Proceedings of the European Dialysis and Transplantation Association*, **12**, 441–451

HUTCHINGS, M. V., SWENEY, P., FERNANDO, O. N. and CONSTABLE, A. R. (1984) Measurement of glomerular filtration rate without blood sampling: Validation in renal transplant patients. *British Journal of Radiology*, **57**, 347–349

JACKSON, B. T. and MANNICK, J. A. (1964) Serial blood flow in first set renal homotransplants undergoing rejection. *Surgery, Gynecology and Obstetrics*, **119**, 1265–1270

JOEKES, A. M., CONSTABLE, A. R. and HYNE, B. E. B. (1974) Renogram monitoring in kidney transplant rejection. In: *Radionuclides in Nephrology—Proceedings of 3rd International Symposium, Berlin, April 1974*, K. Zum Winkel, M. O. Blaufox and J. L. Funck-Brentano (eds.), Stuttgart: Georg Thieme, p. 181

JOHNSON, R. W. G., MALLICK, N. P., GOOI, T. H., COHEN, G. L. and ORR, W. McN. (1977) Improvement in patient and graft survival after cadaveric renal transplantation. Abstract of paper presented to a meeting of the Surgical Research Society. *British Journal of Surgery*, **64**, 831

KIM, Y. C., MASSARI, P. U., BROWN, M. L., THRALL, J. H., CHANG, B. and KEYES, J. W. (1977) Clinical significance of ^{99m}technetium sulphur colloid accumulation in renal transplant patients. *Radiology*, **124**, 745–748

KINCAID-SMITH, P. and HUA, A. S. P. (1974) Beta-adrenergic blocking agents in renal failure. *British Medical Journal*, **3**, 520

KIRCHNER, P. T., GOLDMAN, M. H., LEAPMAN, S. B. and KIEPFER, R. F. (1978) Clinical application of the kidney to aortic blood flow index (K/A ratio). *Contributions to Nephrology*, **11**, 120–126

KLINGENSMITH, W. C. III, DATU, J. A. and BURDICK, D. C. (1978) Renal uptake of ^{99m}Tc S colloid in congestive heart failure. *Radiology*, **127**(1), 185–187

KLINTMALM, G. B. G., IWATSUKI, S. and STARZEL, T. E. (1981) Nephrotoxicity of cyclosporin A in liver and kidney transplant patients. *Lancet*, **1**, 470

KLINTMALM, G. B. G., KLINGENSMITH, W. C. III, IWATSUKI, S., SCHROTER, G. P. J. and STARZEL, T. E. (1981) Tc^{99m} DTPA and I^{131} hippuran findings in cyclosporin A nephrotoxicity in liver transplant recipients. Abstract of paper presented at 28th Annual Meeting of Society of Nuclear Medicine. *Journal of Nuclear Medicine*, **22**(6), P37

KRISTIANSEN, J. H., FREDERIKSEN, P. B. and JEPPESEN, P. (1982) The determination of glomerular filtration rate (GFR) with a portable cadmium telluride (CdTe) detector. In: *Radionuclides in Nephrology*, A. M. Joekes *et al.* (eds.), London: Academic Press, pp. 335–339

KUMAR, B. and COLEMAN, R. E. (1976) Significance of delayed ^{67}Ga localisation in the kidneys. *Journal of Nuclear Medicine*, **17**, 872–875

LAASONEN, L. and KOCK, B. (1978) Angiography and isotope renography in acute rejection of renal transplants. *Scandinavian Journal of Urology and Nephrology*, **12**, 79–82

LEITHNER, C., SINZINGER, H., ANGELBERGER, P. and SYRE, G. (1980) In^{111} labelled platelets in chronic kidney transplant rejection. *Lancet*, **2**, 213–214

LEITHNER, C., SINZINGER, H., SCHWARZ, M. and POHANKA, E. (1982a) Radiolabelled platelets and prostacyclin in diagnosis and treatment of transplant rejection. *Proceedings of the European Dialysis and Transplantation Association*, **19**, 529–535

LEITHNER, C., SINZINGER, H., POHANKA, E., SCHWARZ, M., KIETSCHMER, G. and SYRE, G. (1982b) Recurrence of haemolytic uraemic syndrome triggered by cyclosporin A after renal transplantation. *Lancet*, **1**, 1470

LEONARD, J. C., BAUMANN, W. E., PEDERSON, J. E. and ROY, J. B. (1980) ^{99m}Tc technetium sulfur colloid scanning in diagnosis of renal transplant rejection. *Journal of Urology*, **123**, 815–818

MACLEOD, M. A. and SAMPSON, W. F. D. (1982) An evaluation of a portable cadmium telluride detector and data storage system as a continuous monitor of renal transplant function. In: *Radionuclides in Nephrology*, A. M. Joekes *et al.* (eds.), London: Academic Press, pp. 341–346

MAGNUSSON, G., COLLSTE, L., FRANKSSON, C. and LUNDGREN, G. (1967) Radiorenography in clinical transplantation. *Scandinavian Journal of Urology and Nephrology*, **1**, 132–151

MILMAN, N. and DAHLGER, J. (1980) Effects of aminoglycoside antibiotics on iodohippurate accumulation in rabbit renal cortical slices. In: *Proceedings of IVth International Symposium on Radionuclides in Nephrology, Boston*, Basel: S. Karger, pp. 156–161

MUDGE, G. (1980) *Kidney International*, **18**, 540–552

PRESCOTT, M. C. (1982) MD Thesis, Victoria University of Manchester

PRESCOTT, M. C., TESTA, H. J., LAWSON, R. S. and JOHNSON, R. W. G. (1982) The effect of cyclosporin A on the results of radionuclide investigations of kidney function in renal transplant recipients. In: *Radionuclides in Nephrology*, A. M. Joekes *et al.* (eds.), London: Academic Press, pp. 275–279

ROSENTHALL, L., MANGEL, R., LISBONA, R. and LACOUCIERE, Y. (1974) Diagnostic applications of radiopertechnetate and radiohippurate imaging in post renal transplant complications. *Radiology*, **111**(2), 347–358

ROSSING, N., BOJSEN, J. and FREDERIKSEN, P. L. (1978) The glomerular filtration rate determined with ^{99m}Tc DTPA and a portable cadmium telluride detector. *Scandinavian Journal of Clinical and Laboratory Investigation*, **38**, 23–28

SALAMAN, J. R. (1970) Use of radioactive fibrinogen for detecting rejection in human renal transplants. *British Medical Journal*, **2**, 517–521

SALAMAN, J. R. (1972a) A technique for detecting rejection episodes in human transplant recipients using radioactive fibrinogen. *British Journal of Surgery*, **59**(2), 138–142

SALAMAN, J. R. (1972b) Renal allograft rejection in the rat studied with ^{125}I fibrinogen. *Transplantation*, **14**(1), 74–78

SAMPSON, W. F. D., MACLEOD, M. A. and WARREN, D. (1981) External monitoring of kidney transplant function using ^{99m}Tc (Sn) DTPA. *Journal of Nuclear Medicine*, **22**(5), 411–416

SINGH, A. and COHEN, W. N. (1980) Renal allograft rejection—sonography and scintigraphy. *American Journal of Roentgenology, Radium Therapy and Nuclear Medicine*, **135**(1), 73–77

STAAB, E. V., KELLY, W. D. and LOKEN, M. K. (1969) Prognostic value of radioisotope renograms in kidney transplantation. *Journal of Nuclear Medicine*, **10**(3), 133–135

SWANSON, M. A., CHATTERJEE, S. and DENARDO, S. J. (1979) ^{123}I-fibrinogen scintigraphy in the diagnosis of allograft rejection. *Journal of Nuclear Medicine*, **20**(6), P619

TAUXE, W. N., MAHER, F. T. and TAYLOR, W. F. (1971) Effective renal plasma flow: Estimation from theoretical volumes of distribution of intravenously injected ^{131}I ortho-iodohippurate. *Mayo Clinic Proceedings*, **46**, 524–531

TAUXE, W. N., DUBOVSKY, E. V., KIDD, T., DIAZ, F. and SMITH, L. R. (1982) New formulas for the calculation of effective renal plasma flow. *European Journal of Nuclear Medicine*, **7**(2), 51–54

THOMPSON, F. D. and JOEKES, A. M. (1974) Beta-blockade in the presence of renal disease and hypertension. *British Medical Journal*, **2**, 555–556

WARREN, D. J., SWAINSON, C. P. and WRIGHT, N. (1974) Deterioration in renal function after beta-blockade in patients with chronic renal failure and hypertension. *British Medical Journal*, **2**, 193–194

YEBOAH, E. D., CHISHOLM, G. D., SHORT, M. D. and PETRIE, A. (1973) Detection and prediction of acute rejection episodes in human renal transplants using radioactive fibrinogen. *British Journal of Urology*, **45**, 273–280

11 Paediatric problems

P. J. English

Techniques

In recent years, paediatric clinicians have become more aware of the important role that nuclear medicine can play in the investigation and follow-up of children with urinary tract disorders. This has stemmed not only from the specific functional information that radionuclide studies can provide but also from an appreciation of their low radiation dose and absence of systemic side-effects. These factors make them particularly attractive in the paediatric field, where serial assessment is often required. Now, many children with urinary tract problems can be followed up safely using radionuclide studies in place of conventional radiology, but the initial assessment of the urinary tract or the need for detailed anatomical information usually requires intravenous urography or ultrasound.

The nuclear medicine techniques available for investigating the urinary tract in children are similar to those used in adults and are described fully in Part I. With the widespread availability of modern gamma camera/computer systems, probe renography now has a very limited place in paediatric practice and will not be discussed further here. Gamma camera renography, using either ^{99m}Tc-DTPA or ^{123}I-OIH, is the best overall test for studying the functional integrity of the urinary tract. In children under the age of 3 years this is carried out in the supine position (infants can actually lie on the camera), but in older children the supine, prone or sitting positions may be used, with the camera at the patient's back. The test is difficult to perform in a fractious and unco-operative child, so a mild sedative such as trimeprazine (Vallergan) syrup 3 mg/kg administered 1 hour beforehand is often helpful, particularly when investigating children under the age of 5 years.

Experienced personnel with expertise in handling young children can also do much to allay a child's fears, and a parent or familiar nurse present during the test can offer further reassurance. Mechanical restraints are not recommended as they usually result in a frightened, frustrated child and cannot, in any case, prevent wriggling beneath them. However, some degree of manual restraint will be necessary if satisfactory images are to be obtained in a child who insists on constantly moving.

Extravasation of the administered dose can be prevented in young children by using a 23- or 25-gauge butterfly needle followed by a flushing dose of normal saline. Generally an arm vein is suitable, but if it is desirable to visualize the inferior vena cava (e.g. when investigating an abdominal mass or suspected renal vein thrombosis) a vein in the foot should be used for the injection. In some neonates, a scalp vein is occasionally the only suitable injection site. If there is any likelihood that a diuresis renogram will be necessary, the butterfly needle should be left *in situ* until frusemide has been given, usually at 10–20 minutes from the start of the test. Where this is likely to be difficult technically, the diuretic should be given at the same time as the radiopharmaceutical.

If indicated, indirect micturating cystography can be performed at the end of the renogram study to assess the presence of vesico-ureteric reflux. This will depend on a co-operative child and is only valid if frusemide has not been given. Equivocal results can also occur if there is poor clearance of tracer from the kidney areas. This is not a problem with direct radionuclide micturating cystography which can be performed successfully in children of all age groups and is generally regarded as the more accurate test (Conway and Kruglik, 1976). However, it has the disadvantage that urethral catheterization is required. A No. 8 infant feeding tube can be used for this purpose, and the bladder is filled with a solution of 20–40 MBq (0.5–1.0 mCi) ^{99m}Tc-pertechnetate in 500 ml distilled water or normal saline at room temperature until the child becomes uncomfortable. The child should be allowed to void in his or her usual position with the camera positioned at the back to include the kidney regions and bladder. Reflux is looked for during filling and micturition by storing 5-second images during these phases.

Although functioning renal parenchyma can be visualized from the early images during an ^{123}I-OIH or ^{99m}Tc-DTPA study, more accurate detection of segmental cortical lesions is obtained using a static imaging agent. In children ^{99m}Tc-DMSA is the most commonly used of these agents, and has been shown to be particularly useful in the detection of renal scars where its sensitivity is greater than intravenous urography (Merrick *et al.*, 1980). This high detection rate is achieved by taking posterior and posterior-oblique views. Although 400 000 counts is desirable for each image, fewer counts should be accepted in a restless child. Scars can be missed when an image is distorted by excessive movement. This should be recognized at the time so that the scan can be repeated immediately; the child will incur no extra radiation dose.

Nuclear medicine techniques for estimating total renal function are particularly useful in children because urine specimens are not required. Both the effective renal plasma flow and glomerular filtration rate (GFR) can be estimated accurately by these techniques (*see* Chapter 5). Measurement of the GFR is more popular with clinicians and can be calculated from a single injection method using either ^{51}Cr-EDTA or ^{99m}Tc-DTPA. In children it is desirable to reduce the number of venepunctures to a minimum so that methods of analysis based on a single blood sample or, at most, two blood samples after the initial injection are the most suitable. It is customary to relate the result to body surface area by assuming an average adult value of 1.73 m^2.

Dosage in paediatric studies

In all radionuclide studies in children, the radiation dose absorbed should be kept to a minimum. As discussed in Chapter 19, the adult dose may be reduced in proportion to body weight, although it is clearly important that the amount of activity administered should be sufficiently high for accurate counting statistics.

In the case of clearance measurements, sufficient activity must be present in the plasma samples to permit an accurate assessment of each sample in a practicable measurement time. The activity per unit volume of a sample is inversely proportional to the volume of dilution and, hence, is similarly related to body weight. The quantity administered to a patient may therefore be adjusted in proportion to body weight provided that samples of sufficient volume can be obtained.

For successful organ imaging a given count density is required, and smaller organs

TABLE 11.1. Dosage in paediatric studies

Procedure	Radiopharmaceutical	Dose per kg body wt		Minimum dose	
		(MBq)	(μCi)	(MBq)	(μCi)
Gamma camera renography	^{123}I-OIH	0.2	5.4	3	80
Gamma camera renography	^{99m}Tc-DTPA	1.0	27	4	100
Renal imaging with perfusion study	^{99m}Tc-gluconate	5.5	150	25	750
Renal imaging	^{99m}Tc-DMSA	1.0	27	3	80

with the same uptake should permit the use of a smaller dose. Dosages are often quoted per unit body weight but this can underestimate the quantity required in very young children. Hence, there is a lower limit beyond which the administered dose should not be reduced if meaningful results are to be obtained (*see Table 11.1*).

Assessment of the neonate

The physiology of the infant kidney differs from that of the adult in several ways. Blood-flow and glomerular filtration rate are lower in relation to the body surface area. For instance, at 4 weeks of age, the mean GFR is only 48 ml/min per 1.73 m^2 and only approaches adult values by 12 months (Barrett and Chantler, 1975). Proximal tubular function is also immature, and infant kidneys, especially in the neonate, are less able to handle a sodium load. It is for these reasons that intravenous urography is of little value in the first few days of life and can even be dangerous. There is failure to concentrate the contrast medium and the high sodium load and osmotic diuresis can lead to renal failure in an ill child or cause further deterioration if renal function is already compromised.

Urinary tract investigations in the new-born are best carried out using ultrasound scanning, gamma camera scintigraphy and, if necessary, X-ray micturating cystography. An ultrasound scan should be performed first. In renal failure this will establish the presence of the kidneys and determine whether the collecting systems are dilated. If there is any suggestion that the upper tracts are dilated, a micturating cystogram will be necessary. Individual renal function can be assessed by gamma camera scintigraphy using either ^{123}I-OIH or ^{99m}Tc-DTPA. Unlike the intra-venous urogram, good kidney images are demonstrated in the young neonate provided that the renal function is not severely impaired. In the presence of acute tubular necrosis good perfusion to the kidneys is seen if a first circulation study is performed, followed by continuous renal accumulation of the tracer and absent excretion. By contrast, renal vein thrombosis results in poor perfusion and uptake by the affected kidneys. Repeat tests can be used in both conditions to detect any recovery in renal function.

Renal masses in the neonate can result from a variety of causes (Gordon, 1982). These include: renal vein thrombosis, polycystic and multicystic kidneys, nephroblastoma, medullary necrosis and hydronephrosis. Their assessment requires an integrated diagnostic approach. Ultrasound will determine if the mass or masses are solid or cystic and, in the case of the latter, whether there is also dilatation of the ureter(s) and/or distension of the bladder to suggest vesico-ureteric reflux or lower tract obstruction. Gamma camera scintigraphy may be helpful in elucidating the nature of a renal mass. The presence of a hydronephrotic kidney is often well demonstrated by showing a rim of functioning cortical tissue in the early images followed by tracer accumulation in the dilated pelvicalyceal system later in the study. If activity is also clearly seen in the ureters, a pelviureteric junction obstruction can be excluded. However, the specialized radionuclide methods for assessing the presence or absence of upper urinary tract obstruction (*see* Chapter 8) have not so far been validated in the neonate. It must also be remembered that recovery of individual kidney function can be dramatic in the neonate and that nephrectomy should not be recommended solely on the basis of an *apparently* non-functioning kidney.

Vesico-ureteric reflux

Vesico-ureteric reflux usually arises because of a primary defect at the uretero-vesical junction (primary reflux) but may also be caused by the effects of other urinary tract pathology such as a neuropathic bladder or posterior urethral valves (secondary reflux). Grades of reflux range from mild, with filling of the lower ureter only, to severe where there is reflux into a dilated pelvicalyceal system. Primary reflux most commonly occurs in infancy and has a tendency to spontaneous resolution with increasing age, particularly in those cases where the ureters remain undilated (Normand and Smellie, 1979). It is uncommon in asymptomatic children but is found in 30–50% of children with a history of urinary tract infection (Smellie and Normand 1966; Wein *et al.*, 1972).

The clinical importance of reflux is its association with chronic pyelonephritic scarring (reflux nephropathy), a common cause of hypertension and renal failure in children. Experimental evidence suggests that scarring may be caused by intrarenal reflux of infected urine in kidneys possessing compound renal papillae that present a flat or concave surface to the calyx (Ransley and Risdon, 1978). These compound papillae are usually found in the polar regions—particularly the upper—which are also the areas of the kidney in which scarring is most frequently observed. New or progressive scarring rarely occurs in primary reflux if the urine can be kept sterile. For this reason, medical treatment is usually advised in low-grade reflux but there is uncertainty at the present time as to whether more severe degrees of reflux should be treated conservatively or by ureteric re-implantation (Report of the International Reflux Study Committee, 1981).

Initial screening for vesico-ureteric reflux is best performed by an X-ray micturating cystogram, especially in males, when any lower urinary tract pathology such as urethral valves can be detected at the same time. However, radionuclide cystography, with its lower radiation dose, is an attractive alternative for follow-up studies in both sexes, where the main question is whether reflux is present or not. The indirect method of radionuclide cystography is easy to perform and is well tolerated but lacks the sensitivity of the direct method. However, it is adequate for repeat studies in a co-operative child with good renal function. The direct method is more appropriate in the initial assessment of girls, in young children and in those cases where renal function is compromised. It has also been shown that the latter method can be combined usefully with continuous cystometric recording of bladder function (Maizels *et al.*, 1978).

Accurate assessment of reflux nephropathy in children is essential, as the presence of even a single scar is associated with an increased risk of hypertension in later years (Wallace *et al.*, 1978). ^{99m}Tc-DMSA scanning is a particularly sensitive method for detecting small scars which show up as focal areas of cortical loss, usually in the polar regions of the kidney. The scan should be used as part of the initial assessment of all children with vesico-ureteric reflux and can be repeated at intervals during childhood to assess renal growth, differential function and the development of any new or progressive scarring.

Pelviureteric junction obstruction is sometimes associated with vesico-ureteric reflux and, when suspected, can be confirmed by gamma camera diuresis renography. This test is also useful for ensuring the adequacy of upper tract drainage after ureteric re-implantation. Occasionally after this type of surgery the ureter may drain freely when the bladder is empty but be obstructed with bladder filling due to kinking at the point of entry into the bladder (Gibbons and Gonzales, 1983). This situation can only be detected if the diuresis renogram is performed both with an empty and with a full bladder.

Congenital anomalies of the kidneys

These often remain undetected throughout life but can cause diagnostic problems in both paediatric and adult patients. Radionuclide studies can be helpful in their assessment.

Absent kidney

Unilateral renal agenesis affects approximately 1 in 1500 of the population and is sometimes associated with other abnormalities such as imperforate anus (Emanuel *et al.*, 1974). It is usually suspected from an incidental finding on intravenous urography but should be confirmed by means of a radionuclide study. Gamma camera scintigraphy using either ^{99m}Tc-DTPA or ^{123}I-OIH will fail to show any evidence of cortical function. A first circulation study may help to distinguish a congenitally absent kidney from a non-functioning one in which some perfusion is preserved. Delayed images using a static imaging agent such as ^{99m}Tc-DMSA may also help to demonstrate the presence of a poorly functioning kidney.

Ectopic kidney

The incidence of ectopic kidney is about 1 in 900. In most cases an ectopic kidney results from incomplete ascent of the kidney from the pelvis during early fetal life. Rare forms include thoracic kidney and crossed renal ectopia. Patients with ectopic kidneys are usually asymptomatic but the solitary pelvic kidney, in particular, has an increased incidence of hydronephrosis and calculus formation. Location of the ectopic renal tissue on intravenous urography can be difficult when the kidney overlies the bony pelvis but is easily detected by gamma camera scintigraphy (*Figure 11.1*). If there is slow excretion of the tracer from the pelvic kidney, the presence of obstruction can be determined by administering intravenous frusemide and analysing the resultant diuresis renogram.

Although depth differences are insignificant in children when the kidneys are in their normal position, analysis of relative renal function from the posterior views of a gamma camera study may be inaccurate in ectopic kidneys. If accurate differential function is

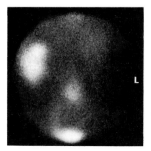

Figure 11.1A Renal scan using ^{99m}Tc-gluconate in the anterior projection showing normal right kidney and pelvic left kidney

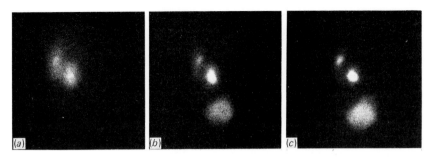

Figure 11.1B Analogue images from ^{123}I-OIH renogram in a case of crossed renal ectopia: (*a*) to (*c*) images at 0–5, 5–10 and 10–15 minutes

required, the effects of renal depth difference can be reduced by taking the geometric mean of count rates from anterior and posterior views (Powers *et al.*, 1981). This is easily performed during a ^{99m}Tc-DMSA scan but will require two studies if a gamma camera renogram is used for this purpose.

Horseshoe kidney

Horseshoe kidney has an incidence of approximately 1 in 400 and, because it is frequently associated with other congenital anomalies, is often discovered in childhood. It is caused by partial fusion of the developing metanephric masses during early fetal life: the kidneys are usually joined at the lower poles although, in a small number of patients, the isthmus connects both upper poles instead. The isthmus prevents proper ascent of the kidneys and usually reaches a final position across the third or fourth lumbar vertebra. The diagnosis is suspected on intravenous urography by finding medially directed calyces and laterally displaced ureters, although the true picture can sometimes be confused with rotation of the kidneys. However, assessment of a horseshoe kidney by gamma camera renography, or by imaging using a static renal agent, often clearly demonstrates the presence of a functioning isthmus. This will occasionally be seen in the posterior projection but is more clearly visualized in the anterior views (*Figure 11.2*).

The incidence of hydronephrosis, calculus formation and infection is increased in horseshoe kidneys. In the presence of such complications gamma camera studies will be useful in assessing the relative renal function of each kidney mass and in evaluating the likelihood of obstruction when the renal pelvis is dilated.

Renal cystic disease

A multicystic kidney usually presents at birth as an abdominal mass. These kidneys have very little function and, on renal static imaging, characteristically show absent perfusion and large 'cold' areas throughout the parenchyma with little or no excretion. Although the scan may sometimes enable a distinction to be made between a multicystic and hydronephrotic kidney (Ash *et al.*, 1982), its main role in these cases is to assess the relative renal function.

Polycystic disease can be of either the infantile or adult varieties. Patients are usually referred because of palpable renal masses, but the adult variety may also present with complications of the disease such as pain, haematuria, infection, hypertension or renal failure. Although the diagnosis is usually made by intravenous urography and ultrasound, the condition can also be recognized by renal static imaging where the presence of multiple 'cold' areas will be seen on both the vascular and parenchymal

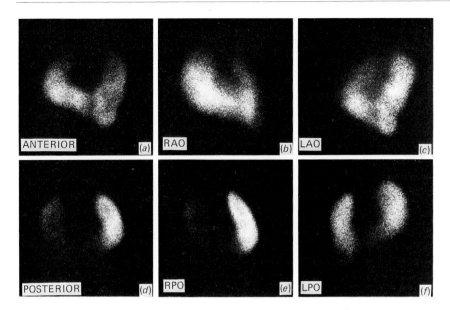

Figure 11.2 Renal scan using ^{99m}Tc-DMSA in a case of horseshoe kidney.
Computer images: (*a*) anterior; (*b*) right anterior oblique; (*c*) left anterior
oblique; (*d*) posterior; (*e*) right posterior oblique; (*f*) left posterior oblique

studies. Gamma camera renography, by evaluating underlying renal function, is useful
for follow-up.

Duplication of the upper urinary tract

Duplicated ureters occur in approximately 1 in 125 of the population. However, a
higher incidence is seen in urological departments, with between 6 and 8% of patients
estimated to have this anomaly (Thompson and Amar, 1958; Meller and Eckstein,
1982). The condition is more common in females and is bilateral in almost 25% of cases.
Incomplete duplication (bifid ureter), where the ureters join before entering the bladder,
is twice as common as the complete variety where both ureters empty into the bladder
independently.

In incomplete duplication, the bifurcation most often occurs below the level of the
sacroiliac joint. Vesico-ureteric reflux is uncommon with this variety but reflux of urine
may occur from one stem of the bifid ureter into the other (uretero-ureteric reflux). The
'seesaw' type is where urine passes from one moiety to the other and back again and
may or may not be associated with urinary stasis (*Figure 11.3*). In the 'up and down'
type, urine is propelled either from an active to a passive moiety or between the renal
pelvis and ureteric confluence (*Figure 11.4*) (*see* Chapter 4). These urodynamic
phenomena can easily be demonstrated by gamma camera scintigraphy which enables
areas of interest to be defined within the kidney, so that separate renograms for each
moiety can be derived (O'Reilly *et al.*, 1978) (*see Figure 2.3*). In assessing 34 incomplete
duplications in children by ^{99m}Tc-DTPA, Meller and Eckstein (1982) demonstrated
'seesaw' reflux in 13 cases and 'up and down' reflux in a further two cases. Surgery may
be necessary if uretero-ureteric reflux is associated with persistent renal pain or
recurrent urinary infections.

In complete duplications, the orifice of the upper pole ureter is usually nearer the
bladder neck, and in a more medial position than that of the lower pole ureter. Reflux

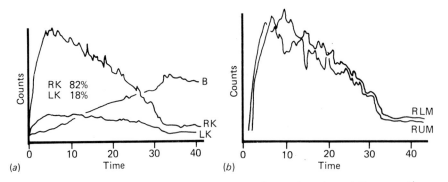

Figure 11.3 (*a*) Derived renogram curves showing fluctuations in activity suggestive of reflux on right (LK = left kidney; RK = right kidney; B = bladder); (*b*) differential renograms from upper and lower moieties of right kidney demonstrating seesaw reflux (RLM = right lower moiety; RUM = right upper moiety)

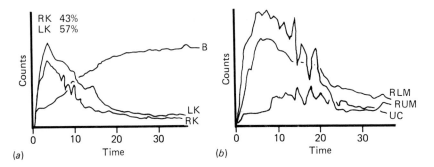

Figure 11.4 (*a*) Derived renogram curves showing fluctuations in activity suggestive of reflux on right (LK = left kidney; RK = right kidney; B = bladder); (*b*) differential study showing smooth excretion from lower moiety but reflux activity between upper moiety and ureteric confluence (RLM = right lower moiety; RUM = right upper moiety; UC = ureteric confluence)

into the lower pole ureter is the most common complication in this variety of duplication. The upper ureter may also be prone to reflux if it drains in an ectopic position. If the orifice of this ureter is the site of a ureterocele, reflux or obstruction to both ureters can occur. In the assessment of complete duplications, the use of radionuclides is complementary to conventional radiology and ultrasound. Vesico-ureteric reflux, particularly into the lower moiety, is often seen as 'saw-tooth' waves on the renogram trace and can usually be confirmed by either direct or indirect radionuclide micturating cystography (*see Figures 4.2* and *4.3*). However, the main role of gamma camera studies is to assess renal function and in particular to determine the relative contribution of each moiety. Heminephrectomy is generally indicated if scanning confirms a poorly functioning pyelonephritic or dysplastic segment.

Pelviureteric junction obstruction

This condition is discussed further in Chapter 8. In children it occurs more commonly in boys and affects the left kidney more than the right (Johnston *et al.*, 1977). Genuine obstruction at the pelviureteric junction must be distinguished from non-obstructive, atonic dilatation of the renal pelvis. In children as well as adults, gamma camera diuresis renography, using either ^{123}I-OIH or ^{99m}Tc-DTPA, has been shown to be a valid test for this purpose (Koff *et al.*, 1980; English *et al.*, 1982). Some form of pyeloplasty is indicated if the renal pelvis is obstructed, although rarely nephrectomy may have to be considered in a poorly functioning kidney. This latter operation should not be undertaken solely on the basis of a low relative renal function obtained from the renogram, but should also depend on the clinical judgement of the surgeon: in some cases kidney function can improve after the obstruction has been relieved. For post-pyeloplasty assessment diuresis renography is generally more useful than intravenous urography and should be the test of choice (Lupton *et al.*, 1979).

Megaureters

It is now firmly established that wide ureters in children seen on intravenous urography can occur in the absence of either obstruction or vesico-ureteric reflux (Whitaker and Johnston, 1975). Appropriate clinical management of these cases depends, therefore, on defining the cause of the ureteric dilatation (*Figure 11.5*).

Vesico-ureteric reflux should be looked for routinely, and in boys the lower urinary tract must be screened at the same time for evidence of obstruction due to posterior urethral valves (*see* earlier section on vesico-ureteric reflux). In the absence of lower urinary tract obstruction, gamma camera diuresis renography can be used to distinguish primary obstructive megaureter, due to a functional block in the region of the ureterovesical junction, from other causes of ureteric dilatation. Although vesico-ureteric reflux can be associated with a pelviureteric junction obstruction and will also

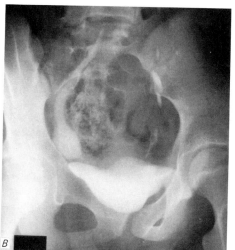

Figure 11.5a and b IVU in case of right primary megaureter

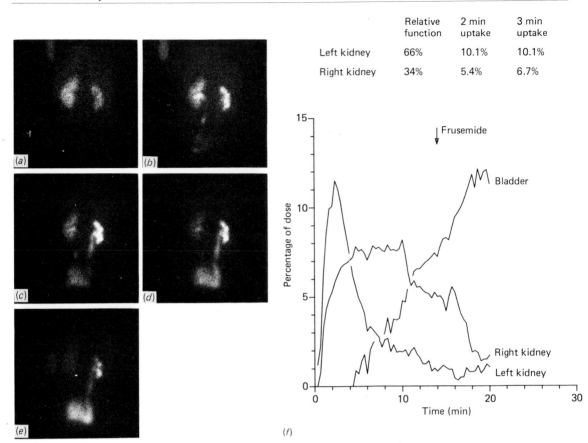

	Relative function	2 min uptake	3 min uptake
Left kidney	66%	10.1%	10.1%
Right kidney	34%	5.4%	6.7%

Figure 11.5C Diuresis renogram in the same patient; frusemide injected 20 minutes after radiopharmaceutical: (*a*) to (*e*) analogue images at 0–2$\frac{1}{2}$, 2$\frac{1}{2}$–5, 5–10, 10–15 and 15–20 minutes; (*f*) derived renogram curves. Note rapid response to frusemide

demonstrate an obstructive diuresis renogram curve, such a case will show absent activity in the ureter on scintigraphy unlike the progressive accumulation of tracer that occurs in primary obstructive megaureter.

Follow-up studies in children with dilated ureters will depend on the underlying pathological entity. For example, in the case of a boy with posterior urethral valves, gamma camera studies will be required to assess renal function after surgical valve ablation, as well as monitoring any complications such as continuing vesico-ureteric reflux or secondary ureterovesical obstruction. In cases where ureteric re-implantation is necessary (e.g. primary obstructive megaureter and some cases of vesico-ureteric reflux) gamma camera diuresis renography is the method of choice for assessing whether there is free drainage of the upper tracts postoperatively. Radionuclide cystography and scanning with ^{99m}Tc-DMSA are useful for following the progress of patients with vesico-ureteric reflux who are treated either conservatively or by surgery. It is clear that in most children with megaureters, prolonged follow-up is necessary. The lower radiation dosage associated with radionuclide studies offers a distinct advantage over routine follow-up with conventional radiology.

Renal trauma

The kidneys in children are less protected than in the adult and are, therefore, more prone to injury (Johnson, 1982). Also, in a significant number of injured kidneys in children, a pre-existing renal abnormality is present, for example hydronephrosis. Intravenous urography is generally employed as the initial test in suspected renal trauma but may give unsatisfactory images of the kidneys due to overlying bowel gas or faecal content. This is not a problem with gamma camera renography which is useful as a quick, non-invasive screening test in the emergency situation. It enables the integrity of the renal vasculature to be assessed as well as giving information on renal function (particularly of the non-traumatized kidney), possible urinary extravasation and any co-existing renal abnormalities. If the clinical situation is less acute, a static imaging agent such as ^{99m}Tc-DMSA allows better visualization of the renal cortex for detecting segmental defects. The subject of renal trauma is discussed further in Chapter 12.

References

ASH, J. M., ANTICO, V. F., GILDAY, D. L. and HOULE, S. (1982) Special considerations in the paediatric use of radionuclides for kidney studies. Seminars in Nuclear Medicine, XII(4), 345–369

BARRATT, T. M. and CHANTLER, C. (1975) Clinical assessment of renal function. In: Pediatric Nephrology, M. I. Rubin and T. M. Barrett (eds.), Baltimore: Williams and Wilkins, pp. 55–83

CONWAY, J. J. and KRUGLIK, G. D. (1976) Effectiveness of direct and indirect radionuclide cystography in detecting vesico-ureteric reflux. Journal of Nuclear Medicine, 17, 81–87

EMANUEL, B., NACHMAN, R., ARONSON, N. and WEISS, H. (1974) Congenital solitary kidney. A review of 74 cases. American Journal of Diseases of Children, 127, 17–19

ENGLISH, P. J., TESTA, H. J., GOSLING, J. A. and COHEN, S. J. (1982) Idiopathic hydronephrosis in childhood—a comparison between diuresis renography and upper tract morphology. British Journal of Urology, 54, 603–607

GIBBONS, M. D. and GONZALES, E. T. (1983) Complications of antireflux surgery. Urologic Clinics of North America, 10(3), 489–501

GORDON, I. (1982) Renal diagnostic imaging. In: Paediatric Urology, D. Innes Williams and J. H. Johnston (eds.), London: Butterworth Scientific, pp. 11–26

JOHNSTON, J. H., EVANS, J. P., GLASSBERG, K. I. and SHAPIRO, S. R. (1977) Pelvic hydronephrosis in children: A review of 219 personal cases. Journal of Urology, 117, 97–101

JOHNSTON, J. H. (1982) Urinary tract injuries. In: Paediatric Urology, D. Innes Williams and J. H. Johnston (eds.), London: Butterworth Scientific, pp. 369–380

KOFF, S. A., THRALL, J. H. and KEYES, J. W. (1980) Assessment of hydro-ureteronephrosis in children using radionuclide urography. Journal of Urology, 123, 531–534

LUPTON, E. W., TESTA, H. J., LAWSON, R. S., CHARLTON EDWARDS, E., CARROLL, R. N. P. and BARNARD, R. J. (1979) Diuresis renography and the results of pyeloplasty for idiopathic hydronephrosis. British Journal of Urology, 51, 449–453

MAIZELS, M., WEISS, S., CONWAY, J. J. and FIRLIT, C. F. (1979) The cystometric nuclear cystogram. Journal of Urology, 121, 203–205

MELLER, S. T. and ECKSTEIN, H. B. (1982) The value of renal scintigraphy in reduplication. In: Radionuclides in Nephrology, A. M. Joekes, A. R. Constable, N. J. G. Brown and W. N. Tauxe (eds.), London: Academic Press, pp. 229–236

MERRICK, M. V., UTTLEY, W. S. and WILD, S. R. (1980) The detection of pyelonephritis scarring in children by radioisotope imaging. British Journal of Radiology, 53, 544–556

NORMAND, I. C. S. and SMELLIE, J. (1979) Vesico-ureteric reflux: The case for conservative management. In: Reflux Nephropathy, J. Hodson and P. Kincaid-Smith (eds.), New York: Masson, pp. 281–286

O'REILLY, P. H., LAWSON, R. S., SHIELDS, R. A., TESTA, H. J., CHARLTON EDWARDS, E. and CARROLL, R. N. P. (1978) A radioisotope method of assessing uretero-ureteric reflux. British Journal of Urology, 50, 164–168

POWERS, T. A., STONE, W. J., GROVE, R. B., PLUNKETT, J. M., KADIR, S., PATTON, J. A. and BOWEN, R. D. (1981) Radionuclide measurement of differential glomerular filtration rate. Investigative Radiology, 16, 59–64

RANSLEY, P. G. and RISDON, R. A. (1978) Reflux and renal scarring. British Journal of Radiology, Supplement 14

Report of the International Reflux Study Committee. (1981) Medical versus surgical treatment of primary vesicoureteral reflux: A prospective international reflux study in children. Journal of Urology, 125, 277–283

SMELLIE, J. and NORMAND, I. C. S. (1966) The clinical features and significance of urinary tract infection in childhood. *Proceedings of the Royal Society of Medicine*, **59**, 415–416

THOMPSON, I. M. and AMAR, A. D. (1958) Clinical importance of ureteral duplication and ectopia. *Journal of the American Medical Association*, **168**, 881–886

WALLACE, D. M., ROTHWELL, D. L. and WILLIAMS, D. I. (1978) The long term follow-up of surgically treated vesico-ureteric reflux. *British Journal of Urology*, **50**, 479–484

WEIN, A. J. and SCHOENBERG, H. W. (1972) A review of 402 girls with recurrent urinary tract infection. *Journal of Urology*, **107**, 329–331

WHITAKER, R. H. and JOHNSTON, J. H. (1976) A simple classification of wide ureters. *British Journal of Urology*, **47**, 781–787

12　Renal and urinary tract trauma

L. Rosenthall

For the purposes of management renal injuries may be classified as minor, major and critical. Parenchymal damage without tears of the capsule or pelvicalyceal system is defined as minor; parenchymal damage and tears in the capsule, pelvicalyceal system, or both represent a major injury; disruption of the renal pedicle or shattering of the renal parenchyma and capsule should be considered as critical or catastrophic injuries. Damage to the kidney and its collecting system can result from blunt, penetrating or iatrogenic injuries, of which blunt trauma accounts for about 80% (Waterhouse and Gross, 1969; Kaufman and Brisman, 1972). Approximately two-thirds of patients with blunt trauma have renal injury only and one-third have multiple organ involvement. The reverse occurs with penetrating injuries due to gunshot wounds and stabbing, where 80% are likely to have multi-organ injury (Scott, Carleton and Goldmann, 1969). Iatrogenic injuries can result from complications of surgery, renal biopsy, retrograde pyelograms and interventional radiological procedures. Ten per cent of adults and 25% of children with renal injuries may have underlying pre-existing abnormalities, such as cysts, tumours, renal enlargement, hydronephrosis and horseshoe kidneys, which make them more susceptible to disruption.

Six imaging modalities are available to assess renal trauma. These are: intravenous urography with drip infusion and tomography, computed tomography, ultrasonography, angiography, magnetic resonance imaging and radionuclide imaging. All have their advocates, and it is still controversial which individual study or combination of studies is most fruitful in a given situation (Smalley and Banowsky, 1971; Lang, 1975; Kay, Rosenfield and Aimm, 1980; Berger and Kuhn, 1981; Schmoller, Kunit and Frick, 1981; Federle et al., 1982). The modalities used will depend on the instrumentation available in a diagnostic centre, local expertise in interpreting a particular modality, whether the patient's physical condition can negotiate a given imaging device, cost-effectiveness of the modalities available, safety of the procedure, radiation dose and the information content of the study in the specific clinical situation.

Radionuclide imaging can provide information on the state of overall and regional blood perfusion, overall and regional parenchymal function, and urinary extravasation. Perirenal haematomas may be disclosed by virtue of a photon-deficient zone in the early perfusion images. Several radiopharmaceuticals can be used. ^{99m}Tc-glucoheptonate (GHA) yields data on perfusion, drainage and distribution of function within the kidney; ^{99m}Tc-dimercaptosuccinic acid (DMSA) can be utilized to assess perfusion and distribution of function, but not drainage; ^{99m}Tc-diethylenetriamine penta-acetic acid (DTPA) yields information on perfusion, function and drainage, but is not well suited to the assessment of regional distribution within the kidney; ^{131}I-OIH assesses function and drainage. ^{123}I-OIH is superior to the ^{131}I-labelled counterpart, because the higher photon flux allows for improved visualization of renal function and drainage, particularly in damaged kidneys. ^{99m}Tc-labelled colloid or erythrocytes have the potential to reveal active bleeding sites, but they have not been fully explored in the context of renal trauma.

Technique

^{99m}Tc-GHA may be used to obtain perfusion, drainage and multiprojection static images. To this end, about 550 MBq (15 mCi) is injected intravenously as a bolus and immediately followed by serial 3-second exposure images for the first 30 seconds to visualize perfusion of the kidneys. At 1 minute a static image is taken, and then images are procured every 3 minutes for 30 minutes to study the drainage phase. At 2 hours, when drainage is, for the most part, complete and the remaining GHA is fixed in the renal cortex, posterior and oblique images are obtained to examine the distribution of function. This should be supplemented with an anterior image especially if the kidneys have disparate intensities, because retroperitoneal haematomas may displace a kidney forward and reduce its apparent count rate.

^{99m}Tc-DTPA is eminently suited for perfusion and drainage evaluation, but static images may be misleading: none of it is fixed to the cortex, and the transit through the parenchyma may be too rapid to disclose small areas of functional deficit. As with ^{99m}Tc-GHA, about 550 MBq (15 mCi) ^{99m}Tc-DTPA is used.

Another approach employs a combination of ^{99m}Tc-GHA for perfusion and delayed static images, and OIH for function and drainage. A bolus injection of ^{99m}Tc-GHA is administered for perfusion and a static 'blood pool' image is taken at 1 minute. This is immediately followed by an intravenous injection of about 8 MBq (200 μCi) ^{131}I-OIH, and serial 3-minute images are obtained from 0 to 30 minutes. At 2–3 hours a single, delayed ^{131}I-OIH posterior image is obtained just prior to posterior and oblique static ^{99m}Tc-GHA images of the kidneys. There should be minimal interference of the two radionuclides, because the energies from ^{131}I and ^{99m}Tc can be separated electronically.

Interpretation

Renal contusion

Simple contusion without parenchymal disruption is characterized by an overall decrease in perfusion and function by radionuclide imaging (*Figures 12.1* and *12.2*). There is an absence of significant traumatic deformity. In mild contusions the kidney may appear larger than the opposite side, whereas more severe degrees of trauma may portray a smaller kidney. Mild forms may show either a slight decrease in perfusion and function or no effect on the radiopharmaceutical kinetics by visual inspection.

Parenchymal disruption

This is caused by intrarenal bleeding or laceration, and it produces a focal deficiency of perfusion and function (*Figures 12.3* and *12.4*). It is best appreciated by multi-projection images of ^{99m}Tc-GHA or ^{99m}Tc-DMSA in the delayed phase. Radionuclide

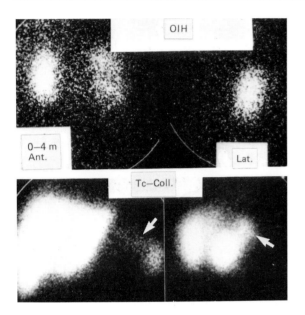
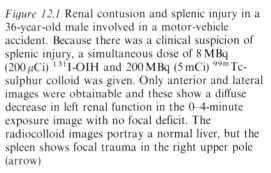

Figure 12.1 Renal contusion and splenic injury in a 36-year-old male involved in a motor-vehicle accident. Because there was a clinical suspicion of splenic injury, a simultaneous dose of 8 MBq (200 μCi) ^{131}I-OIH and 200 MBq (5 mCi) ^{99m}Tc-sulphur colloid was given. Only anterior and lateral images were obtainable and these show a diffuse decrease in left renal function in the 0–4-minute exposure image with no focal deficit. The radiocolloid images portray a normal liver, but the spleen shows focal trauma in the right upper pole (arrow)

features of contusion may be seen elsewhere in the injured kidney. Late sequelae of these lesions on follow-up radionuclide studies may be: unchanging intrarenal mass lesions such as haematomas or necrotic cystic areas, renal atrophy or hydronephrosis. There can be restoration of the contused parts of the kidney, but no change in the defect caused by the haematoma. Radionuclide imaging may therefore help in both initial evaluation and long-term monitoring of these patients.

Non-visualized kidney

A non-visualized kidney in all three phases represents either a critical injury or absence of the kidney (*Figure 12.5*). Some other modality, such as ultrasonography, should be invoked to make the distinction before the patient is submitted to more invasive procedures.

Urinary extravasation

Serial radionuclide imaging is a sensitive method of disclosing urinary extravasation. This can be shown with ^{99m}Tc-GHA, ^{99m}Tc-DTPA and OIH. The ^{99m}Tc compounds are preferred, because the high photon flux can reveal small leaks, although in practice this attribute is not of overriding importance.

Large urinomas visibly displace adjacent background radioactivity. Early in the sequence of images this results in a photon-deficient zone. At this stage the differential diagnosis may be either a haematoma or a urinoma. With time, the urinoma fills with radioactivity, whereas the haematoma remains photon-deficient (*Figure 12.6*) (Rosenthall, 1983).

Leaks in the vicinity of the kidney may sometimes be confused with parenchymal uptake or radioactivity in the ureter. It is therefore necessary to continue the examination until the kidney and urinary tract wash out and a fixed focus remains (*Figure 12.7*). Extravasation in the pelvic region can be another source of confusion, because it may be difficult to discern bladder contents from adjacent extravasated

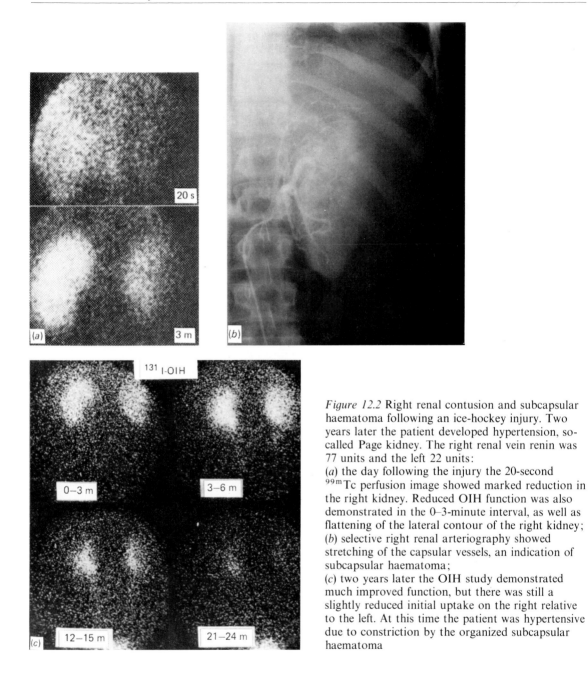

Figure 12.2 Right renal contusion and subcapsular haematoma following an ice-hockey injury. Two years later the patient developed hypertension, so-called Page kidney. The right renal vein renin was 77 units and the left 22 units:
(*a*) the day following the injury the 20-second ^{99m}Tc perfusion image showed marked reduction in the right kidney. Reduced OIH function was also demonstrated in the 0–3-minute interval, as well as flattening of the lateral contour of the right kidney;
(*b*) selective right renal arteriography showed stretching of the capsular vessels, an indication of subcapsular haematoma;
(*c*) two years later the OIH study demonstrated much improved function, but there was still a slightly reduced initial uptake on the right relative to the left. At this time the patient was hypertensive due to constriction by the organized subcapsular haematoma

urine. A comparison of pre- and post-voiding images usually facilitates the distinction (*Figure 12.8*).

Injured kidney and active haemorrhage

Detection of active bleeding of the injured kidney is not commonly made by the radiopharmaceuticals employed for renal assessment. The best opportunity for

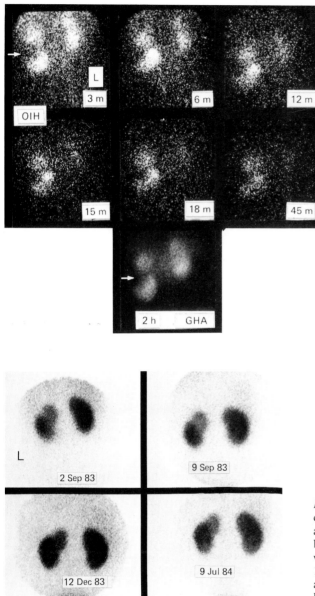

Figure 12.3 Intrarenal haematoma transecting the right kidney following a motor-vehicle accident. The patient was clinically stable and there was no surgical intervention. Shown are selected anterior images of the serial 3-minute exposure OIH study up to 45 minutes. The normal left kidney has virtually washed out by 18 minutes. On the right there is a functional defect in the middle third of the organ (arrow), but the two halves exhibit good initial concentration and drainage without extravasation of urine. However, there is prolonged parenchymal transit, at least 45 minutes, consistent with contusion. The delayed ^{99m}Tc-GHA image at 2 hours shows the haematoma more clearly by virtue of the greater number of counts accumulated

Figure 12.4 Parenchymal injury to the upper third of the left kidney following a motor-vehicle accident. Surgical exploration was not considered because the clinical indicators were stable. There was no evidence of parenchymal restoration after 10 months, and in all possibility it will remain as a permanent scar. Areas of contusion would have been repaired by that time

disclosure seems to be in the perfusion phase where it is viewed as an extrarenal collection (Berg, 1982). After the radiotracer is concentrated in the parenchyma the extrarenal collection may be confused with urinary extravasation. The only positive way of visualizing active bleeding is by radiolabelled colloid or erythrocyte imaging. This area of application has not been explored actively in the renal context even though good success has been achieved in locating occult gastrointestinal bleeding (Winzelberg, Froelich and McKusick, 1981).

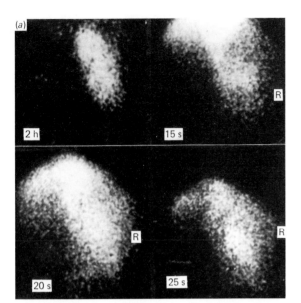

Figure 12.5 Critical injury of the left kidney induced by a motor-vehicle collision. The patient was imaged in the anterior projection because she could not be moved:

(*a*) there is absent perfusion of the left kidney on the ^{99m}Tc first-pass transit study. Additionally, there is failure to visualize the abdominal aorta below the level of the right kidney in the 0–25-second interval. The 2-hour delayed cortical scan also fails to demonstrate left renal function;

(*b*) right transfemoral aortography demonstrated absent left renal vasculature, an aortic defect at the orifice of the left renal artery presumed to be a thrombus (open arrow) and saddle thrombi at the bifurcation of the aorta (arrows). The saddle thrombi probably altered the intra-aortic pressure sufficiently to prevent radionuclide visualization of the aorta

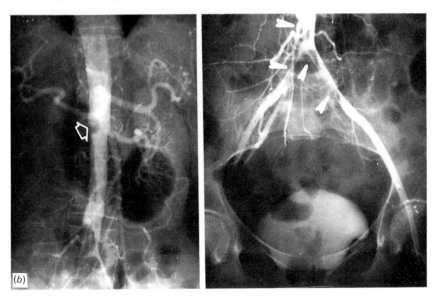

Kidney, liver and spleen trauma

All three organs may be affected, and there is a particularly high association of trauma to the left kidney and spleen. These organs are amenable to simultaneous imaging. This is accomplished by assessing renal perfusion with a bolus injection of ^{99m}Tc colloid, and 10 minutes later the integrity of the liver and spleen is evaluated by static imaging. Upon completion of the latter, sequential OIH images are obtained for appraisal of function and drainage (*see Figure 12.1*).

Arteriovenous fistula

Intrarenal arteriovenous fistulae usually occur as a result of penetrating injuries. They

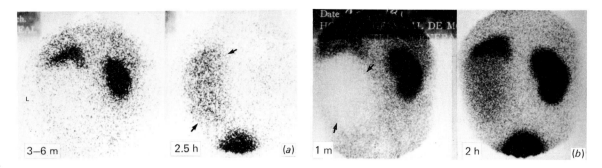

Figure 12.6 Large urinoma in a 9-year-old male following an accident:
(*a*) selected ^{131}I-OIH images obtained in the posterior projection. In the 3–6-minute image the inferior three-quarters of the left kidney shows no evidence of function. At 2 hours the normal right kidney and left renal remnant have washed out, but there is now a large collection of radioactivity on the left side, diagnostic of a urinoma (arrow);
(*b*) ^{99m}Tc-glucoheptonate image at 1 minute and delayed image at 2 hours. There is a large photon-deficient zone initially, which could be caused by either haematoma or urinoma (arrows). However, at 2 hours the previously photon-deficient zone contains radioactivity which is characteristic of a urinoma

are a not infrequent consequence of renal needle biopsy but most heal spontaneously. A large arteriovenous shunt is best appreciated in the radionuclide first-pass transit study as an early focus of high perfusion which waxes and wanes. Many of these are treated by transcatheter therapeutic blockage, and the radionuclide perfusion study can monitor the efficacy of this management (*Figure 12.9*).

Renal vein thrombosis

Renal vein thrombosis *per se* does not cause total renal failure because the presence of collateral venous run-off tends to decompress the congestion and sustain renal function. There are variable degrees of reduced perfusion and cortical concentration of ^{99m}Tc-GHA and ^{99m}Tc-DMSA (*Figure 12.10*). The radiohippurate series demonstrates impaired, but not absent, uptake followed by a prolonged intraparenchymal transit time (Nielander, Bode and Heidendal, 1983).

Fifty to 80% of all renal trauma cases are minor and are treated conservatively unless there are other associated lesions which require surgery. Critical renal trauma demands surgery to salvage the kidney in a pedicle injury or to control bleeding in a shattered kidney. The management of major trauma is more controversial; some advocate a conservative approach if the clinical status of the patient remains stable, whereas others favour early surgical management to preserve as much functioning renal tissue as possible and to explore the abdomen for other sites of injury (Wein, Arger and Murphy, 1977; Thompson, Latourette and Montie, 1977; Case, 1979; Bergqvist *et al.*, 1980; Gibson *et al.*, 1982).

Radionuclides have a clear role to play in the categorization and assessment of such trauma. Unfortunately few prospective or comparative studies are available in the literature, although some authors have reported their experience with these procedures. Using ^{99m}Tc-DTPA ascorbate in its three phases (i.e. perfusion, a static picture which mainly represents blood pool within 2 minutes and delayed static images), Berg was able to detect 51 renal injuries that were later confirmed by aortography (Berg, 1974). There was no statement about the false negative rate, the number of injuries missed by scan but detected either by aortography or surgery. Perhaps a more pragmatic parameter would be the number of renal injuries which were

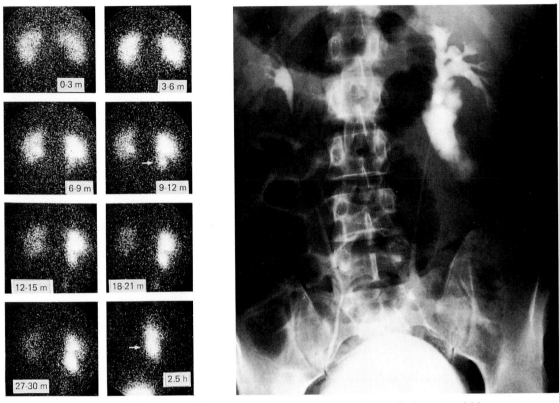

Figure 12.7 Urine extravasation following puncture of the proximal ureter during a renal biopsy attempt. Serial OIH images demonstrate normal function bilaterally and a collection just inferior to the right renal pelvis commencing in the 9–12-minute time frame (arrow), which gets progressively larger. To be sure that it did not represent a segment of dilated ureter, a delayed 2.5-hour image was obtained. At that time the collection was larger and showed a higher concentration of radioactivity (arrow). The intravenous urogram confirmed the radionuclide findings

not detected by scan, but were of surgical significance. Chopp and his colleagues investigated a group of 24 patients, all of whom had three-phase radionuclide images with ^{99m}Tc-GHA, high-dose intravenous urography with nephrotomography and aortography. Seventeen patients had abnormal aortograms. Sixteen were positive with ^{99m}Tc-GHA (94% sensitivity) and 11 with intravenous urography (64% sensitivity). There was one false-positive scan in a patient whose study was performed immediately after a selective arteriogram, and it was postulated that the contrast material adversely affected function and produced a mottled image. Additional information, such as arteriovenous fistula, was procured by aortography in six of the 17 patients compared with the combined information output of intravenous urography and radionuclide imaging (Chopp, Heckmat-Ravan and Mendez, 1980).

In Lisbona's review of seven iatrogenically induced arteriovenous fistulae following hysterectomy (two), nephrectomy (one), and renal biopsy (four), all portrayed the typical high-intensity blush on first-pass transit. Six of the seven were confirmed by arteriography and the seventh was asymptomatic, but had classic signs and a

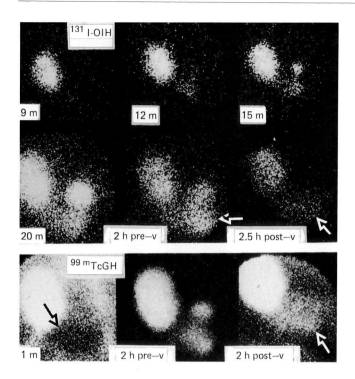

Figure 12.8 This patient received a kidney transplant from a live donor, but the urine output was less than expected. Serial OIH images demonstrated normal renal function, but the accumulation of radioactivity in the area of the urinary bladder was unusual in configuration. The suspected diagnoses were extravasation, bladder clots or bladder diverticulum. A comparison of the pre-void and post-void images showed a large residual collection consistent with urinary extravasation (white arrows). It was later found to emanate from the site of surgical anastomosis. Similar findings were obtained with the ^{99m}Tc-glucoheptonate study. Additionally, the urinoma produced a photon-deficient zone in the 1-minute image (black arrow)

characteristic first-pass perfusion study (Lisbona *et al.*, 1980). Further iatrogenic injuries may be found in renal artery catheterization which can be complicated by segmental or complete renal infarction. Embolization may occur as a result of catheter manipulation elsewhere, such as the heart. Although complete infarction is readily disclosed by intravenous urography as an absence of concentration of contrast material, acute segmental infarction is usually missed. This is due to filling of the calyces which are related to the infarcted segment by a flow of contrast material from adjacent calyces and pelvis. Lisbona reported nine patients with segmental renal infarcts, in whom ^{99m}Tc-GHA disclosed all, in contrast to intravenous urography which diagnosed only two (Lisbona, Derbekyan and Rosenthall, 1981).

Throughout this book the inherent advantages of radionuclide methods of urological investigation have been emphasized. Such qualities, however, are of even more value where the clinician is presented with a seriously injured patient and the need for quick results. In this situation the renal scan provides a dynamic radionuclide angiogram for the assessment of renovascular status followed by a static study for both anatomical and functional assessment of parenchyma and excretory pathways. This test can be performed with the patient prone, supine or on his side. It requires no particular preparation and is unaffected by bowel gas or faecal content. Images are obtainable in the presence of generalized renal dysfunction or allergy to contrast media. Such studies thus fill an important gap between clinical and IVU assessment and more invasive studies in trauma victims.

References

BERG, B. (1974) Radionuclide studies after urinary tract injury. *Seminars in Nuclear Medicine*, **4**, 371–393

BERG, B. C. (1982) Nuclear medicine and complementary modalities in renal trauma. *Seminars in Nuclear Medicine*, **12**, 280–300

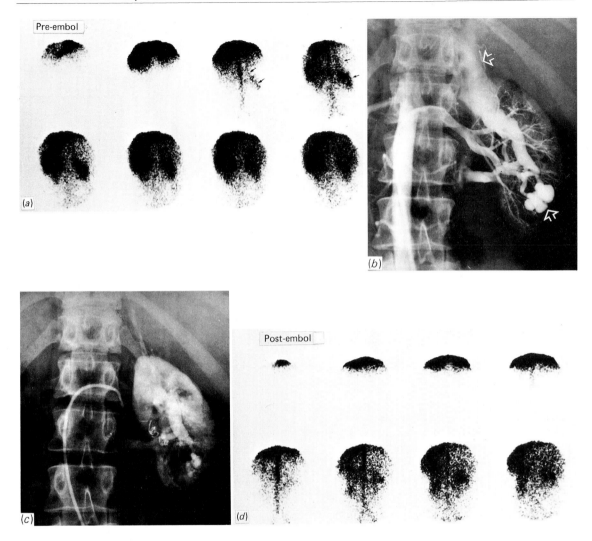

Figure 12.9 Arteriovenous fistula following a right renal biopsy:
(a) ^{99m}Tc-glucoheptonate first-pass perfusion study obtained at 3-second intervals demonstrates a focal high transit on the right side characteristic of a shunt. Arrows indicate the shunt and early venous return;
(b) following the radionuclide perfusion study, an aortogram was performed, and this confirmed the presence of an arteriovenous fistula. The arrows indicate the fistula and early venous visualization;
(c) the catheter was then advanced into the right renal artery and the afferent artery to the fistula was embolized. A post-embolic arteriogram demonstrates a small fistula and marked improvement in the circulatory dynamics;
(d) the post-embolic radionuclide perfusion study is normal

BERGER, P. E. and KUHN, J. P. (1981) CT of blunt abdominal trauma in childhood. *American Journal of Roentgenology, Radium Therapy and Nuclear Medicine*, **136**, 105–110

BERGQVIST, D., GRENABO, H., HEDELIN, H. *et al.* (1980) Long-time follow-up of patients with conservatively treated blunt renal injuries. *Acta chirurgica Scandinavica*, **146**, 291–294

CASE, A. S. (1979) Immediate radiological evaluation and early surgical management of genitourinary injuries from external trauma. *Journal of Urology*, **122**, 772–774

CHOPP, R. T., HECKMAT-RAVAN, H. and MENDEZ, R. (1980) Technetium-99m glucoheptonate renal scan in diagnosis of acute renal injury. *Urology*, **15**, 201–206

(a)   25 July   29 July

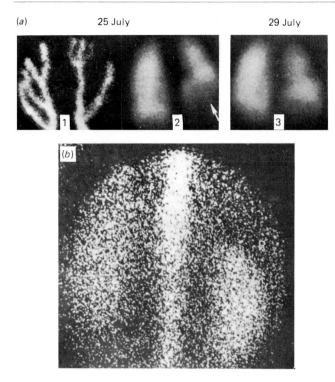

Figure 12.10 Post-traumatic renal vein thrombosis and nephrotic syndrome. This patient was hit by an automobile and suffered internal injuries and multiple fractures. The development of a nephrotic syndrome prompted several investigational procedures: (*a*) Frame 1: a radionuclide venogram obtained by simultaneous bilateral pedal vein injection of ^{99m}Tc-macroaggregates of albumin demonstrates collateral flow in the anterior abdominal wall. This indicates obstruction of the iliac veins, inferior vena cava or both; Frame 2: a posterior image of the lungs obtained with the pedal injections shows an embolus in the right lung base (arrow); Frame 3: four days later the lung scan depicts partial resolution of the embolus; (*b*) one frame of the ^{99m}Tc first-pass transit study shows good perfusion of both kidneys, better on the right than the left. Unlike renal artery occlusion, the collateral venous circulation sustains renal function to variable degrees

FEDERLE, M. P., CRASS, R. A., JEFFREY, B. *et al.* (1982) Computed tomography in blunt abdominal trauma. *Archives of Surgery*, **117**, 645–650

GIBSON, S., KUZMAROV, I. W., McCLURE, D. R. *et al.* (1982) Blunt renal trauma: The value of a conservative approach to major injuries in clinically stable patients. *Canadian Journal of Surgery*, **25**, 25–26

KAUFMAN, J. J. and BRISMAN, S. A. (1972) Blunt injuries of the genito-urinary tract. *Surgical Clinics of North America*, **52**, 747–760

KAY, C. J., ROSENFIELD, A. T. and AIMM, M. (1980) Gray-scale ultrasonography in the evaluation of renal trauma. *Radiology*, **134**, 461–466

LANG, E. K. (1975) Arteriography in the assessment of renal trauma. *Journal of Trauma*, **15**, 553–566

LISBONA, R., DERBEKYAN, V. and ROSENTHALL, L. (1981) Observations on renal scanning and intravenous urography in acute segmental infarction. *Clinics in Nuclear Medicine*, **6**, 253–257

LISBONA, R., PALAYEW, M. J., SATIN, R. *et al.* (1980) Radionuclide detection of iatrogenic arteriovenous fistulas of the genitourinary system. *Radiology*, **134**, 201–203

NIELANDER, A. J. M., BODE, W. A. and HEIDENDAL, G. A. K. (1983) Renography in diagnosis and follow-up of renal vein thrombosis. *Clinics in Nuclear Medicine*, **8**, 56–59

ROSENTHALL, L. (1983) Radionuclide evaluation of renal disease. In: *Recent Advances in Nuclear Medicine*, Vol. 6, John H. Lawrence and H. Saul Winchell (eds.), New York: Grune and Stratton, pp. 117–175

SCHMOLLER, H., KUNIT, G. and FRICK, J. (1981) Sonography in blunt renal trauma. *European Urology*, **7**, 11–15

SCOTT, R., CARLETON, C. E. and GOLDMAN, M. (1969) Penetrating injuries of the kidney: An analysis of 181 patients. *Journal of Urology*, **101**, 247–253

SMALLEY, R. H. and BANOWSKY, L. H. W. (1971) Evaluation of renal trauma by infusion urography. *Journal of Urology*, **105**, 620–622

THOMPSON, I. M., LATOURETTE, H., MONTIE, J. E. *et al.* (1977) Results of non-operative management of blunt renal trauma. *Journal of Urology*, **118**, 522–524

WATERHOUSE, K. and GROSS, M. (1969) Trauma to the genito-urinary tract: A 5 year experience with 251 cases. *Journal of Urology*, **101**, 241–246

WEIN, A. J., ARGER, P. H. and MURPHY, J. J. (1977) Controversial aspect of blunt renal trauma. *Journal of Trauma*, **17**, 662–666

WINZELBERG, G. G., FROELICH, J. W., McKUSICK, K. A. *et al.* (1981) Radionuclide localisation of lower abdominal haemorrhage. *Radiology*, **139**, 465–469

13 Lower urinary tract problems

P. H. O'Reilly and D. Holden

Surgery to the lower urinary tract is often necessary to correct obstruction at the level of prostate, bladder neck or urethra. The aim of such operations is to allow efficient voiding and complete bladder emptying by a process of normal micturition. Assessment usually includes clinical, urographic and endoscopic examinations. It is well known, however, that irritative symptoms of outlet obstruction such as frequency, urgency and urge incontinence (as opposed to obstructive symptoms such as hesitancy and a poor urinary stream) can also occur in detrusor instability; this may be the result of obstruction, but can also occur without it. Surgery without further assessment of bladder function in such cases will inevitably give poor results, and urodynamic studies are now recommended for many patients.

Interest over the years in the use of radionuclides in lower urinary tract studies has been limited. Mulrow *et al.* (1961) used ^{131}I-labelled Diodrast to measure residual urine volumes, and Rosenthall (1963) later improved on this technique using ^{131}I-OIH. Winter (1964) suggested that the estimation of residual volume might be the final step in radioisotope renography, and Strauss and Blaufox (1970) reported their experience of the use of ^{131}I-OIH and probe detectors to measure both residual urine and urinary flow rates. In spite of these studies, nuclear medicine methods, particularly modern gamma camera techniques, have not become widely used to study the lower urinary tract. This is, perhaps, understandable. Urodynamics has become established in its own right as a definitive urological subject with its own mechanical equipment and technology. Yet following renography, the bladder contains a quantity of radioactive urine which might allow gamma camera studies to be applied very conveniently to various aspects of lower urinary tract function. This chapter describes briefly some of these applications.

Urine flow rate

Urinary flow rates can be measured by a variety of different mechanical techniques. These include the continuous measurement of the weight of urine voided (Kaufman, 1957; Bowley and Legg, 1971), the measurement of the flow rate of air displaced from a closed vessel in which the urine was collected (Holm, 1962; Gierup, Ericsson and Okmian, 1969), the use of an electromagnetic flowmeter attached to a collecting funnel (Cardus, Quesada and Scott, 1963) and the application of a rotating disc connected to a

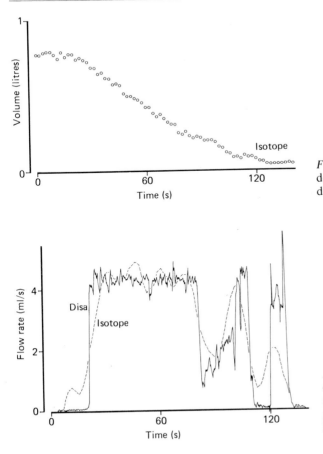

Figure 13.1 Radionuclide voiding study showing decreasing bladder counts with respect to time to derive urinary flow rates

Figure 13.2 Radionuclide flow rate study compared with mechanical (Disa) flow rate apparatus. Maximum flow rate correlation is good but quick instantaneous fluctuations are less well effected by the radionuclide technique

transducer chamber and a collecting vessel, working on the principle that the amount of electrical energy required to maintain the disc velocity constant is proportional to the urine mass flow rate (Rowan *et al.*, 1977).

Following radionuclide renography using ^{123}I-OIH or ^{99m}Tc-DTPA, flow rate can be measured on a dynamic gamma camera study by observing the rate of decreased counts from the bladder region as the patient voids. This activity–time curve represents bladder volume and its derivative measures flow rate (*Figure 13.1*). The curves are calibrated by measuring the activity in the known voided volume. Unfortunately the methodology is rather complicated and somewhat time consuming, and the resulting curves do not show the same detail and instantaneous fluctuations in rate which the mechanical flow rate apparatus is capable of producing (*Figure 13.2*). These are eradicated in the smoothing process necessary to eliminate statistical fluctuations during derivation of the curves. Simpler and more efficient means to measure flow rates exist, but radionuclides can be useful where sophisticated urodynamic apparatus is not available.

Residual urine volume

Residual urine volumes can be estimated directly by urethral catheterization, and indirectly by post-micturition urogram films or ultrasound. Gamma camera images of the bladder before and after micturition will also allow an indirect, non-invasive assessment of residual urine. Counts remaining in the post-micturition picture are measured and calibrated by reference to the activity in the measured voided volume. It is a useful further measurement after renography. Unfortunately, it is not accurate in the patient with a large bladder who voids only a small amount of urine and retains a large residual volume; here the statistical error on the small change in bladder counts leads to large uncertainties in the residual volume. For a valid radionuclide residual estimation, the voided volume needs to be at least as large or preferably larger than the residual volume. In clinical practice, the difference between a residual of 800 and 900 ml may not be vital, and its presence will be clinically obvious; in contrast, the difference between a residual of 30 ml and 130 ml will not be clinically obvious, but can be of far more pathological significance. At this end of the scale, the radionuclide procedure is accurate to within approximately 10 ml (O'Reilly *et al.*, 1981).

The cystometric nuclear cystogram

Radionuclide procedures may be combined with cystometry. Maizels and colleagues reported the use of the 'cystometric nuclear cystogram' in 1979 and emphasized its value in children with vesico-ureteric reflux. This centre had already reported the value of nuclear cystograms, direct and indirect, in the management of such children, and their advantages over standard radiological techniques. During the direct method the patient already has a catheter *in situ*, and it seems logical to supplement the reflux urodynamic data with cystometry. This is particularly relevant, as many children with reflux will also have voiding abnormalities manifested clinically by urgency, incontinence, enuresis or infrequent irregular micturition. These can be clarified simultaneously by the pressure studies. The only difference to the reflux cystogram is in the additional measurement of intravesical pressures during bladder filling and straining. Post-voiding cystogram and renal images are obtained, and the residual volume can be calculated by the method described above. The incorporation of the cystometrogram into the nuclear cystogram enhances the clinical information, especially in neurogenic problems and childhood voiding abnormalities. Assessment of the bladder pressure at which reflux occurs may give some prognostic information on the likelihood of spontaneous cessation of the problem (*Figure 13.3*).

Radionuclide studies in obstructive uropathy of infravesical origin (high pressure chronic retention)

Some patients with bladder outlet obstruction develop bilateral chronic obstructive uropathy with hydronephrosis and dilatation of the ureters. This may affect patients with urethral stricture, bladder neck dysfunction or prostatic hypertrophy. The reason why it should happen to some patients with these conditions and not to others is not known, but it only occurs in those cases which have a large post-micturition residual volume of urine which rests in a bladder *continually* under an abnormally high pressure even after micturition. Mitchell (1955) was the first to define two clear groups of patients with chronic retention of urine—those with low pressure residuals who rarely develop upper tract changes, and those with high pressure residuals who do. George and colleagues (1983, 1984) confirmed this thesis and were the first to use radionuclide techniques to investigate the urodynamic features of such infravesical obstruction.

High pressure chronic retention (HPCR) develops slowly and is asymptomatic until

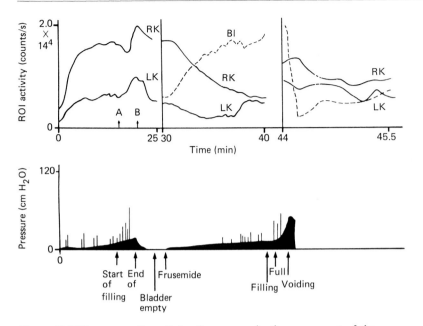

Figure 13.3 The composite activity–time curves in the upper part of the figure show, with varying time bases, the renogram phase (for 25 minutes) followed by the diuretic phase (from 30 to 40 minutes) followed by the micturition phase (from 44 to 45.5 minutes).

The bladder pressure data are recorded on the lower graph. Bilateral reflux is seen during bladder filling and is associated with a significant detrusor pressure rise (63 cm H_2O). At a later stage, following administration of 20 mg frusemide and further filling, left reflux alone occurred at a pressure of 27 cm H_2O. This study clearly demonstrated bilateral reflux, but, in combination with the urodynamic data, it was possible to be quite specific about the conditions under which the reflux occurred in each kidney

complicated by infection, incontinence or uraemia. It is possible to find cases in which the presence of a tense, palpable bladder has been detected in the absence of symptoms and in which upper tract changes are minimal (*Figure 13.4*), cases with moderate upper tract dilatation (*Figure 13.5*) and patients *in extremis* with severe hydronephrosis and advanced uraemia (*Figure 13.6*).

Patients with early disease have non-dilated upper tracts. Renography in such cases is usually normal since renal pelvic and ureteric peristaltic transport mechanisms are intact, and the pressures they generate can overcome the opposing intravesical pressures. Once upper tract dilatation has become sufficiently severe to prevent peristalsis coapting the walls of the dilated ureter, bolus formation becomes impossible and urine transport can only occur with the help of the subsidiary forces which are available. These are hydrostatic pressure in the column of urine between the kidney and bladder when the patient is vertical, and the small decrease in the elevated resting bladder pressure which occurs for a short time after micturition when the bladder becomes less distended and wall tension decreases (Holden, 1984).

Renography has accurately and graphically demonstrated the dependence of such patients on these forces, and helped to clarify the mechanisms of renal function and urine transport in this particular form of bilateral obstructive uropathy. In moderately advanced cases, the effect of posture on urine transport is vividly demonstrated (*Figure 13.7*). Supine renography demonstrates no elimination, but

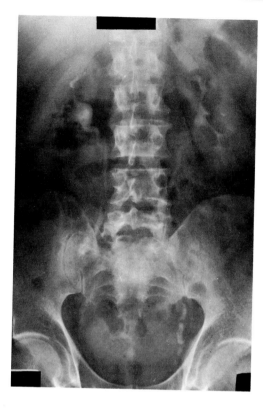

Figure 13.4 Mild high-pressure chronic retention. Large bladder residual urine but minimal upper tract dilatation confined to lower ureteric spindle

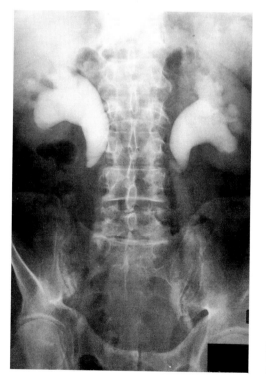

Figure 13.5 Moderate high-pressure chronic retention with large bladder and intermediate degree of ureteric dilatation and hydronephrosis

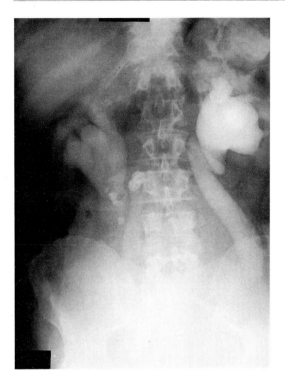

Figure 13.6 Severe high-pressure chronic retention with huge bladder and gross ureteric and pelvicalyceal dilatation

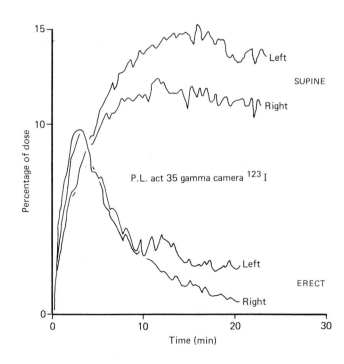

Figure 13.7 The effect of posture on renography in moderate HPCR. Supine renography shows a rising curve suggestive of obstruction. Erect renography in the same patient is normal

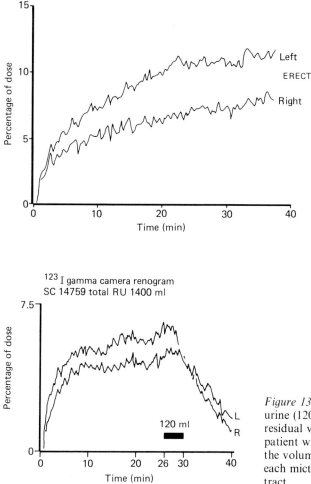

Figure 13.8 Erect renography in advanced HPCR fails to achieve efficient transport

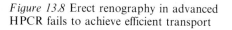

Figure 13.9 The effect of withdrawing a small aliquot of urine (120 ml) by suprapubic aspiration from the large residual volume (approximately 1400 ml) in the erect patient with severe HPCR. Removal of less than 10% of the volume, about the amount voided by the patient at each micturition event, allows drainage from the upper tract

changing to the erect position allows efficient drainage of radionuclide from the renal areas. As bladder pressure rises, upper tract dilatation increases and renal function deteriorates. The radionuclide patterns change, and a rising curve is seen even when renography is performed in the erect position (*Figure 13.8*). If, however, the vertical patient is allowed to void during renography or a small aliquot of urine is removed from the bladder by suprapubic aspiration, both of which result in a decrease in bladder pressure, tracer will be seen to be eliminated from the upper tracts (*Figure 13.9*). The same result can be obtained by performing the study *immediately* after micturition in the supine position, then changing the patient to the erect position (*Figure 13.10*).

Once upper tract dilatation is extreme and renal function grossly impaired, radionuclide uptake will be diminished and curve interpretations will be difficult, although some degree of excretion may still be detected following bladder drainage in the erect patient (*Figure 13.11*).

The use of radionuclide studies in this group of patients has illustrated and clarified the means by which patients with bilateral upper tract dilatation continue to transport urine when the main transport mechanism, peristaltic bolus transport, has failed. Such studies are currently giving investigative urologists considerable insight into the causes

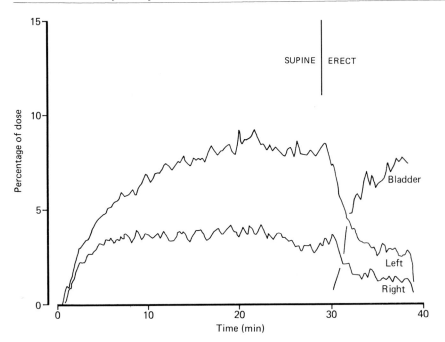

Figure 13.10. Drainage stimulated by a change from the supine position to the erect immediately after micturition in severe HPCR, producing the same conditions and result produced in *Figure 13.9*

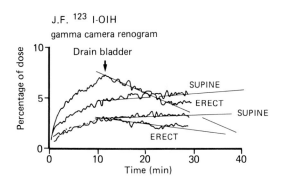

Figure 13.11 Renography in advanced HPCR. Poor function allows only poor uptake of tracer. Bladder drainage allows some, though less than optimal, drainage from the upper tract in the erect position but not the supine

of renal damage in infravesical obstruction and the compensatory methods which preserve renal function in the presence of compromised urine transport in obstruction. Radionuclides have as vital a part to play in such urological research as they have in clinical practice.

References

BOWLEY, A. R. and LEGG, W. R. C. (1971) A new uroflowmeter—an instrument for the estimation of liquid volume and rate of flow. *Medical and Biological Engineering*, **9**, 139–142

CARDUS, D., QUESADA, E. M. and SCOTT, F. B. (1963) Use of electromagnetic flowmeter for urine flow measurements. *Journal of Applied Physiology*, **18**, 845–847

GEORGE, N. J. R., O'REILLY, P. H., BARNARD, R. J. and BLACKLOCK, N. J. (1983) High pressure chronic retention. *British Medical Journal*, **286**, 1780–1783

GEORGE, N. J. R., O'REILLY, P. H., BARNARD, R. J. and BLACKLOCK, N. J. (1984) Practical management of patients with dilated upper tracts and chronic retention of urine. *British Journal of Urology*, **56**, 9–12

GIERUP, J., ERICSSON, N. O. and OKMIAN, L. (1969) Micturition studies in infants and children. *Scandinavian Journal of Urology and Nephrology*, **3**, 1–8

HOLDEN, D. (1984) The factors responsible for maintenance of renal function in humans with wide ureters and vesico-ureteric junction obstruction. Communication ISDU Igls, Austria

HOLM, H. H. (1962) A uroflowmeter and a method for combined pressure and flow measurement. *Journal of Urology*, **88**, 318–321

KAUFMAN, J. J. (1957) A new recording uroflowmeter: a simple automatic device for measuring voiding velocity. *Journal of Urology*, **78**, 99–102

MITCHELL, J. P. (1955) MS Thesis, University of London

MULROW, P. J., HUVOS, A. and BUCHANAN, D. L. (1961) Measurement of residual urine with I-131-labelled Diodrast. *Journal of Laboratory and Clinical Medicine*, **57**, 109–113

O'REILLY, P. H., LAWSON, R. S., SHIELDS, R. A., TESTA, H. J. and CHARLTON EDWARDS, E. (1981) Radionuclide studies of the lower urinary tract. *British Journal of Urology*, **53**, 266–269

ROSENTHALL, L. (1963) Residual urine determination by roentgenographic and isotope means. *Radiology*, **80**, 454–459

ROWAN, D., McKENZIE, A. L., McNEE, S. G. and GLEN, E. S. (1977) A technical and clinical evaluation of the disc uroflowmeter. *British Journal of Urology*, **49**, 285–291

STRAUSS, B. S. and BLAUFOX, M. D. (1970) Estimation of residual urine and urine flow rates without urethral catheterisation. *Journal of Nuclear Medicine*, **11**, 81–84

WINTER, C. C. (1964) Radioisotope uroflowmetry and bladder residual test. *Journal of Urology*, **91**, 103–106

14 Nephrological applications of radionuclides

M. Donald Blaufox, Eugene Fine, Richard Sherman and Stephen Scharf

Nuclear medicine methods have achieved only limited acceptance in nephrology in spite of their potential usefulness and versatility. Nevertheless, radionuclide procedures have several important applications in this field, and the purpose of this chapter is to place these techniques in perspective. Although hypertension may be regarded as a surgical disease when it has a renovascular origin, it is included in this discussion since the majority of patients with hypertension are the responsibility of the nephrologist or general physician.

Assessment of renal size

The assessment of renal size is of considerable importance to the nephrologist in many conditions and especially in renal insufficiency. Normal size is usually compatible with recent onset and potential reversibility of the renal condition while small kidneys suggest long-standing disease. Enlargement of the kidneys may occur in diabetes (*Figure 14.1*), amyloidosis, polycystic disease and other nephrological conditions listed in *Table 14.1*.

Plain radiographic films of the abdomen or intravenous urography with nephrotomography will often demonstrate the size of each kidney. Unfortunately poor preparation, overlying bowel contents, impaired concentration or contraindications due to renal impairment limit their general value. Since ultrasound can provide information on renal size independently of renal function and without any radiation hazard to the patient it is usually considered to be the procedure of choice. Where a simple estimate of renal length and calyceal pattern is required, this is entirely justified. Timmermans (1975) found ultrasound estimates of renal size to differ from actual (nephrectomy) size by less than 15% in 9 of 10 cases examined.

In spite of its obvious value, however, the information provided by ultrasound is entirely structural, and it is often useful to combine an estimate of renal size with evaluation of underlying function. Radionuclides can provide such information.

As a result of the prolonged renal transit time of ^{131}I-orthoiodohippurate (OIH) in renal failure (Blaufox and Conroy, 1968) this agent provides a useful image even by rectilinear scanning. In 18 of 19 patients with advanced renal failure (mean blood urea 34 mmol/l (BUN 96 mg/dl), creatinine 0.67 mmol/l (7.6 mg/dl)) successful visualization has been reported by Freeman *et al.* (1969). Other reports confirm the value of [131]I-

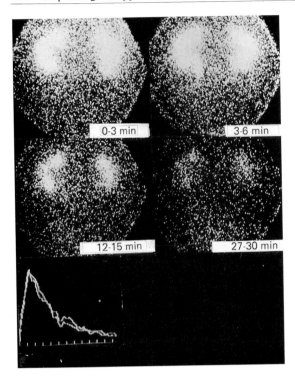

0-3 min   3-6 min

12-15 min   27-30 min

Figure 14.1A Normal renal images with derived renogram curve

OIH in assessing renal size in the presence of severe renal impairment (Schoutens *et al.*, 1972). It has been suggested that renal concentration of OIH occurs with as little as 3% of normal renal function (O'Reilly *et al.*, 1979).

^{99m}Tc, as a chelate, has been used in renal failure. It has been estimated that renal size can be determined with ^{99m}Tc-DTPA in 75% of patients with blood urea over 23 mmol/l (BUN over 65 mg/dl) (Reba *et al.*, 1974). In all but 'very extreme' renal failure ^{99m}Tc-glucoheptonate also has been reported to be imaged (Kohn and Mostbeck, 1979), while DMSA was similarly successful in four of five patients with blood urea over 36 mmol/l (BUN exceeding 100 mg/dl) (Handmaker, Young and Lowenstein, 1975).

Routine radionuclide scanning techniques may underestimate renal size because of the renal position. Lateral scanning of the kidneys has been recommended when this possibility exists (Kohn and Mostbeck, 1979; Bradley-Moore *et al.*, 1982). Virtually any agent is adequate for estimation of renal size in patients whose kidney function is good. ^{99m}Tc-glucoheptonate or DMSA are preferred because of better resolution and the potential for multiple views. In the presence of renal failure ^{131}I-OIH appears to be the single most reliable agent, with good uptake and minimal interference from surrounding organs. The overriding usefulness of ^{131}I-OIH lies in its important prognostic and functional information, discussed below.

Acute renal failure

Acute tubular necrosis

It is often possible to diagnose acute tubular necrosis (ATN) from its clinical features, characteristic urinalysis and blood and urine chemistries. Nuclear medicine procedures

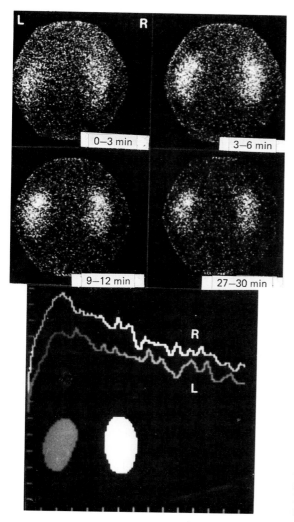

Figure 14.1B An example of mild chronic renal insufficiency in a 50-year-old diabetic male. The kidneys in this instance are not small, and there is an asymmetrical reduction in renal function

TABLE 14.1

Renal size	Condition
Normal	Acute renal failure
	Acute glomerulonephritis
	Acute pyelonephritis
Reduced	Chronic renal failure
	Chronic glomerulonephritis
	Chronic pyelonephritis
	Renal artery stenosis
	Hypoplastic kidney
Increased	Amyloidosis
	Polycystic kidney
	Renal vein thrombosis
	Urinary tract obstruction
	Diabetes

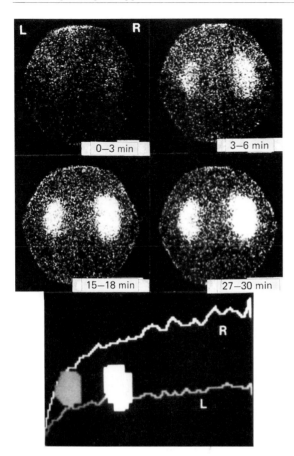

Figure 14.2 ^{131}I-OIH renogram with progressive cortical accumulation during the entire study. No movement of activity to the renal pelvis is seen. The scan pattern is typical of ATN. Asymmetrical renal size was an incidental finding in this case. The renal regions of interest are shown overlaid on the time–activity curves generated from them

have a role in providing supporting evidence, in facilitating recognition of disorders mimicking ATN and in providing important prognostic information.

Difficulty in distinguishing ATN from chronic parenchymal renal disease in patients with advanced renal failure rarely occurs. However, the relatively prompt uptake of labelled OIH in most patients with ATN, compared with the poor, delayed uptake found with advanced chronic renal failure, is a useful diagnostic point (*Figure 14.2*) (Hattner, Maltz and Holliday, 1977). This difference is of particular importance in evaluating patients after renal transplantation.

The presence or absence of renal uptake of OIH in patients with severe renal failure (acute or chronic) is reported to be of value in predicting recovery of renal function. The poor prognosis of patients with acute renal failure and non-visualization on ^{131}I-OIH scanning was confirmed by Sherman and Blaufox (1980a) who reported that all seven patients in their study with this finding failed to recover renal function. In another study, Harwood *et al.* (1976) reported that after 6 months 10 patients with 'prominent' renal uptake had a mean creatinine clearance of 80 ml/min, while the clearance of seven patients with 'faint' uptake was 39 ml/min and that of seven with no renal image apparent was 25 ml/min. Three patients in the no renal image group required chronic haemodialysis, while none did so in the prominent renal image group. The differing prognosis of these groups with similar clinical presentation could not be determined from clinical and laboratory data. Delayed imaging of the kidney does not appear to be very helpful since the prognosis is equally poor in all kidneys which are not imaged by 30 minutes (Sherman and Blaufox, 1980a).

Renal blood flow in ATN has been shown by ^{133}Xe washout to be reduced to approximately one-third of normal (Hollenberg *et al.*, 1968). Some people with ATN retain nearly normal blood-flow. The hepatorenal syndrome (Epstein, Berk and Hollenberg, 1970), cortical necrosis (Kleinknecht *et al.*, 1973) and renal arterial occlusion (Bell, McAfee and Makhuhli, 1981) may be confused with ATN clinically, but differ pathophysiologically in that extreme reduction in renal blood-flow is characteristic. Although the xenon washout technique has provided valuable physiological information, it cannot be used as a routine method. None of the radionuclide methods clinically used yields the same quantitative data.

It has been suggested by Schlegel and Lang (1980) that the 'nuclear filtration fraction' may be of value in acute renal failure. The glomerular filtration rate (^{99m}Tc-DTPA) and renal plasma flow (^{131}I-OIH) were estimated based on 1–2 minute renal uptake of the radionuclides. The 'nuclear filtration fraction' GFR/RPF was found to be increased in ATN, decreased in 'pre-renal' states and normal with post-renal obstruction. Although this approach may provide potentially useful information, it has not yet been confirmed by other investigators.

Renal gallium uptake may sometimes be observed in ATN. George *et al.* (1975) described 12 patients with renal transplants and ATN whose kidneys accumulated the radionuclide. Kumar and Coleman (1976) reported these findings in three patients with ATN, two of whom were renal transplant patients. The extent and intensity of the renal uptake was not described in either report. Though ATN is frequently listed as a cause of renal gallium uptake (Kahn, 1979), other reports of this in the patient without a renal transplant are scarce (Staab and McCartney, 1978). It can probably be concluded safely that intense gallium uptake of the type associated with pyelonephritis or interstitial nephritis probably does not occur in ATN. The importance of grading of gallium uptake cannot be overemphasized. The significance of minor degrees of uptake is doubtful.

Overall the major role of renal imaging in ATN appears to be its important prognostic information. Clearly patients with renal failure and non-visualization on the OIH renal scan fall into a poor prognosis group. It is extremely important to recall when this technique is used that urinary tract obstruction may also produce non-visualization of the kidneys. Although the significance of non-visualization in other conditions is consistent, it cannot be relied on in obstructive disease where recovery may be possible even with no uptake at all of isotope (Sherman and Blaufox, 1980b). Therefore in all cases of non-visualization of the kidney on renal scan, the presence of urinary tract obstruction should be investigated by ultrasound. If obstruction is present, percutaneous nephrostomy should be considered. Recovery of the ability to concentrate radiohippuran in this situation appears to correlate well with the recovery of the kidney (*Figure 14.3*).

Acute pyelonephritis

The role of radionuclides in urinary tract infection is not clear at the present time. Although most investigators reserve radionuclide imaging in infection for a secondary role after intravenous urography, some suggest a more prominent use. Handmaker (1982) described a pattern of striated 'flares' of decreased activity in patients with pyelonephritis imaged with ^{99m}Tc-DMSA. In a review of more than 60 patients he suggested that renal scanning had a greater sensitivity than conventional procedures (*Figure 14.4*).

^{67}Ga localizes non-specifically in acute inflammation and may indicate the presence of an infected kidney. All 17 patients with 'overt signs of pyelonephritis' studied by Kessler *et al.* (1974) showed uptake of gallium at 24–78 hours. In 11 cases the

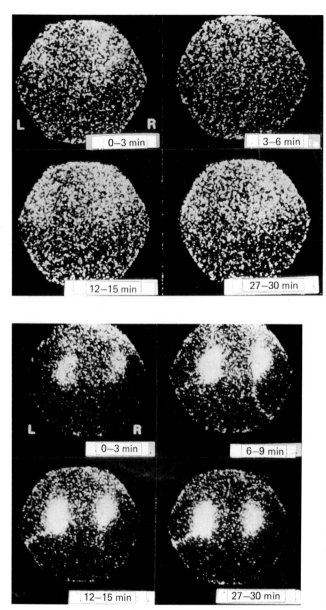

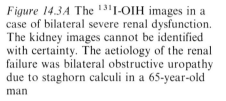

Figure 14.3A The ^{131}I-OIH images in a case of bilateral severe renal dysfunction. The kidney images cannot be identified with certainty. The aetiology of the renal failure was bilateral obstructive uropathy due to staghorn calculi in a 65-year-old man

Figure 14.3B Due to the patient's poor medical condition at the time of presentation, a definitive operative procedure was not immediately performed. Instead, bilateral percutaneous nephrostomies were placed. This study, obtained several days after the nephrostomy placement, demonstrates striking improvement in renal function bilaterally. Radioactivity can be seen in the nephrostomy tubes

uptake was unilateral. There was no uptake in four culture-negative patients with radiological evidence of chronic pyelonephritis. Patients at high risk of infection such as those on immunotherapy or chemotherapy may have a high false positive rate because of alterations in carrier proteins. This problem is not great in unilateral uptake since normal kidneys usually appear symmetrical and unilateral or segmental uptake is usually abnormal.

The possibility has been raised that ^{67}Ga can be helpful in differentiating between upper and lower tract infection. Hurwitz *et al.* (1976) used 24-hour gallium imaging in 49 patients who had pyelonephritis confirmed or excluded by conventional testing. Among 25 with demonstrated upper tract infection, 22 had renal uptake of gallium. In

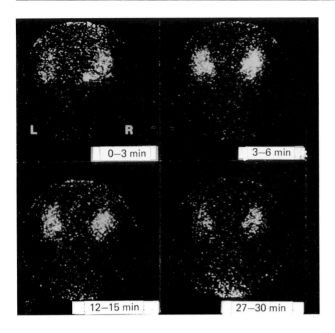

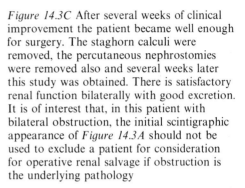

Figure 14.3C After several weeks of clinical improvement the patient became well enough for surgery. The staghorn calculi were removed, the percutaneous nephrostomies were removed also and several weeks later this study was obtained. There is satisfactory renal function bilaterally with good excretion. It is of interest that, in this patient with bilateral obstruction, the initial scintigraphic appearance of *Figure 14.3A* should not be used to exclude a patient for consideration for operative renal salvage if obstruction is the underlying pathology

contrast, four of 24 with only lower tract infection had false positive scans. Gallium uptake was not normally found at 24 hours by these workers; this contradicted other reports. It seems more likely that, with current technology, renal images may be seen normally as late as 48 hours (Hauser and Alderson, 1978). Regardless of technique, renal gallium uptake which increases from the 24- to 48-hour scan, is unilateral, focal or as intense as that of the liver is usually abnormal (Staab and McCartney, 1978; Hauser and Alderson, 1978). Absence of renal uptake in the presence of active infection suggests the possibility of lower rather than upper urinary tract involvement.

In patients with urinary tract infections gallium scanning appears to be a promising, non-invasive method of diagnosing upper tract infection (*Figure 14.5*). In addition, the procedure appears useful in recognizing unsuspected pyelonephritis or renal abscess in patients with fever of undetermined origin and in localizing renal infection in patients with polycystic kidney disease (Kahn, 1979). Although most cases of urinary tract infection are easily managed with routine diagnostic methods, there is a role for nuclear medicine in selected cases.

Acute interstitial nephritis

Recognition of acute interstitial nephritis (non-infectious) may be straightforward when the characteristic features are present but is more difficult if these features are absent. It is often mistaken for ATN. Wood and colleagues (1980) first noted the intense, diffuse, 48-hour uptake of gallium in three patients with biopsy evidence of this disorder. Linton and colleagues (1980), reporting on nine patients with acute interstitial nephritis due to drugs, described the same finding on gallium scanning. In addition, they studied patients with other renal disorders including six patients with ATN in whom there was no uptake of the radionuclide. These authors suggested that gallium scanning may help distinguish patients with acute interstitial nephritis from those with ATN, and other forms of renal disease (*Figure 14.6*).

R.P. 27♀

6 Sep 74   L/R=1.27

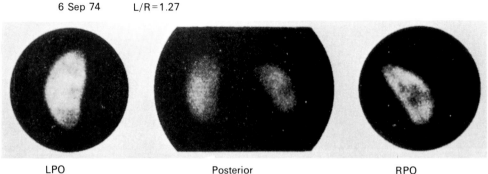

LPO   Posterior   RPO

11 Nov 74   L/R=1.13

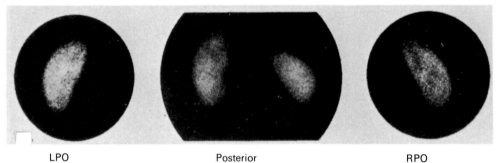

LPO   Posterior   RPO

Figure 14.4 A ^{99m}Tc-DMSA study of a 27-year-old woman with right flank pain, pyuria and fever. Early in September the right kidney demonstrates a mid-renal defect, which most prominently displays the flare pattern on the right posterior oblique (RPO) view. The follow-up in mid-November shows a return to normal appearance. (Reproduced with permission of H. Handmaker, 1982)

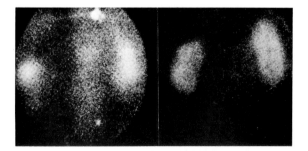

Figure 14.5 On the left is the posterior view obtained 48 hours after injection of ^{67}Ga-citrate. The patient was a 48-year-old male with back pain, pyuria and fever. Normally the kidneys would not be visualized. By contrast, this patient with acute bilateral pyelonephritis demonstrates bilateral, intense, focal ^{67}Ga uptake within the kidneys. On the right is the corresponding glucoheptonate study

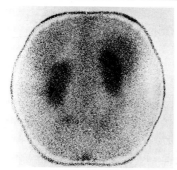

Figure 14.6 46-hour posterior image of ^{67}Ga uptake in the kidneys in a 30-year-old male with interstitial nephritis proven by biopsy

Renal artery embolism

Renal artery embolism should be considered as a cause of acute renal failure, particularly in patients with atrial fibrillation or acute myocardial infarction. Radionuclide studies can play a major diagnostic role in this disorder.

Early reports on patients with renal artery embolism noted the good correlation of ^{99m}Tc-pertechnetate flow studies with renal arteriography (Freeman *et al.*, 1971). Lessman *et al.* (1978) reported on 17 cases with renal artery embolism, 15 of whom had acute renal failure. ^{99m}Tc-pertechnetate perfusion scanning showed unilateral or bilateral absence of renal perfusion in nine of ten cases studied and the remaining patient had bilateral perfusion defects. In the eight patients who also underwent angiography the findings were virtually identical.

Even when renal artery embolism does not completely interrupt renal blood-flow, renal failure may occur in association with multiple parenchymal infarcts. ^{131}I-OIH was diagnostic in this situation in a patient with endocarditis and renal failure (Schoutens, Dupois and Toussant, 1972). More recently ^{99m}Tc-DTPA (Sanders, Menon and Sanders, 1978), ^{99m}Tc-glucoheptonate (Khan, 1979) and ^{99m}Tc-DMSA (Arnold *et al.*, 1975) have been used and advocated for recognition of this problem.

When the diagnosis of acute renal failure due to renal artery embolism is under consideration, radionuclide renal scanning may be of considerable value in recognizing as well as excluding the diagnosis (*Figure 14.7*). Arteriography may not be necessary unless there are plans for surgical intervention (Hartenbower *et al.*, 1970; Atkins and Freeman, 1973; Lessman *et al.*, 1978).

Chronic renal failure

Chronic pyelonephritis

Recognition of chronic non-obstructive pyelonephritis in the adult is not always simple, since a positive urine culture and pyuria are non-specific. The classic changes on urography (calyceal blunting and deformity with depression of the overlying cortex) are seen most commonly in childhood as a result of vesico-ureteric reflux (Hodson, 1967). Adults with pyelonephritis may have advanced histological damage without an apparent abnormality on urography (Saunders and Corriere, 1974). The problem is further compounded by the continuing debate of the criteria for diagnosis of pyelonephritis and the fact that the end-stage kidney shares a common histological appearance with many other disease entities (*Figure 14.8*).

The use of radionuclides is supported even by [197]Hg chlormerodrin studies (Davies *et al.*, 1972). In one such investigation 50 patients with the clinical diagnosis of chronic pyelonephritis and normal urography were reviewed. Despite the poor image

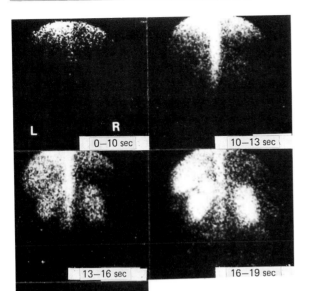

Figure 14.7 A rapid-sequence flow study after bolus injection of 370 MBq (10 mCi) ^{99m}Tc-glucoheptonate. While the gross appearance of activity is symmetrical between the two kidneys, a subtle defect is present in the left upper pole. Delayed static images (at 2 hours after injection) show the defect clearly. This patient had a renal arterial embolus with infarction in the region of the defect. The peripheral wedge-shaped appearance is typical

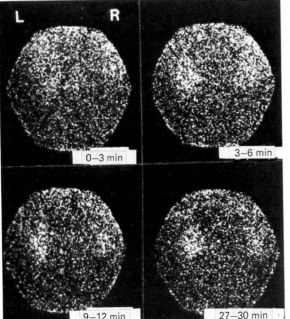

Figure 14.8 The typical appearance of chronic renal insufficiency is demonstrated on these ^{131}I-OIH images. The kidneys are small and have a very poor initial uptake of radiotracer as a result of a significant reduction in renal function. The serum creatinine was 0.49 mmol/l (5.5 mg/100 ml). Note the gradual and progressive accumulation of radiotracer within the kidneys during the course of the study. Activity could be shown to reach the bladder

resolution of obsolete equipment and an imaging agent no longer in use, localized renal defects were seen in 10 patients.

McAfee (1979) reported on 31 patients with chronic pyelonephritis (seven with renal insufficiency) who had urography and renal scans with ^{99m}Tc-glucoheptonate and ^{131}I-OIH and had abnormalities in at least one of these studies. Although the overall sensitivity to renal morphological abnormalities in this study was greater with urography than with scanning, focal parenchymal damage was seen better with nuclear imaging in eight patients and glucoheptonate was reported to be more useful than OIH. ^{99m}Tc-DMSA is also shown to be of great value in the assessment of cortical scarring in pyelonephritis (Handmaker, Young and Lowenstein, 1975; Kahn, 1979; O'Reilly, Shields and Testa, 1979).

An advantage over urography is that renal scans can demonstrate intraparenchymal abnormalities which do not deform the collecting system or renal outline. Nuclear imaging, therefore, may be a useful supplement to urography for detection of renal damage due to chronic pyelonephritis.

Renal lymphoma

Renal insufficiency is a common complication of malignant lymphomas and results from hypercalcaemia, uric acid nephropathy, glomerulopathies, dehydration, urinary tract obstruction, amyloidosis or lymphomatous infiltration of the kidneys (Richmond et al., 1962). Gallium scanning will detect lymphomatous organ involvement, including that of the kidney, with a sensitivity of from 30% to 77%, depending upon the specific lymphoma and the imaging equipment used (Frankel et al., 1975; Turner et al., 1978). A false positive rate of about 5% has been reported. Again, the many factors which affect gallium uptake by the kidney make interpretation of bilateral uptake difficult. A multinodular pattern of renal involvement which is sometimes detectable on scanning (Shirkhoda, Staab and Mittelstraedt, 1980), is ten times more common at autopsy than diffuse involvement (Richmond et al., 1962), making the pattern of gallium uptake useful. Although gallium is of use in selected cases, it is unlikely to be of general value with its variable sensitivity and false positive rates. The role of nuclear medicine in renal masses other than lymphoma is discussed in Chapter 9.

Hypertension

Probably the first clinical application of nuclear medicine in nephrology was in patients with hypertension. Although at present this application is less useful than that in many other diseases such as obstructive uropathy, the high world-wide prevalence of hypertension and the many misconceptions of the role of nuclear medicine in its management justify a detailed discussion.

Most people with elevated blood pressure suffer from essential hypertension. Untreated elevations of blood pressure are responsible for the failure of several organ systems, probably as a result of direct damage to blood vessels. These complications include: stroke due to associated cerebrovascular disease, renal failure as a consequence of nephrosclerosis, claudication from peripheral vascular disease, heart failure as a result of left ventricular hypertrophy and coronary artery disease as the result of direct damage to the coronary arteries.

Table 14.2 lists the major causes of secondary or 'curable' hypertension. The question that must be addressed is how can one find these patients, recognizing that they represent only a very small fraction of all of the hypertensive population.

Essential hypertension is not usually associated with any symptoms. Therefore,

TABLE 14.2. Causes of secondary hypertension

Endocrine	Cushing's syndrome
	Conn's syndrome
	Phaeochromocytoma
	Hyperthyroidism
Vascular	Coarctation of the aorta
	Renal artery stenosis
Renal	Congenital renal disease
	Diabetes
	Glomerulonephritis
	Gout
	Interstitial nephritis
	Obstructive uropathy
	Polycystic kidney disease
	Pyelonephritis
	Renin-secreting tumours
	Vasculitis
Drugs	Amphetamines
	Oestrogens and oral contraceptives
	Steroids
Miscellaneous	Increased intracranial pressure
	Licorice
	Toxaemia of pregnancy
	Lead poisoning

symptomatic disease should alert the physician to the possibility of secondary hypertension or of the development of end-organ damage. It is often difficult to determine if end-organ damage is the consequence or the cause of hypertension. For this reason, the interpretation of renal radionuclide studies in hypertension presents a considerable problem.

Renovascular hypertension and its prevalence

Partial obstruction of the renal artery is a cause of decreased renal perfusion at a reduced pressure and results in increased production of renin. Consequent increases in angiotensin and aldosterone produce fluid retention, vasoconstriction and sustained hypertension. Once the physiological variables are stabilized, peripheral plasma renin activity is frequently elevated, but it can be normal. The usual screening tests for renovascular hypertension (RVH) are listed in *Table 14.3*. Their complex inter-relationship is a major problem in interpreting such tests.

It is important to consider prevalence of the disease before adopting a diagnostic algorithm for renovascular hypertension so that these expensive and invasive tests can be used in a productive manner.

Renovascular hypertension is the most common form of secondary hypertension. The prevalence of secondary hypertension is variously reported as 0–30% and depends not only on the source of the study population but also on the definition of hypertension in that population and its severity (Gifford, 1969; Imura, 1973; Berglund, Andersson and Wilhelmsen, 1976; Rudnick *et al.,* 1977; Davis *et al.,* 1979). Several recent studies have demonstrated a substantial benefit from treating patients with diastolic blood pressures between 90 and 95 mmHg. About 70% of the hypertensive population have diastolic blood pressures between 90 and 104 mmHg (Hypertension Detection and Follow-up Program, 1979). The prevalence of renovascular disease in this group is probably well below 1%.

Population-based studies typically have found a low prevalence of secondary

TABLE 14.3. Diagnostic tests for renovascular hypertension

Test	Comments	Reference
Peripheral plasma renin activity	Helpful if very high	Wallach et al. (1975)
Intravenous urography	Rapid sequence; films obtained every minute for 5 minutes	Bookstein et al. (1972)
Renography and renal scintigraphy	Convenient and useful screening test	Blaufox et al. (1982)
Renal vein renin	Helpful in lateralization of lesion and predicting response to surgery	Marks and Maxwell (1975)
Angiography	Required for definitive diagnosis and surgery. Digital intravenous angiography may simplify the procedure and reduce morbidity	Buonocore et al. (1981)
Blood pressure response to angiotensin competitor	Has not gained widespread clinical utility	Brunner et al. (1973)
Blood pressure response to converting enzyme inhibition	Has not gained widespread clinical utility	Case et al. (1977)

hypertension. In the Hypertension Detection and Follow-up Program (1979), 9.1% of patients with severe hypertension (diastolic BP 115 mmHg) may have had renovascular hypertension. However, the apparent prevalence in the entire group, including mild and moderate hypertensives, was only 0.13%. Recent data demonstrate a higher prevalence of renovascular hypertension in patients with severe disease. In one study, 31% of all patients presenting with a diastolic blood pressure greater than 125 mmHg or grade 3 or 4 retinopathy were discovered to have renovascular hypertension. When white patients were analysed separately from black (in whom severe hypertension is common), the figure was over 40%. In general, it may be assumed that only 5–10% of hypertensive patients in a hospital-based population have identifiable causes for their disease and even fewer in a general population. An identifiable cause, in a given patient, signals to the referring physician the potential for cure. Unfortunately, in many cases this potential cannot be realized. The clinical characteristics of individual patients may give some guidance to the potential for surgical cure (*Table 14.4*). Diagnostic tests

TABLE 14.4. Clinical characteristics of essential hypertension and renovascular hypertension cured by surgery*

	Essential hypertension	Renovascular hypertension
Duration of hypertension		
< 1 year	12	24
> 10 years	15	6
Age of onset (> 50 years)	9	15
Family history of hypertension	71	46
Fundi (grade 3 or 4)	7	15
Bruit		
Abdomen	9	46
Flank	1	12
Abdomen or flank	9	48
BUN (> 20 mg/100 ml)	8	15
Serum K (< 3.4 mEq/litre)	8	16
Serum CO_2 (> 30 mEq/litre)	5	17
Urinary casts	9	20
Proteinuria (trace or more)	32	46

* 131 cases in each group, matched by age, sex, race and diastolic blood pressure. Only the statistically significant differences are presented, from Simon et al. (1972, p. 1211)

have additional value if they can prognosticate the likelihood for cure of hypertension upon further intervention—and if they provide information about the level of function of the involved kidney. The remainder of this review aims at developing an approach to the hypertensive patient to utilize the available diagnostic and prognostic nuclear medicine procedures. These procedures should be placed in their proper perspective with respect to other non-nuclear tests.

Renal imaging in renovascular hypertension

In renovascular hypertension virtually any pattern may be observed, but the most useful one is decreased and delayed accumulation and excretion of radiotracer seen on the affected side (*Figure 14.9*). Prolonged transit time may be seen as a result of decreased urine flow secondary to increased water reabsorption on the affected side. Bilateral ureteric catheterization for split renal function evaluation may demonstrate decreased urine volume with decreased sodium concentration on the affected side (Connor *et al.*, 1960). If it is chronically affected the involved kidney may be small and the renal blood-flow significantly reduced. In some cases, even the scintigraphic pattern cannot distinguish among various aetiologies for asymmetric renal dysfunction. Not all cases of obstruction demonstrate the collecting system either. Therefore, obstruction or chronic unilateral pyelonephritis may be interpreted falsely as suggestive of renovascular hypertension (*Figure 14.10*) (Kenny *et al.*, 1975). Asymmetric renal function is also more common in patients with essential hypertension. Making things

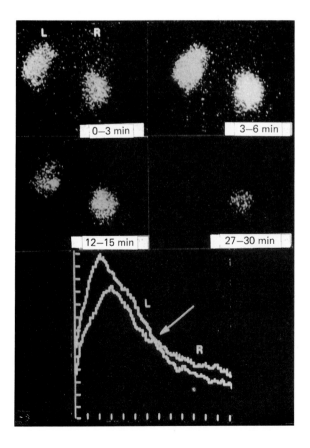

Figure 14.9A This 32-year-old woman had a right flank bruit and severe hypertension, refractory to medical management. The ^{131}I-OIH images demonstrate excellent bilateral uptake but with a smaller right kidney with proportionally fewer counts than the left. Sequential images reveal normal left-sided excretion but modest cortical retention in the right. The renogram curve shows a delayed and decreased peak of activity on the right, as well as delayed excretion, with a 'cross-over' of the curves shown at the arrow. Although not diagnostic, these findings suggest the possibility of renal artery stenosis on the right

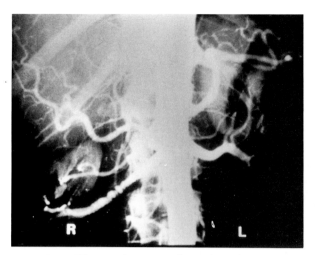

Figure 14.9B The arteriogram performed on the patient studied in *Figure 14.9A* revealed fibromuscular dysplasia of the right renal artery

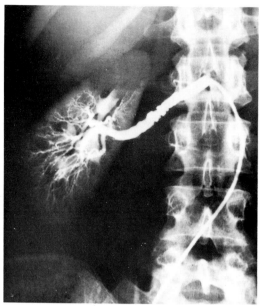

Figure 14.9C After percutaneous transluminal angioplasty, the repeat arteriogram on the patient studied in *Figures 14.9A* and *B* showed some reduction in the degree of stenosis of the right renal artery. Blood pressure medications were still required, but less intensively than before the procedure, and with greater efficacy of blood pressure control

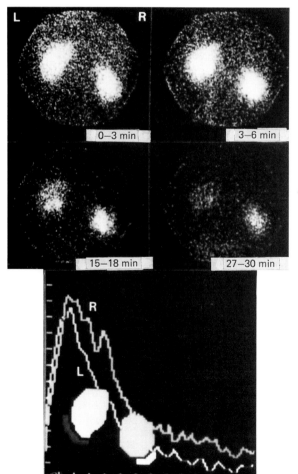

Figure 14.9D A postoperative ^{131}I-OIH study was obtained in which the differences in the images are subtle in comparing this with *Figure 14.9A*. However, the renogram curve demonstrates significantly improved uptake with a modest prolongation of transit through the right kidney

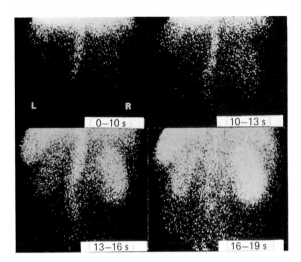

Figure 14.10 This posterior radionuclide angiogram demonstrates a small left kidney with delayed and decreased appearance of radiotracer within it. This suggests decreased flow to the left kidney. This study was obtained in a 65-year-old man with intermittent left-sided obstruction and presumed superimposed chronic pyelonephritis. Asymmetrical flow can result from renal disease other than renal artery stenosis, which is a probable explanation for many false positive studies in patients with hypertensive disease

even more complicated is the fact that these conditions may occasionally cause secondary hypertension themselves (Belman, Kropp and Simon, 1968). False negative scans may be seen also. Most series report sensitivities of approximately 80–85% and specificities in the same range for the diagnosis of renovascular hypertension (Maxwell, Lupu and Taplin, 1968; Nordyke, Gilbert and Simmons, 1969; Farmelant, Sachs and Burrows, 1970a, b; Keane and Schlegel, 1972; Secker-Walker, Sheperd and Cassell, 1972; Wall, Hilario and Whalen, 1972; Maxwell, 1975).

Although false positive rates of 10–15% are usually reported, this is more a reflection of the lack of specificity of the test than its inaccuracy. That is, although these 10–15% of patients do not have renovascular hypertension, they probably do have an asymmetry of renal function. There is a wide number of conditions resulting in unilateral renal disease (*Table 14.5*).

There is growing interest in the use of angiotensin converting enzyme inhibitors to enhance the sensitivity of radionuclide studies in the diagnosis of renal artery stenosis (Drew *et al.*, 1984; Oei *et al.*, 1984; Nally *et al.*, 1985; Aburano *et al.*, 1985; Sfakianakis *et al.*, 1985; Wenting *et al.*, 1985). In normal subjects these agents cause peripheral arterial vasodilation and lower peripheral vascular resistance. In patients with essential hypertension, effective renal plasma flow may increase, while the glomerular filtration rate does not change after administration of converting enzyme inhibitors. In patients with renovascular disease the effects may be more complex. Some investigators report a marked decrease in filtration fraction of the affected kidney after angiotensin converting enzyme inhibitors are given. There is a suggestion that these changes may

TABLE 14.5. Differential diagnosis of unilateral decrease in renal perfusion

Renal artery stenosis
Renal vein thrombosis
Parenchymal renal disease
Collecting system obstruction
Compression of hilar vessels
Perirenal abscess
Perirenal haematoma
Ptosis

Adapted from McAfee *et al.* (1977)

enhance the functional difference between a normal and abnormal kidney caused by renal artery stenosis. This approach may increase the sensitivity of radionuclide studies. We look forward to further investigation of the diagnostic role of this class of compounds.

The use of ^{123}I-OIH, with the additional aid of functional imaging, may provide another means to improve the diagnostic utility of OIH for the detection of renovascular hypertension. Various parenchymal renal disorders, and virtually all kidneys with end-stage renal failure, regardless of aetiology, are associated with hypertension, usually due to fluid retention. OIH renograms have some application, however limited, in the evaluation of parenchymal renal dysfunction. The major use for OIH in the end-stage disease is to detect the existence of functional renal tissue when other modalities identify merely a shrunken kidney. ^{99m}Tc-DTPA studies, which depend upon glomerular filtration for renal visualization (see below), are generally less sensitive in identifying functional renal tissue reliably in renal failure.

Other parenchymal disorders associated with hypertension, such as polycystic kidneys, are best identified by morphological studies. Rarely, as mentioned above, chronic obstruction may present as hypertension (Belman, Kropp and Simon, 1968).

A diagnostic approach to the hypertensive patient

It appears from the combined epidemiological statistics that hypertension is associated with a correctable lesion in only 5–10% of hypertensives in high-risk groups. Screening tests clearly must be inexpensive and convenient in order to be practical. Furthermore, these tests should be sensitive enough to detect disease in a high percentage of those who have it and indicate absence of disease in those who do not.

At various times in the past 20 years many of the tests listed in *Table 14.3* have been proposed to screen all hypertensives in order to identify those with correctable hypertension. It should be apparent that none of these tests is appropriate for mass screening. They are all too expensive, some are too invasive and few are convenient. For example, it has been proposed that all hypertensive patients have an IVU or a renogram to screen for possible renovascular hypertension (Melby, 1975a, b). The results of screening with nuclear medicine techniques and IVU are summarized in *Tables 14.6* and *14.7*.

If the cost of both procedures—as well as the potential morbidity and even the mortality associated with contrast injections—are ignored, one still arrives at the conclusion that these are too inconvenient to be screening procedures.

The following approach is suggested for the evaluation of hypertensive patients. The schema outlined below is summarized by the flowsheet (*Figure 14.11*).

1. All hypertensives should have a complete history and physical examination.
2. Without undue expense, inconvenience or complexity, every hypertensive patient should have blood specimens obtained for a complete blood count, blood urea and serum creatinine, serum electrolytes, cholesterol and uric acid. A urinalysis (gross and microscopic) should be performed. Finally, a chest X-ray and ECG should be obtained. The history and physical examination and the simple blood tests can help segregate patients into two groups, those with potentially correctable hypertension and those with probably essential hypertension:

    (a) Aortic coarctation should be suspected on the basis of the physical examination. The chest X-ray obtained will confirm this suspicion.
    (b) The history and physical examination will often give clues as to presence or absence of the other correctable hypertensive disorders. Episodic hypertension by history, with flushing, palpitations and headache suggest phaeochromocytoma. Signs of acromegaly, cafe au lait spots, neurofibromata, multiple

TABLE 14.6. Nuclear medicine tests in renovascular hypertension

(A) ^{99m}Tc *perfusion studies*

	True negatives		Specificity	
	Visual	*Quantitative*	*Visual*	*Quantitative*
Essential HTN ($n = 33$)	27/33	29/33	42/54 = 85%	29/33 = 88%
Controls ($n = 21$)	19/21	—		

	True positives		Sensitivity	
RVH ($n = 18$) (16 quantified)	17/18	13/16	94%	81%

Adapted from Keim *et al.* (1979)

(B) ^{131}I-OIH *studies*

Study	True positives	False positives
Renogram	85	10
Urogram	78	11
Both	91	18

From McNeil *et al.* (1975)

TABLE 14.7. The IVU in the diagnosis of renal artery stenosis

Series	Sensitivity*	Specificity*
Bookstein *et al.* (1972)	83% (138 RAS)	88.6% (771) (essential HTN)
Maxwell *et al.* (1964)	93% (42 RAS)	83% (121) (61 normotensive)
Wilson *et al.* (1963)	72% (128 RAS)	92% (125) (60 hypertensive)
Stewart *et al.* (1962)	86% (22 RAS)	75% (105)
Thornbury *et al.* (1982)	60.2% (197 RAS)	—

* Number of cases in parentheses

endocrine disorders, thyroid nodularity, and family history help increase suspicion of phaeochromocytoma. Laboratory examination revealing hypo- or hypercalcaemia in the absence of renal disease suggests co-existing hyperparathyroidism or medullary carcinoma of the thyroid, respectively. These are associated with familial multiple endocrine neoplasia syndromes of which phaeochromocytoma is often a feature.

(c) Stigmata of hyperthyroidism or Cushing's syndrome also are apparent from history and physical examination. Suspicion of hyperthyroidism requires an additional blood specimen for a T4 determination. Cushing's syndrome is more likely, as is hyperaldosteronism if hypokalaemia is present. Further blood tests for morning cortisols or renin determinations, respectively, should be obtained. The patient should not be taking diuretics at this stage of the evaluation, of course.

(d) An abdominal bruit suggests renal artery stenosis and the possibility of RVH. Evidence upon initial patient presentation of severe end-organ damage such as grade 3 or 4 hypertensive retinopathy, or renal dysfunction without other apparent cause is associated with a 30% likelihood for RVH. Severe diastolic hypertension (diastolic blood pressure greater than, or equal to, 130 mmHg) is also associated with a 30% likelihood for renovascular hypertension. Failure of

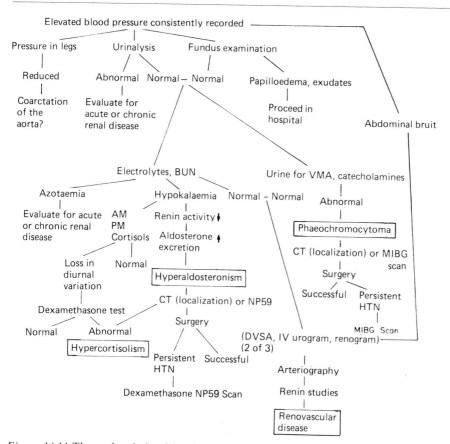

Figure 14.11 The authors' algorithm for the diagnostic evaluation of hypertension

the blood pressure to respond in a patient with good compliance to antihypertensive therapy also suggests the possibility of renovascular hypertension.

3. Palpable abdominal masses may reveal polycystic kidneys. Family history as well as laboratory evidence of renal dysfunction also argue for further morphological renal evaluation.

From the above schema we see that most of the correctable forms of hypertension are immediately suggested by the history, physical examination and initial blood and laboratory examinations. Hypercortisolism, hyperaldosteronism or phaeochromocytoma are suggested by the initial examination and laboratory work and confirmed by radioimmunoassay. Pre-surgical adrenal localization is probably best performed by CT scan at the present time. However, radionuclide procedures have a relevant role in the detection of adrenal remnants and metastases from phaeochromocytoma (*see* Chapter 9). The situation is quite different if the initial laboratory work and evaluation suggest renovascular hypertension. With the above screening schema, the likelihood for renovascular hypertension is approximately 30% before further testing.

The next diagnostic step would be either a radioisotope renogram and IVU or an intravenous digital angiogram. The best available data do not distinguish clearly among these examinations on the basis of sensitivity or specificity, all values being approximately 80–85%.

Since none of the procedures by themselves ensures diagnostic certainty, it may be necessary to perform two of the above tests. From a pre-test likelihood of disease of 30%, two positive tests (e.g. renogram and digital angiogram) raise the likelihood to over 93%, while two negative tests drop the likelihood of disease well under 5%. Two positive tests are then followed by split renal vein renin determinations before arteriography (with or without angioplasty, as indicated). Two negative tests effectively rule out renovascular hypertension. A positive and a negative test or equivocal results may indicate the need for an arteriogram.

No matter which work-up is chosen, radionuclides are extremely valuable for follow-up. All patients submitted to surgery for renovascular hypertension should have gamma camera renograms, preoperative for baseline and then for follow-up of the surgical result. This is especially important in patients undergoing balloon dilatation where several procedures may be necessary before success is achieved.

Regardless of the individualized approach, there is a significant role for the use of nuclear medicine procedures in the evaluation of the hypertensive patient.

References

ABURANO, T., TAKAYAMA, T., NAKAJIMA, K. *et al.* (1985) Split renal function in patients with hypertension following continued Captopril treatment. *Journal of Nuclear Medicine*, **26**, P73

ARNOLD, R. W., SUBRAMANIAN, G., McAFEE, J. G. *et al.* (1975) Comparison of ^{99m}Tc complexes for renal imaging. *Journal of Nuclear Medicine*, **16**, 357–367

ATKINS, H. L. and FREEMAN, L. M. (1973) The investigation of renal disease using radionuclides. *Postgraduate Medical Journal*, **49**, 503–516

BELL, E. G., McAFEE, J. G. and MAKHULI, Z. N. (1981) Medical imaging of renal diseases—suggested indications for different modalities. *Seminars in Nuclear Medicine*, **11**, 105–127

BELMAN, A. B., KROPP, K. A. and SIMON, N. M. (1968) Renal pressor hypertension secondary to unilateral hydronephrosis. *New England Journal of Medicine*, **278**, 1133–1136

BERGLUND, G., ANDERSSON, O. and WILHELMSEN, L. (1976) Prevalence of primary and secondary hypertension: Studies in a random population sample. *British Medical Journal*, **2**, 554–556

BLAUFOX, M. D. and CONROY, M. (1968) Measurement of renal mean transit time of hippuran ^{131}I with external counting. *Journal of Nuclear Medicine*, **12**, 107–116

BLAUFOX, M. D., KALIKA, V., SCHARF, S. and MILSTEIN, D. (1982) Applications of nuclear medicine in genitourinary imaging. *Urological Radiology*, **4**, 155–164

BOOKSTEIN, J. J., ABRAMS, H. L., BUENGER, R. E. *et al.* (1972) The role of urography in unilateral renovascular disease. *Journal of the American Medical Association*, **220**, 1225–1230

BRADLEY-MOORE, P. R., NAGEL, J. S., CANO, R. A. *et al.* (1982) Kidney size measurement—mathematical solution to problems of angulation on two axes (abstract). *Journal of Nuclear Medicine*, **23**, P111

BRUNNER, R. R., GARVAS, H. and LARAGH, J. H. (1973) Angiotensin II blockade in man by Sar^{1}-ala^{8}-angiotensin II for understanding and treatment of high blood pressure. *Lancet*, **2**, 1045–1048

BUONOCORE, E., MEANEY, T. F., BORKOWSKI, G. P. *et al.* (1981) Digital subtraction angiography of the abdominal aorta and renal arteries: Comparison with conventional angiography. *Radiology*, **139**, 281–286

CASE, D., WALLACE, J. M., KEIM, H. J. *et al.* (1977) Possible role of renin in hypertension as suggested by renin-sodium profiling and inhibition of converting enzyme. *New England Journal of Medicine*, **296**, 641–646

CONNOR, T. B., THOMAS, W. C. Jr, HADDOCK, L. and HOWARD, J. E. (1960) Unilateral renal disease and its detection by ureteral catheterization studies. *Annals of Internal Medicine*, **52**, 544–559

DAVIES, E. R., ROBERTS, M., ROYLANCE, J. *et al.* (1972) The renal scintigram in pyelonephritis. *Clinical Radiology*, **23**, 370–376

DAVIS, B. A., CROOK, J. E., VESTAL, R. E. *et al.* (1979) Prevalence of renovascular hypertension in patients with grade III or IV hypertensive retinopathy. *New England Journal of Medicine*, **301**, 1273–1276

DREW, H., LaFRANCE, N., BENDER, W. *et al.* (1984) Renal function in patients with renovascular hypertension following inhibition of angiotensin converting enzyme. *Journal of Nuclear Medicine*, **25**, P36

EPSTEIN, M., BERK, D. P. and HOLLENBERG, N. K. (1970) Renal failure in the patient with cirrhosis. *American Journal of Medicine*, **49**, 175–185

FARMELANT, M. H., SACHS, S. E. and BURROWS, B. A. (1970a) The influence of tissue background activity on the apparent renal accumulation of radioactive compounds. *Journal of Nuclear Medicine*, **11**, 112–117

FARMELANT, M. H., SACHS, S. E. and BURROWS, B. A. (1970b) Prognostic value of radioisotope renal function studies for selecting patients with renal arterial stenosis for surgery. *Journal of Nuclear Medicine*, **11**, 743–748

FRANKEL, R. S., RICHMAN, S. D., LEVENSON, S. M. *et al.* (1975) Renal localization of gallium-67 citrate. *Radiology*, **114**, 393–397

FREEMAN, L. M., GOLDMAN, S. M., SHAW, R. K. *et al.* (1969) Kidney visualization with ^{131}I-ortho-iodohippurate in patients with renal insufficiency. *Journal of Nuclear Medicine*, **10**, 545–549

FREEMAN, L. M., MENG, C. H., RICHTER, M. W. *et al.* (1971) Patency of major renal vascular pathways demonstrated by rapid blood flow scintigraphy. *Journal of Urology*, **105**, 473–481

GEORGE, E. A., CODD, J. E., NEWTON, W. T. *et al.* (1975) ^{67}Ga citrate in renal allograft rejection. *Radiology*, **113**, 731–733

GIFFORD, R. W. (1969) Evaluation of the hypertensive patient with emphasis on detecting curable causes. *Milbank Memorial Fund Quarterly*, **47**, 170–186

HANDMAKER, H., YOUNG, B. W. and LOWENSTEIN, J. M. (1975) Clinical experience with ^{99m}Tc-DMSA (dimercaptosuccinic acid), a new renal imaging agent. *Journal of Nuclear Medicine*, **16**, 28–32

HANDMAKER, H. (1982) Nuclear renal imaging in acute pyelonephritis. *Seminars in Nuclear Medicine*, **12**(3), 246–253

HARTENBOWER, D. L., WINSTON, M. A., WEISS, E. R. *et al.* (1970) The scintillation camera in embolic acute renal failure. *Journal of Urology*, **104**, 799–802

HARWOOD, T. H., HIESTRMAN, D. R., ROBINSON, R. G. *et al.* (1976) Prognosis for recovery of function in acute renal failure. *Archives of Internal Medicine*, **136**, 916–919

HATTNER, R. S., MALTZ, H. E. and HOLLIDAY, M. A. (1977) Differentiation of reversible ischaemia from end-stage renal failure in nephrotic children with ^{131}I-hippurate dynamic scintigraphy. *Journal of Nuclear Medicine*, **18**, 438–440

HAUSER, M. F. and ALDERSON, P. O. (1978) Gallium imaging in abdominal disease. *Seminars in Nuclear Medicine*, **8**, 251–270

HODSON, C. J. (1967) The radiological contribution toward the diagnosis of chronic pyelonephritis. *Radiology*, **88**, 857–871

HOLLENBERG, N. K., EPSTEIN, M., ROSEN, S. M. *et al.* (1968) Acute oliguric renal failure in man—evidence for preferential renal cortical ischaemia. *Medicine*, **17**, 455–474

HURWITZ, S. R., KESSLER, W. O., ALAZRAKI, N. P. *et al.* (1976) Gallium-67 imaging to localize urinary tract infections. *British Journal of Radiology*, **49**, 156–160

HYPERTENSION DETECTION AND FOLLOW-UP PROGRAM COOPERATIVE GROUP (1979) Five year findings of the Hypertension Detection and Follow-up Program: I. Reduction in mortality of persons with high blood pressure, including mild hypertension. *Journal of the American Medical Association*, **242**, 2562–2671

IIMURA, O. (1973) Actual incidence of secondary hypertension. *Japanese Circulation Journal*, **37**, 1040–1044

KAHN, P. C. (1979) Renal imaging with radionuclides, ultrasound and computed tomography. *Seminars in Nuclear Medicine*, **9**, 43–57

KEANE, J. M. and SCHLEGEL, J. U. (1972) The use of a scintillation camera system for scanning of hypertensive patients. *Journal of Urology*, **108**, 12–14

KEIM, H. J., JOHNSON, P. M., VAUGHAN, D. Jr *et al.* (1979) Computer assisted static/dynamic renal imaging: A screening test for renovascular hypertension. *Journal of Nuclear Medicine*, **20**(1), 11–17

KENNY, R. W., ACKERY, D. M., FLEMING, J. S. *et al.* (1975) Deconvolution analysis of the scintillation camera renogram. *British Journal of Radiology*, **48**, 481–486

KESSLER, W. O., GITTES, R. F., HURWITZ, S. R. *et al.* (1974) Gallium-67 scans in the diagnosis of pyelonephritis. *Western Journal of Medicine*, **121**, 91–93

KLEINKNECHT, D., GRUNFELD, J. P., GOMEZ, P. C. *et al.* (1973) Diagnostic procedures and long term prognosis in bilateral renal cortical necrosis. *Kidney International*, **4**, 390–400

KOHN, H. D. and MOSTBECK, A. (1979) Value of additional lateral scans in renal scintigraphy. *European Journal of Nuclear Medicine*, **4**, 21–25

KUMAR, B. and COLEMAN, R. E. (1976) Significance of delayed ^{67}Ga localization in the kidneys. *Journal of Nuclear Medicine*, **17**, 872–875

LESSMAN, R. K., JOHNSON, S. F., COBURN, J. W. *et al.* (1978) Renal artery embolism. *Annals of Internal Medicine*, **89**, 477–482

LINTON, A. L., CLARK, W. F., DRIEDGER, A. A. *et al.* (1980) Acute interstitial nephritis due to drugs. *Annals of Internal Medicine*, **93**, 735–741

MCAFEE, J. G., THOMAS, F. D., GROSSMAN, Z. *et al.* (1977) Diagnosis of angiotensinogenic hypertension: The complimentary roles of renal scintigraphy and the saralasin infusion test. *Journal of Nuclear Medicine*, **18**(7), 669–675

MCAFEE, J. G. (1979) Radionuclide imaging in the assessment of primary chronic pyelonephritis. *Radiology*, **133**, 203–206

MCNEIL, B. J., VARADY, P. D., BURROWS, B. A. and ADELSTEIN, S. J. (1975) Measures of clinical efficacy. Cost-effectiveness calculations in the diagnosis and treatment of hypertensive renovascular disease. *New England Journal of Medicine*, **293**, 216–221

MARKS, L. S. and MAXWELL, M. H. (1975) Renal vein renin: Value and limitations in the prediction of operative results. *Urologic Clinics of North America*, **2**, 311–325

MAXWELL, M. H. (1975) Cooperative study of renovascular hypertension. *Kidney International*, **8**, S153–S160

MAXWELL, M. H., LUPU, A. N. and TAPLIN, G. V. (1968) Radioisotope renogram in renal arterial hypertension. *Journal of Urology*, **100**, 376–383

MAXWELL, M. H., GONICK, H. C., WIITA, R. and KAUFMAN, J. J. (1964) Use of the rapid sequence intravenous pyelogram in the diagnosis of renovascular hypertension. *New England Journal of Medicine*, **270**, 213–220

MELBY, J. C. (1975a) Extensive hypertensive work-up: Pro. *Journal of the American Medical Association*, **231**(4), 399–401

MELBY, J. C. (1975b) Extensive hypertensive work-up. In rebuttal to Dr Finnerty. *Journal of the American Medical Association*, **231**(4), 404

NALLY, J. V., CLARKE, H. S., GRECOS, G. P. *et al.* (1985) Superior diagnostic value of captopril(CAP)-enhanced non-invasive studies in unilateral renal artery stenosis (uRAS). *Journal of Nuclear Medicine*, **26**, P73

NORDYKE, R. A., GILBERT, F. I. Jr and SIMMONS, E. L. (1969) Screening for kidney disease with radioisotopes. *Journal of the American Medical Association*, **208**, 493–496

OEI, H. Y., GEYSKES, G. G., DORHOUT MEES, E. J. *et al.* (1985) Captopril induced renographic alteration in unilateral renal artery stenosis. *Journal of Nuclear Medicine*, **25**, P36

O'REILLY, P. H., SHIELDS, R. A. and TESTA, H. J. (1979) Renovascular hypertension and renal failure. In: *Nuclear Medicine in Urology and Nephrology*, 1st edn., London: Butterworths, pp. 81–85

RICHMOND, J., SHERMAN, R. S., DIAMOND, H. D. *et al.* (1962) Renal lesions associated with malignant lymphomas. *American Journal of Medicine*, **32**, 184–206

RUDNICK, K. V., SACKETT, D. L., HIRST, S. and HOLMES, C. (1977) Hypertension in a family practice. *Canadian Medical Association Journal*, **117**, 492–497

SANDERS, R. C., MENON, S. and SANDERS, A. D. (1978) The complementary uses of nuclear medicine and ultrasound in the kidney. *Journal of Urology*, **120**, 521–527

SAUNDERS, C. D. and CORRIERE, J. N. (1974) The inability to diagnose chronic pyelonephritis on the excretory urogram in adults. *Journal of Urology*, **111**, 560–562

SCHLEGEL, J. U. and LANG, E. K. (1980) Computed radionuclide urogram for assessing acute renal failure. *American Journal of Roentgenology, Radium Therapy and Nuclear Medicine*, **134**, 1029–1034

SCHOUTENS, A., DUPUIS, F. and TOUSSAINT, C. (1972) ^{131}I-Hippuran scanning in severe renal failure. *Nephron*, **9**, 275–290

SECKER-WALKER, R. H., SHEPERD, E. P. and CASSELL, K. J. (1972) Clinical applications of computer assisted renography, *Journal of Nuclear Medicine*, **13**, 235–248

SFAKIANAKIS, G., KYRIAKIDES, G., JAFFE, D. *et al.* (1985) Single visit captopril renography for the diagnosis of curable renovascular hypertension (RVH). *Journal of Nuclear Medicine*, **26**, P133

SHERMAN, R. A. and BLAUFOX, M. D. (1980a) Clinical significance of nonvisualization with ^{131}I-hippuran renal scan. In: *Radionuclides in Nephrology*, N. K. Hollenberg and S. Lange (eds.), Stuttgart: Thieme, pp. 235–239

SHERMAN, R. A. and BLAUFOX, M. D. (1980b) Obstructive uropathy in patients with nonvisualization on renal scan. *Nephron*, **25**, 82–86

SHIRKHODA, A., STAAB, E. V. and MITTELSTAEDT, C. A. (1980) Renal lymphoma imaged by ultrasound and gallium-67. *Radiology*, **137**, 175–180

STAAB, E. V. and MCCARTNEY, W. H. (1978) Role of gallium-67 in inflammatory disease. *Seminars in Nuclear Medicine*, **8**, 219–234

STEWART, P. H., DEWEESE, M. S., CONWAY, J. *et al.* (1962) Renal hypertension: An appraisal of diagnostic studies and of direct operative treatment. *Archives of Surgery*, **85**, 617–635

THORNBURY, J. R., STANLEY, J. C. and FRYBACK, D. G. (1982) Hypertensive urogram: A nondiscriminatory test for renovascular hypertension. *American Journal of Radiology*, **138**, 43–48

TIMMERMANS, L. (1975) A comparison of radioisotopic and ultrasonic scanning of the kidney. In: *Radionuclides in Nephrology*, K. zum Winkel, M. D. Blaufox and J. L. Funck-Brentano (eds.), Stuttgart: Thieme, pp. 101–106

TURNER, D. A., FORDHAM, E. W., ALI, A. *et al.* (1978) Gallium-67 imaging in the management of Hodgkin's disease and other malignant lymphomas. *Seminars in Nuclear Medicine*, **8**, 205–218

WALL, C. A., HILARIO, E. M. and WHALEN, T. J. (1972) An orderly search for a vascular lesion producing hypertension. *Journal of Urology*, **108**, 511–514

WALLACH, L., NYARAI, I. and DAWSON, K. G. (1975) Stimulated renin: A screening test for hypertension. *Annals of Internal Medicine*, **82**, 27–34

WENTING, G. J., TAN-TJIONG, H. L., DERKX, F. H. M. *et al.* (1984) Split renal function after captopril in unilateral renal artery stenosis. *British Medical Journal*, **288**, P886–P890

WILSON, L., DUSTAN, H. P., PAGE, I. H. *et al.* (1963) Diagnosis of renal arterial lesions. *Archives of Internal Medicine*, **112**, 270–277

WOOD, B. C., SHARMA, J. N., GERMANN, D. R. *et al.* (1980) Gallium citrate Ga-67 imaging in non-infectious interstitial nephritis. *Archives of Internal Medicine*, **138**, 1665–1666

Part 3

Basic principles

15 Physics

R. S. Lawson

The atom

All matter is made up of individual *atoms* of the various *elements* (e.g. hydrogen, H; oxygen, O). Several atoms often bind together to form *molecules* which behave as separate entities (e.g. water, H_2O). Chemistry and biology are concerned with the ways in which atoms combine into molecules, but in this chapter attention will be confined to the physics of the atom itself, irrespective of whether it is in isolation or whether it is part of a complex molecule forming a biological structure.

An atom is roughly spherical, with a diameter of about 2×10^{-10} m. However, almost all the mass of the atom is concentrated in the *nucleus* at its centre, which is only about 10^{-14} m in diameter. The rest of the space is occupied only by a very diffuse cloud of orbiting *electrons*, each of which carries a negative electric charge of one unit. The nucleus is made up of *protons*, which each carry one unit of positive charge, and *neutrons*, which are uncharged. Since the number of electrons in an atom is normally equal to the number of protons, the net charge of the atom in its normal state is zero. A proton and a neutron have approximately the same mass (about 1.7×10^{-24} g) but an electron has a mass of only about 1/2000 of this, so that the contribution of the electrons to the total mass of the atom is negligible. The mass of the atom is proportional to its *mass number*, A, given by

$$A = Z + N$$

where Z is the number of protons and N the number of neutrons in the nucleus. Z is known as the *atomic number* of the atom. It is a measure of the positive charge on the nucleus, which determines the number of negatively charged electrons which normally surround it. Since it is these electrons which determine the chemistry of the atom, all atoms with the same atomic number are practically indistinguishable chemically and so are classed as belonging to the same element. Atoms are classified into different nuclear types, or *nuclides*, according to their atomic number and mass number. Nuclides with the same atomic number but different mass numbers are called *isotopes*. A particular nuclide is usually specified by writing its chemical symbol with its mass number as a superscript and its atomic number as a subscript. Thus $^{123}_{53}I$, $^{127}_{53}I$ and $^{131}_{53}I$ are all isotopes of iodine with 53 protons and 70, 74 and 78 neutrons, respectively. Because the chemical symbol automatically implies a particular atomic number, the subscript is often omitted.

TABLE 15.1. Physical properties of some important radionuclides used in renal studies

Nuclide	Half-life	Decay mode	Principal gamma rays and percentage of decays	Half-value layer for gamma rays (mm)	
				Lead	Tissue
^{131}I	8.06 days	Beta-minus	82% (364 keV)	2.3	63
			7% (637 keV)	5.0	77
			6% (284 keV)	1.4	57
^{125}I	60 days	Electron capture	7% (35 keV)	0.04	23
			115% (27 keV*)	0.02	17
			25% (31 keV*)	0.03	20
^{123}I	13.0 hours	Electron capture	84% (159 keV)	0.35	49
^{99m}Tc	6.03 hours	Isomeric transition	88% (140 keV)	0.25	47
^{67}Ga	78.1 hours	Electron capture	38% (93 keV)	0.08	39
			24% (185 keV)	0.5	51
			16% (300 keV)	1.6	58
^{51}Cr	27.7 days	Electron capture	10% (320 keV)	1.9	61

* Principal emissions from ^{125}I are X-rays

There is always an optimum balance between the numbers of protons and neutrons in a nucleus. With 53 protons the optimum number of neutrons is 74 and so ^{127}I is a stable nuclide. Nuclides with either too few neutrons (e.g. ^{123}I) or too many neutrons (e.g. ^{131}I) are unstable and will eventually change spontaneously into other nuclides which are more stable. This is the process of *radioactive decay* and the nuclides involved are called *radionuclides*. The unstable radionuclide that is decaying is called the *parent* nuclide and the new nuclide that is formed by its decay is called the *daughter*. It is the energy given out in radioactive decay that we make use of in nuclear medicine.

Radioactivity is, therefore, an instability in the arrangement of the protons and neutrons in the nucleus of the atom. However, it is also possible for the atom to radiate energy as a result of the instabilities in the arrangement of its orbiting electrons. An electron in an outer orbit has a higher energy than one in an inner orbit. Since each energy level only has room for a limited number of electrons, in the normal or *ground state*—where the atom has the lowest possible energy—the electrons occupy the lowest few energy levels.

If for some reason one of the outer electrons is raised to a higher energy level, the atom is no longer in its ground state, but in an *excited state*. This excited state will not be stable and the electron will fall back spontaneously to the lowest vacant energy level. In doing so it must lose energy equal to the difference between the two levels, and it does this by emitting a photon of light with the appropriate energy. Alternatively, if one of the innermost electrons from the atom is removed, again there is an unstable excited state, and it decays back to the ground state by allowing electrons from the higher energy levels to cascade down to fill the gap. In the process these electrons must give up their energy as photons. However, because the energy differences between the levels are much greater in this case than in the previous one, these photons are not of visible light, but of *X-rays*. In either case the energy or wavelength of the photons emitted is characteristic of the emitting atom.

It is convenient to measure the energy of the photons emitted in this sort of process in units of *electronvolts*, eV. One electronvolt is the energy that is lost by an electron in falling through a potential difference of one volt. It is equal to 1.6×10^{-19} joules. In these units visible light photons have an energy of a few eV and X-rays an energy of a few thousand eV, written as keV.

In a similar way it is also possible to have different energy levels of the nucleus itself. Since the nucleus is made up of closely packed protons and neutrons, these energy levels cannot be visualized as different orbits, but rather as different arrangements of the nuclear particles. One situation in which the nucleus has too high an energy level is when the ratio of protons to neutrons is not optimum. To minimize the energy of the nucleus and to make it stable again, it is necessary to turn a neutron into a proton or vice versa. This is the process of *beta decay*.

It is also possible for a nucleus to contain the right proportion of protons to neutrons, but in an unstable arrangement, so that it is in an excited state. Like the excited atom, an excited nucleus will decay back to its ground state and in doing so emit its excess energy as a photon. This is *isomeric transition*. Because the nuclear force responsible for the nuclear energy levels is much stronger than the electric force which gives rise to the electron energy levels, higher-energy photons would be expected from the decay of an excited nucleus. In fact, the photon energies are several hundred thousand electronvolts, i.e. several hundred keV, and sometimes up to a million electronvolts, written MeV. Although these photons are not really any different in their nature from X-rays, they have been given a separate name, *gamma rays*. The energies of gamma rays and X-rays do in fact overlap, but the term X-rays is reserved for photons from atomic electron transitions and gamma rays for photons from nuclei.

It is the gamma rays emitted from the decay of an excited nucleus that are so useful in nuclear medicine. As in the case of atomic X-rays, their energies are characteristic of the particular atom involved.

Radioactive decay

Half-life

Nuclear decay is a random process: it is impossible to predict when any individual atom will disintegrate. All that can be said is that there is a certain probability that it will disintegrate in any given time interval. Therefore, if we take a large number of identical atoms, an average number of disintegrations per second can be obtained. The number of disintegrations per second is a measure of the strength of activity of a sample of a radionuclide. An activity of one disintegration per second is called a *becquerel*, Bq. Nuclear medicine usually deals with activities of several million disintegrations per second, i.e. several megabecquerels, MBq. Traditionally, the unit of activity has been the *curie*, Ci, originally defined as the activity of one gram of radium. The curie is equal to 3.7×10^{10} disintegrations per second. The submultiples millicurie (mCi) and microcurie (μCi) are still sometimes encountered:

$1\,\text{mCi} = 37\,\text{MBq}$

$1\,\text{MBq} = 27\,\mu\text{Ci}$

The activity, A, of a radioactive source, measured in disintegrations per second, is equal to the number of radioactive atoms present, N, multiplied by the probability that any one of them will decay in one second. If this probability is called λ, then

$A = \lambda N$

The activity may also be defined as the rate at which N is decreasing. Thus

$$A = -\frac{dN}{dt} = \lambda N \tag{1}$$

The solution of this differential equation gives the activity at any time t as

$$A(t) = A_0\, e^{-\lambda t} \tag{2}$$

where A_0 is the activity at time $t = 0$. This is known as exponential decay and may be

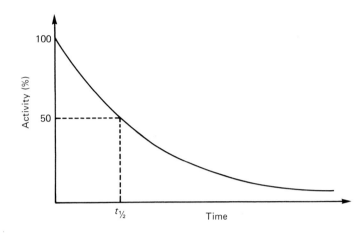

Figure 15.1 The exponential decay of radioactivity

represented graphically as in *Figure 15.1*. While this theory applies to any radioactive material, the steepness of the decay curve (determined by λ) will be different in each case and characteristic of the radionuclide. It is convenient to measure this in terms of the *half-life*, $t_{1/2}$, defined as the time taken for the activity of a given sample to decay to half its original value. It is related to λ as follows:

$$t_{1/2} = \frac{0.693}{\lambda} \tag{3}$$

Note that the activity will halve in each half-life irrespective of when measurements are started. For example, consider a source with a half-life of 6 hours which has an activity of 80 MBq at midday. At 1800 hours the activity will be only half this value, or 40 MBq and by midnight it will be 20 MBq. Therefore in 12 hours (two half-lives) it has decayed to one-quarter of the original activity. After 2 days the activity will be only 0.3 MBq (1/256 of the original activity) but it will still halve during the next 6 hours.

Counting statistics

The random nature of the radioactive process means that there will never be exactly the same number of disintegrations taking place in two successive equal time intervals. Measuring the activity of a sample by counting the number of gamma rays that it gives off in a fixed time will not always give precisely the same result, even assuming that the counting apparatus is perfect. One way to get a more accurate result would be to take four separate measurements and then calculate their average. However, this would give exactly the same result as taking one measurement over a period four times as long. It may be expected, therefore, that the longer the period over which the gamma rays are counted, the more accurate will be the result. It can be shown that if N gamma rays are counted in a given time, then the random statistical nature of the radioactive process will lead to a standard error of the measurement equal to $\sqrt{N}$. The percentage standard error is therefore given by $(\sqrt{N}/N) \times 100$ or $100/\sqrt{N}\%$. A measurement of 10 000 counts would be expected to have a precision of $\pm 1\%$, i.e. there is a 60% probability that the 'true' count lies between 9900 and 10 100.

Beta decay

It has already been stated that nuclides with too many protons or too many neutrons are unstable and will spontaneously try to change into a more stable state through the process of beta decay. This can be divided into three categories: *electron emission* (β^- decay), *positron emission* (β^+ decay) and *electron capture*. The first occurs when there are too many neutrons, and the second and third when there are too many protons.

The first category of beta decay may be regarded as the transformation of one of the excess neutrons into a proton and an electron. In the process a fourth particle is also produced. This particle, called a *neutrino*, has no electric charge and hardly ever interacts with matter, so it is not likely to be able to be detected directly. The transformation may be written as:

$$n \rightarrow p + e^- + \bar{v} \tag{4}$$

where n is a neutron; p is a proton; e^- is an electron; and $\bar{v}$ is a neutrino. If this happens to one of the neutrons in the nucleus of $^{131}_{53}I$, the loss of a neutron and gain of a proton turns it into $^{131}_{54}Xe$. Note that the mass number, 131, has not changed but the atomic number has increased by one, and, hence, turned the iodine atom into a xenon atom. Thus:

$$^{131}_{53}I \rightarrow ^{131}_{54}Xe^+ + e^- + \bar{v} \tag{5}$$

where the '+' superscript indicates that the ^{131}Xe atom is in a positively ionized state because it only has the 53 electrons that the original ^{131}I had instead of the 54 required to make it neutral. The electron and neutrino emitted carry off the excess energy of the nucleus. The electron emitted in this way is commonly referred to as a *beta particle*. A decay scheme of this type is often shown diagrammatically by drawing the nuclear energy levels of the parent and daughter nuclides. The energy levels for the two nuclides are drawn side by side with those for the nuclide of higher atomic number on the right.

A simplified version of the decay scheme for ^{131}I is shown in *Figure 15.2*. The oblique arrows indicate alternative modes of beta decay which result in different excited states of the daughter nuclide. The beta particle energy shown in each case is the maximum possible for that transition, but beta particles will be emitted with a range of energies, because for each transition the available energy is shared with a neutrino. The mean energy of the beta particle is often taken to be approximately one-third of the maximum.

The vertical arrows represent transitions between excited states of the daughter which normally take place immediately after the corresponding beta decay. In each case a gamma ray photon carries off the difference in energies and the percentage probability figures indicate the proportion of disintegrations in which these particular transitions take place. Thus, for example, a gamma ray photon of 364 keV is emitted after 82% of disintegrations of ^{131}I.

The second category of beta decay may be regarded as the transformation of one of

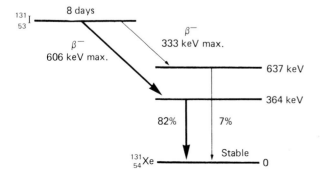

Figure 15.2 The radioactive decay scheme of ^{131}I via beta emission. The decay scheme has been simplified by omitting several less probable transitions

the excess protons:

$$p \rightarrow n + e^+ + \nu \tag{6}$$

where e^+ is a positron (exactly like an electron but with a positive charge) and ν is another sort of neutrino. An example of a nuclide which decays in this way by positron emission is ^{18}F. Thus:

$$^{18}_{9}F \rightarrow {}^{18}_{8}O^- + e^+ + \nu \tag{7}$$

The '$-$' superscript indicates that the ^{18}O atom is left in a negatively charged state with one too many electrons. Note that the mass number has remained unchanged but that the atomic number has decreased by one. As in electron emission, the positrons have a range of energies from zero up to a maximum.

Since the positron produced in a decay of this type is the exact opposite, or antiparticle, of an ordinary electron, it will not travel very far in matter before it comes to a stop and then annihilates with a nearby electron. This produces two gamma rays, each of 510 keV energy, which fly off in opposite directions:

$$e^+ + e^- \rightarrow \gamma + \gamma \tag{8}$$

The third category of beta decay is electron capture. This is a process by which a nucleus can change an excess proton into a neutron by absorbing one of the atomic electrons from an inner orbit:

$$p + e^- \rightarrow n + \nu \tag{9}$$

This mode of decay has some advantages for nuclear medicine, because it does not involve the emission of any electrons or positrons. These emissions are a nuisance, because they are totally absorbed in the body and so increase the radiation dose to the patient without contributing to the detection of the nuclide. The disadvantage is that, because one of the inner atomic electrons is removed, the daughter atom will be produced in an excited atomic state and so it will eventually decay back to its ground state, emitting X-rays in the process.

An example of a nuclide that decays by electron capture is ^{123}I. We can write

$$^{123}_{53}I + \text{atomic electron} \rightarrow {}^{123}_{52}Te^* + \nu \tag{10}$$

$$^{123}_{52}Te^* \rightarrow {}^{123}_{52}Te + \text{X-rays}$$

where the asterisk indicates an excited atomic state. The decay scheme for ^{123}I is shown in *Figure 15.3*.

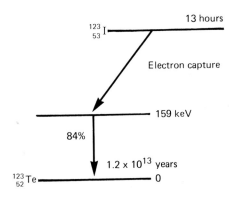

Figure 15.3 The radioactive decay scheme of ^{123}I via electron capture

Alpha decay and fission

Alpha decay and nuclear fission are two related decay processes which only occur for heavy nuclei. In *alpha decay* a heavy, unstable nucleus can decay to a state of less energy by emitting an alpha particle. This is just a combination of two protons and two neutrons—i.e. the nucleus of $^4_2$He. The alpha particles are emitted with definite energies which are characteristic of the particular decay. The daughter nuclide will have an atomic number 2 less than that of its parent and a mass number 4 less. It may be left in an excited nuclear state after the decay, in which case it will decay to its ground state by gamma emission. Alpha-emitting isotopes are not used in nuclear medicine.

In spontaneous *nuclear fission* a heavy nucleus breaks up into two approximately equal fragments of lighter nuclei and one or more spare neutrons. These fission fragments are usually in a highly excited state and will decay with the emission of gamma rays. They are also likely to have excess neutrons, and so are radioactive, decaying by electron emission. Fission is therefore useful to nuclear medicine as a means of producing some of the electron-emitting radionuclides, such as ^{131}I, and ^{99}Mo used in technetium generators.

Isomeric transition: gamma emission

The daughter nuclides of many radioactive decays are left in an excited nuclear state following alpha or beta decay of the parent. In most cases the excited nucleus will immediately decay to its ground state by isomeric transition, emitting one or more gamma ray photons. The process is vital to nuclear medicine, because it is just these gamma rays which are used to detect the presence of a radionuclide in a patient. Gamma emission usually occurs so rapidly (with a half-life of less than 10^{-10} seconds) that it is not separable from the original alpha or beta decay. The energies of the gamma rays produced are characteristic of the nuclear energy levels of the daughter nuclide, but since they are so closely associated with the decay of the parent nuclide, they are often spoken of as if they originated from the parent. For example, ^{131}I is said to have a gamma ray energy of 364 keV when in actual fact it is the ^{131}Xe that results from the beta decay of ^{131}I which produces the gamma ray (*see Figure 15.2*).

For ^{131}I this distinction is not important for practical purposes, because the beta decay is followed immediately by the gamma emission. However, it sometimes happens that certain excited states of the nucleus have lifetimes much longer than normal. These may be several seconds or even hours. A nucleus in one of these states is said to be *metastable*. If as a result of a beta decay the daughter nuclide is left in a metastable state, then it is possible to distinguish the original beta decay of the parent from the subsequent decay of the metastable daughter, which may occur seconds or hours later.

A metastable nuclide may eventually decay by emitting a gamma ray in the usual way, but there is an alternative process which often occurs in the decay of metastable states. This is *internal conversion*. Internal conversion occurs when an excited nuclear state loses its energy by passing it directly to one of the nearby atomic electrons in one of the inner orbits. This electron is then ejected from the atom, carrying away the excess energy of the nucleus which would otherwise have been removed by gamma emission. Internal conversion electrons thus have specific energies, unlike the electrons emitted in beta decay. Since the resulting atom is missing an electron from an inner orbit, internal conversion will always be followed by X-ray emission from the atom as the orbiting electrons rearrange themselves. Internal conversion can also occur when ordinary excited nuclear states decay, but it is far more likely when metastable states are involved.

As far as nuclear medicine is concerned, the most important example of a nuclide that exhibits a metastable state is technetium-99. Since the metastable state behaves just like

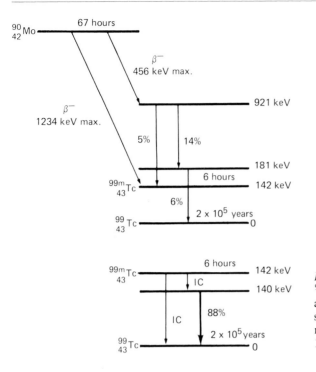

Figure 15.4 The radioactive decay schemes of ^{99}Mo and ^{99m}Tc. ^{99}Mo decays by beta emission, and some of the decays result in the metastable state of ^{99m}Tc. This decays by isomeric transition, resulting in internal conversion electrons and 140 keV gamma rays

a separate nuclide in its own right, it is written with a superscript m: thus, ^{99m}Tc. It is produced by the beta-minus decay of molybdenum-99, as shown in *Figure 15.4*. ^{99}Mo has a half-life of 67 hours and decays by two routes to ^{99m}Tc, which is metastable, having a half-life of 6 hours and lying at an energy of 142 keV above the ground state of ^{99}Tc. In about 1% of the decays the metastable state decays directly to the ground state by internal conversion. Most of the decays, however, are by internal conversion to a slightly lower level at 140 keV. This then decays immediately by gamma emission (88%) or internal conversion (11%) to the ground state and it is this gamma ray that is the principal feature of the decay of ^{99m}Tc. The ground state of ^{99}Tc is not, in fact, stable, but, since it has a half-life of 200 000 years, the quantity of radioactivity produced is totally insignificant.

The 6-hour half-life of ^{99m}Tc is sufficiently long for it to be separated easily from the parent ^{99}Mo. This is easy to achieve chemically, because technetium is soluble in saline but molybdenum is not. This principle is used in the technetium generator to provide technetium in the form of sodium pertechnetate (Na[^{99m}Tc]O$_4$) by flushing saline through a column containing ^{99}Mo which has been decaying for a few hours. The major feature of the emission from ^{99m}Tc is the 140 keV gamma ray. There are no electrons from beta decay and most of the conversion electrons are very low energy. There are also several X-rays from excited electron energy levels following the internal conversion. Nevertheless, ^{99m}Tc approaches very closely to being an ideal radionuclide for nuclear medicine studies, being an almost pure gamma emitter with a suitable energy for detection and having a short half-life.

Interaction of radiation with matter

In a vacuum, and in the absence of electric or magnetic fields, all types of radiation travel uninterrupted in straight lines away from the source. The intensity of the radiation falls off as the inverse square of the distance away from the source, simply because the same number of particles get spread out over a larger area as the distance increases.

When radiation passes through matter, as well as having its intensity reduced by the inverse square law effect, it is further affected by interactions with the material. These are broadly of two types: *scattering* and *absorption*. In a scattering process the radiation is deflected away from its original direction and in doing so gives up some of its energy, but in an absorption process the radiation is stopped completely and gives up all of its energy. The net result of these interactions is to transfer energy from the incident radiation to the atoms of the material. Some of this energy is lost as heat and molecular vibrations, but a lot of it goes into ionizing the atoms by knocking out some of their orbiting electrons. It is this *ionization* by the radiation which is responsible for its damaging effect on biological tissue, but it is also the means by which the radiation can be detected.

When the interaction of radiation with matter is considered, it is important to distinguish between charged particles (i.e. electrons and alpha particles) and photons (i.e. gamma rays and X-rays), because they behave in rather different ways.

When a beam of charged particles passes through matter, each particle undergoes many successive scattering interactions with the atomic electrons—and occasionally with the nuclei—which it encounters. If the particle is an electron it can ionize atoms of the material through which it passes by *electron collision* with the atomic electrons. If an electron passes close to a much more massive nucleus it will be decelerated violently and emit some of its energy as *bremsstrahlung* X-rays which themselves can go on to produce further ionization. Each scattering results in the electron giving up a small amount of its energy, and it will finally come to a stop when it has undergone sufficient interactions to lose all of its energy. An electron of a given energy will thus have a definite *range* that it can travel in a material before it stops. For example, the range of a 600 keV electron (the maximum energy of a beta particle from ^{131}I decay) is about 2.5 m in air and 3 mm in tissue.

Since alpha particles are much heavier than electrons and have two units of charge they produce denser ionization. They can also undergo *nuclear collisions*, producing a recoiling atomic nucleus which produces further ionization of the material. Alpha particles lose energy more rapidly and have a shorter range than electrons. The range of a 1 MeV alpha particle is 5 mm in air and only 0.007 mm in tissue. Neither alpha particles nor electrons have sufficient range in tissue to escape from a patient, and so all of their energy contributes to the radiation dose to the patient and none escapes to be usefully detected externally.

Beams of gamma or X-ray photons interact with matter in a different manner. They tend to undergo only a small number of scatters before they are totally absorbed and pass on all their energy to *secondary electrons* in the material. These secondary electrons produce further ionization of the material, and are soon stopped. Secondary electrons are produced by *Compton scattering* when a photon scatters off an electron with a consequent change in the photon direction and reduction in its energy. The *photoelectric effect* also produces secondary electrons when a photon is completely absorbed by an atomic electron, ejecting it from its orbit and leaving the atom in an ionized and excited state. For gamma rays with an energy above 1 MeV *pair production* is also possible when the gamma ray changes into an electron and positron pair.

As a beam of gamma rays passes through matter, the number of photons in the beam—i.e. its *intensity*—is attenuated as more and more photons are scattered out of the beam by a single Compton event, or suddenly absorbed by the photoelectric effect. This behaviour contrasts with the effect of material on a beam of charged particles, where it is the *energy* of each particle that is attenuated by many successive scatterings until it finally stops. There is not, therefore, any definite range for gamma rays as there is for charged particles. In fact, the number of photons remaining in a gamma ray beam decreases exponentially with increasing distance into the material, and so we can never say that the beam is totally stopped. Instead we usually specify the *half-value layer*, which is the thickness of material needed to reduce the intensity to half its original value. For example, the half-value layer for 140 keV gamma rays is about 0.25 mm of lead or 47 mm of tissue, and for 364 keV gamma rays it is 2.3 mm of lead or 63 mm of tissue.

Further reading

BURCHAM, W. E. (1973) *Nuclear Physics, An Introduction*, London: Longman
EISBERG, R. M. (1961) *Fundamentals of Modern Physics*, New York: John Wiley and Sons
WAGNER, H. N. Jr (ed.) (1968) *Principles of Nuclear Medicine*, Philadelphia: Saunders

16 Instrumentation

R. A. Shields and D. L. Hastings

The instrumentation encountered in diagnostic nuclear medicine is principally that concerned with the detection and measurement of gamma radiation. Any radiation detector must exploit some physical interaction between the radiation and the material of the detector; it must absorb some of the incident energy and convert it into a 'readable' form. The absorption of gamma radiation is at least a two-stage process: the gamma photon first transfers some or all of its energy to *secondary electrons* and these secondary electrons subsequently cause *ionization* or *excitation*. Perhaps the most direct way to detect radiation is by means of an *ionization chamber*, which 'catches' the ions produced in air by attracting them to oppositely charged electrodes. If the air is continuously irradiated (e.g. by placing a radioactive source within it), then the ions flowing between the polarized electrodes constitute a small electric current. Doses of radioactivity dispensed in nuclear medicine laboratories are usually measured by exploiting this principle. A typical 'radioisotope calibrator' produces a current of 10^{-11} A for a dose of 40 MBq of ^{99m}Tc.

The individual electrical pulses corresponding to photon or particle interactions are, in general, too small and are collected too slowly for efficient detection; for this reason the proportional counter and Geiger–Müller counter tubes were developed. These devices are gas-filled tubes which provide internal amplification of the electrical pulses following ionizing events within them. They are used for radiation monitors and for beta particle detection, but they can only absorb a small proportion of incident gamma ray photons, and so have too low a sensitivity for most *in vivo* nuclear medicine techniques.

In fact, there is one type of radiation detector which dominates this field of application: the *scintillation detector*. In this device absorbed radiation energy causes the excitation of electrons into elevated energy levels within a crystal structure or complex molecule. These excited electrons subsequently fall back again, whereupon energy is re-emitted as light photons, or 'scintillations'. Among the many materials, solid and liquid, organic and inorganic, which exhibit this property, the crystal of sodium iodide has the greatest efficiency for conversion of incident gamma ray energy into light. It has become the detector of choice for most nuclear medicine applications.

The sodium iodide scintillation detector

In order to obtain a high and uniform sensitivity, it is necessary to prepare the sodium iodide in a highly pure monocrystalline form containing a controlled quantity of thallium 'activator'. A sophisticated technology has developed so that these crystals may be grown to various sizes up to about 50 cm in diameter (for a gamma camera) and cut to various shapes, normally cylindrical. For the radioactive assay of small samples a hole may be cut out of a single crystal so that the sample may be completely surrounded by detecting material—the *scintillation well detector*. The material is hygroscopic and discolours on exposure to atmosphere; detector crystals are therefore always encapsulated—usually in a thin aluminium can with a hermetically sealed transparent window. A reflective layer between crystal and can ensures that as much as possible of the emitted light passes through the window. Even so, this is a very small amount of light. Each keV of energy lost by a secondary electron in the crystal produces about 20–30 light photons. A gamma ray photon from ^{99m}Tc which is completely absorbed in the crystal gives all its 140 keV of energy to the secondary electrons, which consequently produce a flash containing 3000–4000 photons of light. Most of this light is emitted within half a microsecond. The detection of this flash of light is almost invariably by means of a *photomultiplier tube*—an evacuated glass tube containing a number of electrodes. The assembly is shown in diagrammatic form in *Figure 16.1*. A thin coating of photoemissive material on the inner surface of the front face of the tube constitutes the *photocathode*; it is usually connected externally to ground potential. The most sensitive photocathodes are capable of releasing one electron for the absorption of about 10 light photons, so that the collection of all the light emitted during the scintillation event referred to above should result in the release of 300–400 electrons. The electrons are attracted toward the first *dynode*, because this is connected externally to a positive potential—about 300 V. On hitting the first dynode, each electron may liberate three or four secondary electrons; these are accelerated toward the next dynode; and so on. A typical photomultiplier tube may have ten dynodes, and a gain of 4 at each stage would produce an overall gain of 4^{10} or about one million. The movement of all these electrons through the anode and into the external electronic

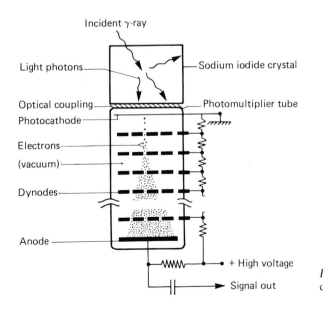

Figure 16.1 The sodium iodide scintillation detector assembly

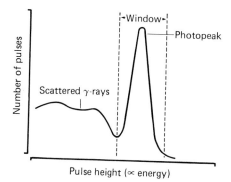

Figure 16.2 Spectrum of pulse heights produced in a scintillation detector by monoenergetic gamma rays

circuit constitutes an electrical pulse which may be measured (the size being proportional to the amount of light collected) and counted.

The assembly of crystal and photomultiplier tube is contained within a light-tight and antimagnetic shield. Sometimes integral assemblies are used, in which the light losses between crystal and photomultiplier are reduced by eliminating the glass window of the crystal's encapsulation and sealing the two components together.

If the scintillation detector is irradiated with monoenergetic gamma rays and the sizes of the pulses produced are measured, they comprise a wide range of heights with a distribution typically such as that shown in *Figure 16.2*. Those gamma ray photons which are totally absorbed in the crystal give rise to the pulses within the *photopeak*, whereas those which are partly scattered give rise to smaller pulses. The spread of pulse heights within the photopeak occurs because of statistical uncertainties at the various stages of the energy conversion processes. The *full width at half maximum* of this distribution peak expresses the ability of the detector to resolve the energies of different incident gamma rays. Typically, this value may be 11% of the pulse height for 140 keV gamma rays, and this percentage is inversely proportional to the square root of the gamma ray energy.

When one uses a radiation detector, it is usually vitally important to reduce as far as possible the number of detected events due to unwanted sources—background radiation, scattered radiation, and so on. We can do this with the scintillation detector by selecting only those pulses which occur within a given range—or *window*—of pulse heights and by adjusting this window to encompass the photopeak.

The major components of a detector system and its associated electronics, sometimes termed a *nucleonic channel*, are shown in *Figure 16.3*. The *high-voltage supply* provides the large potential difference required between cathode and anode of the photomultiplier tube—typically about 1300 V. The intermediate voltages for the dynodes are provided by the resistors of the dynode chain (*see Figure 16.1*), which are sited within the detector assembly housing. The high-voltage supply must be very stable: a drift of 1% could cause a change in gain of the photomultiplier of 7% and consequent shift of the whole pulse height spectrum.

The pulses, once *amplified*, are fed to a *pulse height analyser* which senses whether they come within the permitted range. The operator can normally select both the position and width of this range, either by adjusting 'lower level' and 'upper level' controls, or 'lower level' and 'window width', or 'energy' and '% window', according to the design of the particular instrument. Pulses may then be counted by a *scaler* controlled by a *timer*, or they may be taken to a *ratemeter* to give a continuous indication of count rate. With either system the statistical uncertainties associated with nuclear emission and detection processes will become apparent: a single reading of the scaler when divided by the preset time will give only a single estimate of the count rate, and the ratemeter output will fluctuate to an extent determined by its time constant.

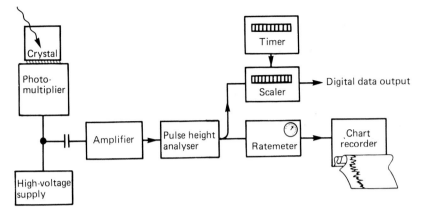

Figure 16.3 Major components of a typical nuclear detection system

Setting the ratemeter to a long time constant reduces the fluctuation but results in the system having a slow response to a change in count rate. In general, one should wait for a period equal to three times the time constant before taking a reading from a ratemeter which is responding to a change in count rate. Any nucleonic system must therefore be set up and its mode of operation determined by careful consideration of the nature of the signals to be detected.

External probe systems

The measurement of radioactivity *in vivo* may be done using scintillation detectors in a variety of configurations. The simplest is the *external probe*, which comprises a detector assembly mounted in a radiation shield with an aperture, or *collimator*, through which the radiation may pass. This will measure uptake of tracer in a region, and may be used to ascertain temporal changes in that uptake, but it will not give information on spatial distribution of activity.

The choice of material and thickness of the shield depends upon the energy of the radiation likely to be encountered; a compromise must normally be reached between the need to exclude unwanted radiation, on the one hand, and the requirements of manoeuvrability and practicality, on the other. The dimensions of the collimator are determined by the field of view required, and also in some cases by the manner in which the field of view should change with distance of the source from the detector.

For renography the following factors should be considered: the normal adult kidney measures approximately 11 × 6 cm, with a mean thickness of 3 cm and a mean depth below the lumbar skin of 5 cm. The vertical position is likely to vary by ±3 cm with postural change, and it is therefore desirable that the vertical field of view of a collimator should encompass such a variation. It should not, however, include an unnecessary proportion of non-renal (background) tissue. The field of view horizontally is further restricted by the need to exclude the contralateral kidney. A design which attempts to satisfy these criteria is shown in *Figure 16.4*. The collimator has a rectangular shape, longer vertically than horizontally. A small radioactive source moved along a line 5 cm away from the front face of the collimator would produce a bell-shaped response profile, and it is usual to measure the *field of view* as the distance between the points at which the detector would give 50% of its maximum response. For the design shown this distance is approximately 17 cm vertically and 9 cm horizontally at 5 cm from the front face. The probe shielding is built of lead 16 mm thick, which

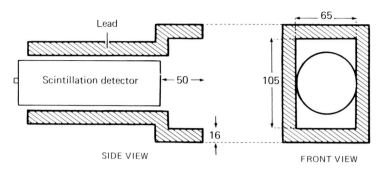

Figure 16.4 A probe design for renography. Dimensions in millimetres

would attenuate a direct beam of the gamma radiation from ^{131}I to 6% of its incident intensity. However, most unwanted photons may be expected to strike the shield at an oblique angle and so take a longer path through the lead; those striking it at 45° would, for example, suffer an attenuation down to 2.5%.

Assemblies of external probes have been designed for many purposes in nuclear medicine, and a typical system for renography, based on the probe design above, is shown in *Figure 2.4*. Such a system should allow adjustment of the position and angulation of each renal probe in its vertical plane, and of the separation of the two planes. It is preferable not to permit angulation in a horizontal plane: this might result in the contralateral kidney being brought into the field of view of a renal probe, with consequent high *cross-talk* on the renogram.

The signal from each probe is fed to a pulse-height analyser, as indicated in *Figure 16.3*. This must be adjusted to respond to pulses from the gamma rays at a given energy. Finally, the ratemeter outputs from several detectors may be sent to a multi-channel chart recorder.

The rectilinear scanner

The need to acquire information about the spatial distribution of activity was originally met by the *rectilinear scanner*. This was the first imaging device, and was the work-horse of most nuclear medicine departments before it was superseded by the gamma camera. A brief description is included here for the sake of completion.

A scintillation detector (typically based on a 125-mm diameter sodium iodide crystal) is supported on a horizontal arm which scans back and forth over an area of the patient (*Figure 16.5*). The detector is shielded by lead and has a collimator comprising multiple tapered channels, so that gamma rays can only reach it directly if they originate from the direction of a small region some distance away: the *focal depth*. The collimator is interchangeable; it must be selected according to the energy of gamma rays (which determines the thickness of lead used) and for a given compromise between the demands of *sensitivity* (large, short holes), *spatial resolution* (small, long holes) and focal depth (degree of taper).

As the detector scans back and forth, it detects the concentration of radioactivity in a small region which 'moves' within the patient through the organ of interest. Between each scan line the detector is moved a small incremental distance in a perpendicular direction, and the rectilinear pattern produced covers an area over the patient. The position of the detector is constantly mapped by a *display system*. The signal from the detector, after pulse-height analysis as previously described, is used to modulate the display.

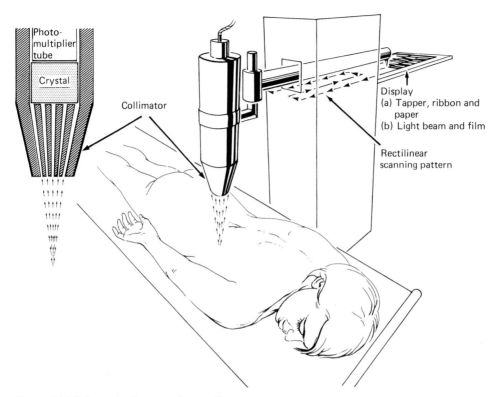

Figure 16.5 Schematic diagram of a rectilinear scanner

In a typical display system the detected scintillations cause marks to be tapped out on paper through an inked ribbon as in a typewriter. In some machines the ribbon is multicoloured and is moved according to the count rate to produce a *colour scan*. Most commonly, a photographic film is exposed to a light beam which is modulated by the detected count rate signal to produce a *photoscan*. It is also possible to use a cathode ray tube display. Whichever form of display is adopted, it can only be an approximate representation of the digital information acquired by the detector, and it is sometimes considered advantageous to record the digital information electronically for subsequent processing and replay.

The scanner's speed, line-spacing and area of view may all be adjusted to suit a given study and patient, but a typical scan may take 15–20 minutes to complete. The resultant single image represents the distribution of activity during that time, and the device cannot, therefore, be used for dynamic studies.

The scintillation camera

The scintillation camera (or gamma camera) was first described by H. O. Anger in 1957. The detector comprises a single large crystal of sodium iodide up to 500 mm in diameter and usually 12.5 mm thick, coupled to an array of photomultiplier tubes, typically 37 of them, as shown schematically in *Figure 16.6*. All the photomultiplier tubes are connected to a complex circuit, termed 'resistor matrix' in the diagram, which is really a kind of analogue computer. After each scintillation in the crystal this circuit produces three simultaneous signals. The x and y signals represent the cartesian co-ordinates of

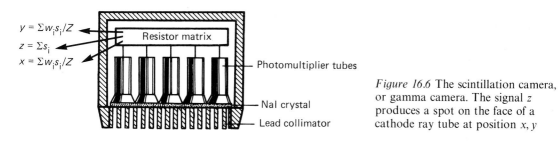

$y = \Sigma w_i s_i / Z$

$z = \Sigma s_i$

$x = \Sigma w_i s_i / Z$

Resistor matrix

Photomultiplier tubes

NaI crystal

Lead collimator

Figure 16.6 The scintillation camera, or gamma camera. The signal z produces a spot on the face of a cathode ray tube at position x, y

the position of the scintillation; each is a pulse whose height is a weighted sum of the pulse heights from the photomultiplier tubes where the weights are predetermined by the position of each tube in the array. The z signal represents the total amount of light emitted and is the simple sum of all the pulses. As with other forms of scintillation detector, the latter is proportional to the energy deposited in the crystal, and it may therefore be used to select detected events corresponding to totally absorbed primary gamma photons from a particular radionuclide.

The x and y signals are used to direct the spot on a cathode ray tube and a picture is built up on the film of an open-shutter camera which views the screen. A second, 'persistence', cathode ray tube may also be used to give an instantaneous visual assessment which is helpful when positioning the patient.

The time taken to record each scintillation may be of the order of $2\,\mu s$, so that very high counting rates can be detected. For a typical static imaging application, however, the detected count rate might be 2000 per second; as approximately 400 000 counts are needed to produce a good picture, this takes a few minutes. A gamma camera is shown in *Figure 16.7*.

The collimator is a vital part of the instrument. Anger's original design incorporated a 'pinhole' collimator whereby the gamma rays formed an inverted image of the

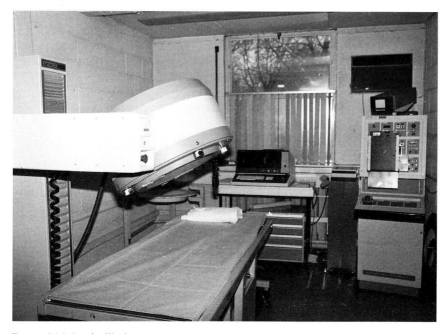

Figure 16.7 A scintillation camera (gamma camera)

distribution onto the crystal in a manner analogous to that of the pinhole camera. This design suffered from low efficiency and a magnification of the image which depended upon the distance of the source. Most later designs have used multiple parallel holes as indicated in *Figure 16.6*. Only gamma rays from a preferred direction (perpendicular to the plane of the detector) may strike the crystal, and thus an image is formed of the projection of the activity distribution in this direction. Alternative designs include the diverging collimator (which extends the field of view) and the converging collimator (which reduces the field of view and can enhance spatial resolution), but both of these introduce spatial distortions.

Even having chosen to use a parallel-hole design, however, it is necessary for the designer of the instrument to provide for changing the collimator, and for most users to store at least two or three collimators. There are two main reasons for this. The first is to be able to select a thickness of lead to match the energy of the gamma rays. Septa of 0.3 mm thickness may be sufficient in a collimator designed for the 140-keV gamma rays of ^{99m}Tc, whereas a thickness of 2 mm may be necessary for the higher energies emitted by ^{67}Ga. It is undesirable to use a collimator designed for high energies with low energy gamma rays because the efficiency of the detector will be sub-optimal, and furthermore the image may have a visible collimator pattern superimposed upon it.

The second major reason for selecting a collimator is to choose a level of trade-off between *resolution* and *sensitivity*. A collimator comprising many small holes will have good resolution, but poorer sensitivity than one with fewer, larger holes. It may be necessary to sacrifice some resolution in the interest of improving the sensitivity (and hence shortening imaging time or enabling reduction of patient dose). Gamma cameras are often supplied with a choice of 'general purpose' and 'high resolution' low-energy collimators in addition to medium- or high-energy collimators.

In contrast to the rectilinear scanner, the resolution of the gamma camera fitted with a parallel-hole collimator is best at the surface of the collimator and falls off gradually with source distance. The shorter the collimator, the more rapidly resolution falls off with distance.

For the gamma camera there exists a further limitation on spatial resolution: the intrinsic resolution of the detector. This arises principally because the detector must make a 'decision' about the position of each scintillation based upon the number of photoelectrons liberated by the photocathodes of each of the relevant photomultiplier tubes. After the detection of a given intensity of scintillation, this number has a statistical uncertainty, and, hence, the estimate of position of any given scintillation is itself subject to error.

In practice, a fine radioactive line source placed in front of the camera would give an image whose variation of intensity could be described by a bell-shaped profile. The full width at half maximum (FWHM) of this line spread function may be as little as 2 mm when measured at the surface of a modern gamma camera detector. However, if a collimator is used and the source is placed 100 mm deep in a large scattering medium, then the FWHM of the line spread function is, at best, about 7.5 mm. This may therefore be taken as a good indication of the limit of resolution of currently available gamma cameras. When attempting to interpret these figures in terms of the minimum size of detectable lesions or features, a number of problems arise: the lesion may be superimposed on normal active tissue or on a radioactive background; the underlying activity may itself be varying; the image produced may be statistically 'noisy'. In general, a better effective resolution can be expected from a technique which involves the detection of positive uptake of tracer than from a technique which demands the detection of a 'cold' region within a sea of activity. Renal space-occupying lesions, for example, detected as cold areas on a renal scan may not be seen if smaller than 15 mm across, whereas the ureters, with only a 1 mm internal diameter, may be demonstrated if filled with a suitable radiopharmaceutical.

The performance of a gamma camera may be described by assessment of the following characteristics.

1. *Uniformity of sensitivity*. This describes the response of the instrument to a uniformly distributed source of activity (a 'flood field'). The standard deviation of 1000 picture elements from a flood image might be $\pm 10\%$ or higher for the Anger camera as described above, because of variations in sensitivity, photomultiplier gain and electronic components. Recent developments, however (*see* below), have reduced this figure to the order of $\pm 3\%$ for modern gamma camera systems.
2. *Spatial resolution*, as indicated above, is a measure of the spread of the image of a line or point source, and may be subdivided into the *intrinsic* resolution of the detector, and the *system* resolution of the instrument including collimator.
3. *Spatial linearity* is a measure of the fidelity by which straight lines across the source are reproduced as straight lines on the image.
4. *Sensitivity* of the system using a given collimator is a measure of the detected count rate in response to unit activity in the source.
5. *Count rate capability* is the ability of the system to detect high count rates from large quantities of activity—important for rapid dynamic studies particularly when all the bolus of injected activity may be in the field of view at one time. It is important to assess this using realistic scattering conditions and energy windows (because gamma rays outside the photopeak may contribute to the loss of response at high count rates). A typical camera may show 10% count loss at about 40 000 counts per second and may actually saturate at about 70 000 cps with normal settings. Some systems incorporate a 'high count rate' switch which permits the detection of much higher count rates at the expense of deterioration of quality of image.
6. *Energy resolution*, as described on page 217, is a measure of the spread of pulse-heights for a given incident gamma ray energy. In a gamma camera the 'energy' signal is the sum of outputs from many photomultiplier tubes. Variations in individual responses can thus lead to poor overall resolution and consequent loss of quality through the inability of pulse-height analysis to separate direct from scattered gamma rays.

Improvements in gamma camera design

During recent years there has been steady improvement in camera performance arising from a number of technical developments. First, the sensitivity has been enhanced by the use of more efficient and specially shaped photomultipliers, and by the development of the light guide interface between crystal and photomultiplier. The use of a thinner crystal (10 mm instead of 12.5 mm) has improved the resolution (by reducing scatter) for low-energy gamma rays without significantly impairing sensitivity. Developments in the electronic amplifiers and pulse-position circuitry have further improved resolution across the field of view, and, by processing pulses faster, have improved count rate capability.

Most significant has been the introduction of microprocessor circuitry to perform two major types of correction to the detected pulses before they contribute to the image. The first is to correct for the variation in pulse-height response across the field of view by means of a stored matrix of correction values (the so-called 'energy correction'). The second is to adjust the computed position co-ordinates of the detected event according to a stored map of known distortions—thus achieving a 'linearity correction'. When these two corrections have been applied the non-uniformity of sensitivity over the field of view may be reduced to the order of $\pm 3\%$, thus rendering redundant the old and unsatisfactory method of uniformity correction by means of a computer-stored map of sensitivity factors.

Although electronics and microprocessor technology continue to advance, the spatial resolution of modern systems is governed by the collimator. With current concepts, therefore, the quality of images produced at depth in a patient is unlikely to improve dramatically.

Display of images

In the standard 'analogue' gamma camera display system, the image appears as a distribution of dots on a cathode ray tube (CRT), integrated over a period of time on photographic film. Some gamma camera systems are now entirely 'digital', which means that the x and y co-ordinates of each scintillation are classified into one of, say, 128 values, and the resulting image comprises a pattern of squares (pixels) of varying density as produced by a computer system (see below). Most studies involve the production of several images; this may be done by changing the photographic film manually between exposures. More conveniently, a multi-formatting device is used which projects successive images onto different parts of a sheet of film. Rapid dynamic sequences are obviously best recorded using a multi-formatter.

The electronic position signals produced by the gamma camera may be fed directly to a digital computer system. Although the main purpose of this is to undertake quantitative analysis of dynamic studies, it also permits a variety of alternative display modes for images. The clinician may study the image information by viewing a CRT screen directly. The images displayed may be adjusted so that the optimum range of intensities is used to present the information. Dynamic studies may be replayed rapidly as cine sequences. In some cases colour is used to represent different levels of intensity.

Emission tomography

Conventional images obtained with a gamma camera are projections of a three-dimensional distribution. The view obtained from, for example, the 'anterior' is formed by gamma rays emitted from all parts of the organ and tissues in front of and behind it. Tomographic techniques aim to reproduce the distribution in a set of layers or 'cuts'. By acquiring a set of images from many projection angles around the patient it is possible to collect sufficient information from the three-dimensional distribution for a computer to reconstruct images of cross-sections. *Figure 16.8* shows one camera system designed to produce such data. It may 'step and shoot' 64 or 128 times in a complete revolution about the supine patient while each image is stored in a computer system. The sequence of images thus acquired may be replayed as a dynamic sequence at a speed far greater than that used for acquisition; these images display the distribution as if the patient is being rotated in front of the camera and can be very helpful in demonstrating the distribution prior to further processing.

If a single profile across the patient is extracted from each image at the same level, then a set of projection data is available from which the computer can reconstruct a transverse axial cross-section. The computation is usually done by modifying each projection by a suitable filter function and back-projecting the modified data onto an image plane in a manner similar to that adopted in X-ray computed tomography (CT) scanning. The algorithm should, however, in the case of radionuclide *emission* tomography, take account of the attenuation suffered by gamma radiation between the source (within the patient) and detector. This is a difficult problem and the solutions are necessarily approximate because they must make assumptions about the pattern of attenuation.

A whole set of parallel transverse sections may be computed, the resulting images being the nuclear medicine equivalent of X-ray CT images. By using a gamma camera the whole set of sections is acquired simultaneously, but it should be noted that the

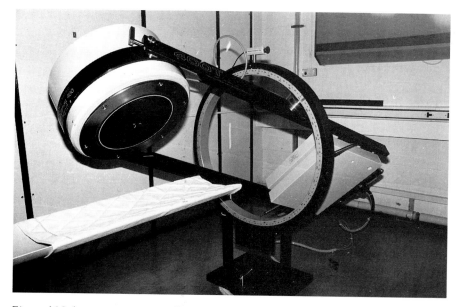

Figure 16.8 A gamma camera on a rotating gantry suitable for emission tomography

complete acquisition in practice takes a minimum of 10 minutes and in many cases may be considerably longer, depending upon the activity concentration and the sensitivity of the camera system. During the acquisition period the distribution of activity should remain sensibly constant; the technique is therefore unsuitable for dynamic studies. It has considerable potential, however, in 'static' situations such as DMSA imaging.

The more sophisticated computer software packages permit the derivation of longitudinal sectional images (sagittal, coronal or oblique) from the reconstructed transverse axial sections.

The technique outlined above is sometimes termed 'single photon emission computed tomography' (SPECT) in order to distinguish it from positron emission tomography (PET) in which the properties of positron-emitting radionuclides are exploited. A positron is stopped close to its point of emission, yielding a pair of gamma ray photons emitted in exactly opposite directions. If both photons are detected simultaneously by opposing detectors, then a 'line of sight' is established for the source. From many such lines an image of the distribution may be reconstructed. Positron imaging equipment is more complex and expensive than that for single photon imaging, and positron-emitting radionuclides are less widely available. Although PET has had significant impact on pure research (notably in neurophysiology and cardiology) it has not yet become a widely adopted routine diagnostic technique.

The nuclear medicine computer system

Data acquired by a gamma camera may be stored and processed by a nuclear medicine computer system. In the system shown in *Figure 16.9* two gamma cameras, in separate rooms, are connected to the computer. The *hardware* associated with each gamma camera comprises a terminal from which data acquisition is controlled, and a monitor for displaying the images. Data analysis may be carried out in another room using a terminal which has associated with it a display monitor from which images may be

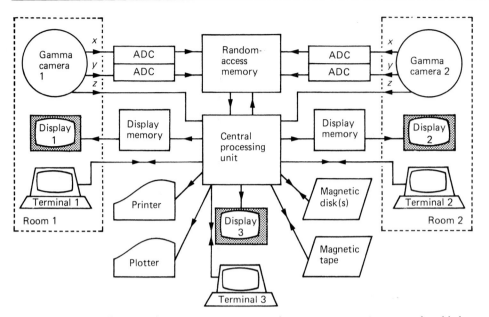

Figure 16.9 Block diagram of a computer system serving two gamma cameras and a third terminal for simultaneous processing

photographed, a printer, and a plotter for output of results in graphical form. Any terminal can direct data storage onto magnetic cartridge disk, floppy disk or magnetic tape.

In order for the system to function a set of programs is required, and these comprise the *software*. In addition to the standard software package supplied by the manufacturer there is usually a facility to accommodate user-written programs.

Acquisition of digital images

The x and y position signals from a gamma camera are both usually analogue representations of the co-ordinates of each scintillation. Two analogue-to-digital converters (ADCs) are used and their outputs are fed directly to the memory of the computer. Each time a scintillation is detected within the preselected energy window the gamma camera sends a z signal which instructs the computer to read the values of the ADC outputs and store one count. Thus, as gamma rays are detected by the camera, x–y co-ordinate pairs representing the positions of scintillations stream into the computer from the ADCs. This information may be stored either in *frame mode* or in *list mode*, the former being the more common.

In *frame mode* a digital image is built up as the counts are acquired. The digital image is a square matrix of individual elements which contains a representation of the field of view of the camera. Typically the matrix may consist of 4096 picture elements, or pixels, in a 64×64 array. The computer sets aside a number of memory locations corresponding to the numbers of pixels and each scintillation in the camera crystal producing a z signal to the computer (i.e. lying within the energy window) causes the contents of the location defined by the x–y pair to be incremented by one. Thus an image is built up with each pixel containing the number of counts acquired at its particular co-ordinates. Upon termination of acquisition the digital image is transferred from memory to one of the storage devices, usually a magnetic disk.

In *list mode* (sometimes termed *serial mode*) no images or matrices result directly from the acquisition. The values of successive co-ordinates are stored in sequential memory locations forming a *list* of x–y pairs. In addition, time markers are inserted in the list data at regular intervals, typically every 1 or 10 msec. The list is transferred to disk on completion of acquisition. The data may subsequently be formatted into one or many images of any matrix size or type and of any time interval within the acquisition period.

Compared with frame mode, list mode acquisition uses large amounts of memory and disk space. For example, in frame mode, a 64×64 image matrix requires 4096 storage locations regardless of how many counts are stored in the image. In list mode, using 1-msec time markers the number of storage locations required is given by the number of counts multiplied by 2 (an x–y pair for each count) plus the length of acquisition in milliseconds. For even a small study of 10-second duration and 200k counts this is approximately 100 times as much storage space as for the equivalent frame mode study. List mode does, however, give flexibility in setting image parameters and is useful for certain applications where rapid first circulation studies over selected time periods are required, such as in nuclear cardiology. List mode acquisition is generally of no use for renal studies.

Two types of frame mode acquisition are employed for renal studies: *static* and *dynamic*.

For a *static* acquisition the computer captures data for a preset time limit or a preset number of counts and then waits for the operator to initiate another acquisition or terminate the patient study. During the intervening wait the operator may wish to reposition the patient for a different view or alter the preset time or count limit. In *dynamic* mode the initiation of one image acquisition automatically follows completion of the previous image, producing a sequence of consecutive frames. The operator specifies a preset frame time and the number of frames. No information is lost between frames because, while one image is being acquired into memory, the previous image is being written to disk. Currently, nuclear medicine computers can acquire up to 100 frames per second. However, such high frame rates would rapidly fill up the storage devices and are rarely required. Most dynamic studies operate with frame times of between 1 second and a few minutes.

Display of digital images

The individual elements of a digital image each contain a value. To enable the human eye to see the image the values are converted to brightness or colour levels by a translation table, which may have from eight to 512 levels.

In *raster* mode each image pixel is displayed as a dot, so the display of a 64×64 matrix requires 4096 dots. The 4096 dot positions are scanned in raster mode by the electron beam of the oscilloscope, and the brightness of each dot depends on the voltage applied to the electron gun. Immediately prior to outputting the image the computer determines the maximum count in the image and allocates this to the highest value in the translation table. If the translation table has 16 intervals the rest of the pixel values are divided into the range and converted to 15 incremental voltage levels. A raster scan must be refreshed 30 times a second by reading the digital matrix from the computer memory. The computer may have a special *remote memory* associated with, and used only for, the display device, allowing it to perform other tasks while the image is displayed.

A special type of raster mode device is a storage display. In this case each pixel is represented by a small area of screen within which many dots may be displayed. Each dot has the same intensity, and the brightness of a particular pixel is determined by the number of dots within the area. The phosphor coating on a storage display screen has a long persistence time so that the image needs to be projected only once although it may take several seconds for the entire display to appear.

The most commonly used form of display in nuclear medicine computer systems is the black-and-white or colour video monitor. These operate in a similar way to a standard television with an electron beam scan of 525 or 625 lines, the intensity of the beam being modulated to produce different brightness levels in the image. The time taken for a complete scan of 625 lines is one-thirtieth of a second, and, like the raster mode display, the image is refreshed 30 times per second. Also like the raster mode, the video display has an associated remote memory into which a digital image is loaded and from which it is continually sent to the video monitor by a video interface. For black-and-white video a single translation table is required to convert the range of count levels into brightness levels. For colour video three translation tables are required for each of three electron guns providing the three primary colours, red, green and blue. Some computer systems offer a facility for modifying the translation tables so that the operator may define a different colour display scale or even, for special applications, a non-linear black-and-white display scale. With more than about 32 levels of colour or intensity the transitions between adjacent levels appear continuous to the human eye.

Hard copy of images may be obtained photographically. Alternatively the image may be plotted on a dot-matrix printer with fine dot resolution. A line printer produces a whole line of characters at a time instead of printing them one by one. Special 'characters' may be generated using the dot density technique in a similar way to that of storage display systems

Matrix size and type

The amount of storage space used by a digital image depends on the matrix size which may range from 32 × 32 to 256 × 256 pixels. It also depends on the matrix type which can be either *word mode* or *byte mode*. In *word mode* images each pixel occupies one full word of computer memory. Most minicomputer systems for nuclear medicine use words of 16 bits, each bit being a 1 or 0 of binary notation. The largest number of levels which can be represented by 16 bits is 2^{16} or 65 536 so the highest possible number of counts which can be stored in one pixel of a word mode image is 65 535 (the first level being 0). In *byte mode* images each pixel occupies only 8 bits (= one byte) so the highest possible number of counts which can be stored in one pixel is $2^8 - 1$ or 255. As soon as 255 is exceeded the count becomes 0 and again continues incrementing. This recycling of count levels can cause strange effects on byte mode images if it is allowed to occur. Some computers, however, automatically allow for byte mode overflow during acquisition by detecting when any pixel reaches the 255 limit and dividing the whole image by 2, after which acquisition continues as normal. The number of times the image is divided is recorded as a scaling factor and stored with the image. In any subsequent analysis a program can use the scaling factor to determine the counts within the image. Byte mode images have the advantage of requiring half the storage space of word mode images using the same matrix size, but the disadvantages are a slight loss of accuracy in determining acquired counts and an increased complexity in performing calculations and manipulations on the images by computer program.

Table 16.1 summarizes the amounts of computer memory and storage required for the eight combinations of matrix size and type. Within the constraint of storage limits, the prime consideration affecting the choice of matrix is the information required from the patient test. A larger matrix size (one with a larger number of elements) gives a better image resolution because the pixels are smaller. This effect is illustrated in *Figure 16.10* where an analogue image from a 400-mm field of view camera is shown digitized into 64 × 64, 128 × 128 and 256 × 256 matrices with pixel widths of 6.25, 3.13 and 1.56 mm respectively. For a given total number of counts in an image there are fewer counts in a smaller pixel and thus a greater variation in pixel counts across the image

TABLE 16.1. Matrix sizes and types for image digitization

Matrix size	Matrix type	Number of elements	Memory required (words)	Pixel width (mm)*
32 × 32	Byte	1 024	512	12.5
32 × 32	Word	1 024	1 024	
64 × 64	Byte	4 096	2 048	6.25
64 × 64	Word	4 096	4 096	
128 × 128	Byte	16 384	8 192	3.13
128 × 128	Word	16 384	16 384	
256 × 256	Byte	65 536	32 768	1.56
256 × 256	Word	65 536	65 536	

* Assuming 400-mm total field of view

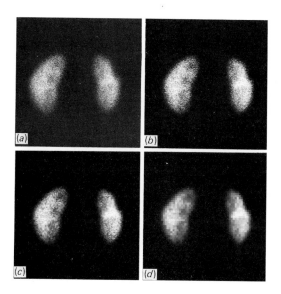

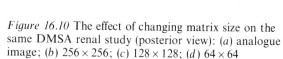

Figure 16.10 The effect of changing matrix size on the same DMSA renal study (posterior view): (*a*) analogue image; (*b*) 256 × 256; (*c*) 128 × 128; (*d*) 64 × 64

due to poorer count statistics. This causes a digital image on a larger matrix size to appear noisier, although on the smaller matrix size of 64 × 64 the individual pixels become visible. Therefore the larger matrix sizes are used for static acquisitions where generally a higher number of counts is acquired and the resolution of detail is important. In a dynamic study where good resolution is not paramount a smaller matrix size of 64 × 64 is usually used, not only because of lower image counts but also because of storage space considerations which lead, in addition, to the choice of byte mode. Dynamic renal studies are usually acquired in 64 × 64 byte mode. Static studies may be acquired in 128 × 128, or 256 × 256 byte mode, unless the computer cannot handle byte overflows or a special analysis program cannot easily process byte mode data, in which cases word mode must be employed.

Storage devices

A computer's memory has the capacity to hold only a few images at any one time, and an external storage device is essential to the successful operation of a nuclear medicine computer system. Three types of storage in common use are:

1. Floppy disk
2. Hard disk
3. Magnetic tape.

The floppy disk is the smallest and most portable of the storage media. The two surfaces of the disk are coated with a magnetic film similar to that used on magnetic tapes. The film can hold digital data in binary form with magnetic domains representing single bits of information. Each of the two disk surfaces may hold approximately 0.6 megabytes of data (1 byte = 8 bits). The disk is loaded into a disk drive which grips the disk at the centre and spins it at 360 rpm. As the disk rotates a read/write head moves radially across the surface to access information. Some floppy disk drives can access both surfaces with a head for each surface, giving a capacity of 1.2 megabytes for double-sided use. The time taken to access a piece of data depends on the previous position of the read/write heads, a typical access time being about 500 msec.

A cartridge disk unit may contain one or several hard disks, each known as a platter. A single platter cartridge is easily and quickly interchangeable whereas a multi-platter unit is often never removed except for servicing, and is sometimes termed a 'fixed' disk. A hard disk is made of aluminium coated with a magnetic film, similar to that of the floppy disk, on which binary data can be recorded. A single platter unit has a capacity of 2.5 or 5 megabytes depending on whether it has a 'low' or 'high' density magnetic coating. Unlike the floppy disk system the read/write head does not come into contact with a hard disk but rides on a cushion of air 1 μm above the surface. Any particle of debris such as smoke can damage the head or scratch the surface and in severe cases may cause a 'head crash'. It is therefore essential that magnetic disks be treated with great care. The access time will depend on the position of the head, but an average value is about 100 msec, five times faster than for a floppy disk. A multi-platter disk drive unit has a read/write head for each platter. The rotation speed is 3600 rpm giving a fast access time of about 40 msec. Storage capacities may be up to 300 megabytes depending on make and model.

A particular design of hard disk drive, known as the *Winchester*, uses a sealed unit enclosing heads and disk surfaces. This overcomes the dust and debris problem, but the disks are not interchangeable.

Magnetic tape is obtainable in lengths of 600, 1200, and 2400 feet with a data density of 800 bytes per inch. This gives a total capacity of 23 megabytes for a 2400-foot tape. The tape drive unit operates at 25 inches per second, so to access data at the far end of the tape may take over 3 minutes.

The different types of storage media are compared in *Table 16.2*. Most computer systems include either single- or multi-platter cartridge disk units. Such units have the fastest access time, which becomes an important factor when processing large amounts of data and when rapid dynamic studies are undertaken (as with some applications in

TABLE 16.2. Comparison of different storage devices

Storage medium	Speed	Typical access time (msec)	Number of magnetic surfaces	Capacity		
				Megabytes	Images 64 × 64 byte mode	Dynamic studies (75 images)
Floppy disk	360 rpm	500	1 or 2	0.6 or 1.2	150 or 300	2 or 4
Cartridge disk (single platter)	1500 rpm	100	2	2.5 or 5.0	600 or 1200	8 or 16
Multi-platter disk	3600 rpm	40	3 to 15	20 to 300	5000 to 75 000	65 to 1000
Magnetic tape	640 mm/s	1 minute	1	23	5750	75

nuclear cardiology). A disk unit is generally regarded as an essential integral feature of the nuclear medicine computer system.

However, cartridge disks, especially the multi-platter type, are also the most expensive of the storage media. The single-platter cartridge disk could easily be filled in one day since only 8 or 16 average-length dynamic studies would reach the total capacity. Even a multi-platter disk would fill up within a week or two in a busy department. For long-term storage the floppy disk or magnetic tape media are best because of their low cost. A 2400-foot magnetic tape can store an average of 75 dynamic studies. The major disadvantage of magnetic tape is long access time; it is therefore normally used only for archival purposes. Although floppy disks cost slightly more than magnetic tape in terms of a cost per image, they are extremely portable and take up little physical storage space.

Data analysis

All computer systems require a master program, or operating system, which controls operations within the central processing unit, and the flow of data to or from any interfaces to which peripheral devices may be connected.

For a nuclear medicine system, the basic requirements of a software package are:

1. The ability to acquire images in a variety of matrix sizes and types both in static mode and in a range of dynamic frame rates.
2. The ability to display the images, with variable contrast on black-and-white or colour monitors in static or dynamic mode.
3. Long-term storage of image data.
4. A facility for generating regions of interest over selected parts of the image and generating curves of counts vs. time for those regions.
5. A method of producing a hard copy of any data analysis.

Other functions may allow manipulation and processing of images and curves. An additional useful feature is the facility to incorporate user-written programs into the system which allows the user to tailor the system to departmental requirements.

Regions of interest may be delineated by the operator by moving a cursor on a displayed image to outline a specific area. The cursor may be moved by certain keys on the keyboard, a joystick or a light pen which appear to draw on the display. *Figure 2.3* showed regions of interest delineated over renal images using a joystick. Several regions may be stored and the counts within each region printed out. For a dynamic study each region count may be determined for each image in the sequence to produce a curve of counts against time. This may be converted to count per pixel or, since the frame rate is known, count rate against time. A curve, or set of curves, may undergo further processing by a user program to extract characteristic parameters and perhaps convert count rate within an organ to percentage of administered radioactivity. The results of such analyses are shown in the many examples of gamma camera renograms in Parts 1 and 2.

Further reading

BELCHER, E. H. and VETTER, H. (1971) *Radioisotopes in Medical Diagnosis*, London: Butterworths
HINE, G. J. (1974) *Instrumentation in Nuclear Medicine*, Vol. II, New York: Academic Press
KUHL, D. E. (ed.) (1983) *Principles of Radionuclide Emission Imaging*, Oxford: Pergamon
WAGNER, H. N. Jr (ed.) (1968) *Principles of Nuclear Medicine*, Philadelphia: Saunders

17 Radiopharmaceuticals

H. J. Testa

A radiopharmaceutical is a radioactive compound used in medicine for the purpose of diagnosis or therapy. It should have a constant composition, and it should be radionuclidically and radiochemically pure; it should also be non-toxic and specific for the organ or system under study.

For diagnostic use the radionuclide should have a short physical half-life; ideally this should be long enough to permit completion of the test but short enough to avoid unnecessary radiation to the patient. Preferably the radionuclide should emit only gamma radiation; for external detection, and in particular for gamma camera studies, the energy of the gamma rays should be in the range of 100–200 keV. The physical characteristics of radionuclides used in this work are listed in *Table 15.1* on page 206.

The choice of a radiopharmaceutical for investigation of the kidney is usually based on one of the classic aspects of renal function: glomerular filtration, tubular reabsorption and tubular secretion. In addition some compounds are useful because they become fixed in the tubular cells. The principal radiopharmaceuticals used in renal studies are summarized in *Table 17.1*. It is important to recognize that the use of a single radiopharmaceutical could serve more than one purpose; for example, labelled sodium ortho-iodohippurate (OIH) can be used to measure effective renal plasma flow, to perform classic renography and to obtain functional images of the kidneys from which several other parameters of renal function may be derived.

Radiopharmaceuticals used for renal perfusion studies

The normal 'renal fraction' (the portion of the cardiac output which passes through the kidneys) is approximately 25%. This represents an average renal blood-flow of the order of 1200 ml/min. This high rate of perfusion allows the production of fast dynamic images of the first passage of a radioactive tracer through the kidneys—radionuclide angiography—by injecting a bolus of radioactivity into an antecubital vein (*see* Chapters 3 and 7).

Any ^{99m}Tc-labelled radiopharmaceutical is suitable for this kind of study including technetium in its ionic form of pertechnetate (TcO_4^-). This is easily obtained by means of a 'generator', which consists of the parent radionuclide, molybdenum-99, adsorbed onto an alumina column and contained within a radiation

TABLE 17.1. Principal renal radiopharmaceuticals

Common name	Full name	Radionuclide	Structure	Physiology	Applications
Technetium	Sodium pertechnetate	^{99m}Tc	$Na^+TcO_4^-$	Diffusible ionic tracer	Perfusion
DTPA	Diethylenetriamine-pentaacetic acid	^{99m}Tc	$(HOOC\cdot CH_2)_2 N\cdot CH_2\cdot CH_2\cdot N(CH_2\cdot COOH)\cdot CH_2\cdot CH_2\cdot N(CH_2\cdot COOH)_2$	Glomerular filtration	1. GFR 2. Perfusion 3. Imaging 4. Renogram 5. Relative function
EDTA	Ethylenediamine-tetraacetic acid	^{51}Cr	$(HOOC\cdot CH_2)_2 N\cdot CH_2\cdot CH_2\cdot N(CH_2\cdot COOH)_2$	Glomerular filtration	GFR
OIH	Sodium ortho-iodohippurate	^{123}I ^{125}I ^{131}I	(iodophenyl)$\cdot CONH\cdot CH_2\cdot COO^-\cdot Na^+$	Tubular secretion	1. Renogram 2. Imaging 3. ERPF
DMSA	Dimercaptosuccinic acid	^{99m}Tc	$HOOC-CH(SH)-CH(SH)-COOH$	Tubular secretion and concentration	1. Imaging 2. Relative function 3. Detection of scarring
Gluconate	D-Gluconic acid	^{99m}Tc	$HO\cdot H_2C-CH(OH)-CH(OH)-CH(H)-CH(OH)-COOH$	Glomerular filtration, tubular reabsorption	1. Imaging 2. Perfusion

| Glucoheptonate GHA | D-Glucoheptanoic acid | ^{99m}Tc | $$\begin{array}{ccccc} H & H & OH & H & H \\ | & | & | & | & | \\ HO\cdot H_2C-C-C-C-C-C-COOH \\ | & | & | & | & | \\ OH & OH & H & OH & OH \end{array}$$ | Glomerular filtration, tubular reabsorption | 1. Imaging 2. Perfusion |
| Gallium | Gallium citrate | ^{67}Ga | $$\begin{array}{c} COOH \\ | \\ HOOC\cdot CH_2-C-CH_2\cdot COOH \\ | \\ OH \end{array}$$ | Protein and neutrophil binding | Detection of inflammatory processes |

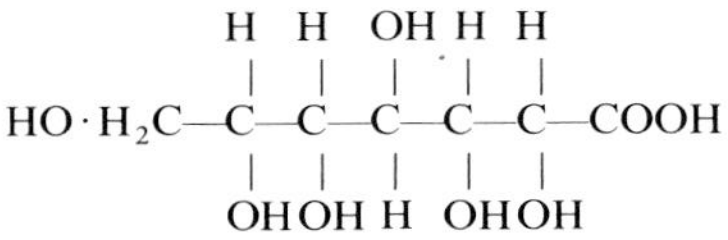

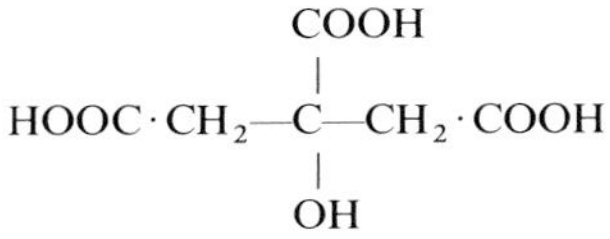

Generally the structures of metal complexes and chelates in solution are poorly understood. There may often be several different forms in equilibrium. Thus only the ligands are shown above. For further information on chelates of DTPA and EDTA, see Noll, Siefert and Munze (1983); on gluconates and glucoheptonates see Russell and Speiser (1980) and Sawyer (1984)

shield. The elution of this column with saline produces a solution containing the daughter, technetium-99m, as pertechnetate. Modern generators are designed so that successive elutions can be carried out in order to provide a re-usable source of sterile material over a period determined by the half-life of the parent (67 hours), giving a useful life of approximately 7 days. The half-life of ^{99m}Tc itself is only 6 hours and this, combined with its monoenergetic gamma radiation of 140 keV and its lack of particulate emission, makes it an excellent choice of radionuclide.

In most circumstances perfusion studies of the kidney are combined with further imaging or renographic procedures. Either ^{99m}Tc-gluconate or ^{99m}Tc-DTPA (see below) is then the radiopharmaceutical of choice. The main clinical application of perfusion studies is in the evaluation of patency of the renal arteries (renal artery stenosis, renal trauma, renal transplantation), in the investigation of aortic lesions which may affect renal perfusion and in some cases of chronic renal failure in which the presence or absence of renal perfusion may suggest whether or not renal dialysis is indicated.

Radiopharmaceuticals used for clearance studies

Glomerular filtration rate

A fraction of the plasma perfusing the kidneys is filtered at the glomeruli; the volume of this ultrafiltrate expressed in ml/minute is defined as the glomerular filtration rate (GFR). The formation of this fluid, which has the same concentration as the plasma, appears to be regulated only by hydrodynamic laws and does not require energy expenditure by the glomerular cells. The compounds used to measure GFR must have a molecular weight of less than 5000 in order to achieve maximum filtration through the glomerular membrane. They should be physiologically inert, non-ionic, be unbound to plasma proteins and should not be reabsorbed or excreted by the renal tubules.

The determination of the GFR using non-labelled substances such as inulin or creatinine was performed in animals and man for many years before radioactive compounds became available (Smith, 1956; Pitts, 1963; Berlyne et al., 1964; Bennett and Porter, 1971). Indeed, the clearance of inulin for measuring GFR has become the standard against which the elimination by the kidney of other substances is assessed. However, the use of non-labelled inulin requires rather cumbersome procedures involving time-consuming spectrophotometric methods and bladder catheterization; it is not surprising to note that, when labelled inulin became available, it was immediately employed to measure GFR. Inulin may be labelled in several ways: ^{14}C-inulin (Cotlove, 1955) emits beta particles, necessitates liquid scintillation counting of samples and precludes techniques involving external detection. The iodinated forms (^{125}I and ^{131}I) have been shown to lack stability in vivo (Bianchi, 1972) and the radionuclide may be eliminated by extrarenal pathways. Chromium-51 is probably the radionuclide of choice, and ^{51}Cr-inulin has been shown to give clearances which correlate well with those obtained using unlabelled inulin (Materson, Johnson and Perez-Stable, 1969).

Labelled radiological contrast media have also been used: diatrizoate—available commercially as Hypaque or Renografin—has been labelled with ^{131}I and used for the measurement of GFR. Iothalamate, labelled with ^{125}I or ^{131}I, has also been validated against inulin clearance. These compounds are partially excreted by an extrarenal pathway, particularly in cases of renal insufficiency (Bianchi, 1972); whereas this does not mitigate against their use in a method which determines both urine and plasma activities, it does invalidate their application to a plasma disappearance method.

The approach which has received most attention in recent years is the use of chelates of radioactive metals. The molecular weight of these compounds is of the order of 400. They are mainly extracted by the kidneys, although a small fraction may be excreted via the biliary system. The chelating agents ethylenediamine tetraacetic acid (EDTA) and diethylenetriamine pentaacetic acid (DTPA) have been labelled with a number of radionuclides, and their success for the measurement of GFR would appear to rest on the stability of the compounds *in vivo*. ^{51}Cr-EDTA has probably received the most attention for this purpose. Its clearance has been shown to correlate well with, but be slightly less than, that of inulin (Garnett, Parsons and Veall, 1967), and its stability and lack of extrarenal clearance make it eminently suitable for plasma disappearance analysis (Chantler *et al.*, 1969).

Chelates of other metals (La, Co, In, Yb) have attracted interest, but none with such potential for convenience and reduction of radiation dose as [99m]Tc. After ^{99m}Tc-DTPA had been introduced for renal imaging (*see* Chapter 3) its use for GFR measurement was precluded by poor stability both *in vitro* and *in vivo* (Hauser, Atkins and Nelson, 1970; Blaufox, Chervu and Freeman, 1975). However, later studies with commercially produced materials have shown very good correlation with ^{51}Cr-EDTA (Hilson, Mistry and Maisey, 1976), and developments in the labelling technique (Chervu *et al.*, 1977; Carlsen *et al.*, 1979) further emphasize this view. Russell and colleagues (1983) have shown that systematic errors are due to protein binding, and that accuracy may be very good if the protein binding is measured and the calculation of GFR performed on the unbound fraction. The ideal characteristics of ^{99m}Tc and the availability of suitable commercial kits now make this compound the tracer of choice for routine clinical estimation of GFR.

Effective renal plasma flow

Effective renal plasma flow (ERPF) is the portion of the renal plasma flow which perfuses the renal secretory tissue, excluding the small fraction which perfuses the perirenal fat, pelvis and capsule (Goldring, Clarke and Smith, 1936). It may be determined by measuring the clearance of a compound such as para-aminohippuric acid (PAH), 80% of which is extracted by the kidneys in the first pass.

It has not been possible to produce a gamma-emitting labelled form of *p*-aminohippuric acid, and by far the most widely used radioactive analogue is *o*-iodohippuric acid (OIH) labelled with ^{131}I or [125]I. Its lower extraction efficiency (66% compared with 80% for PAH) could be a result of its considerably greater degree of plasma protein binding (67% compared with 26% for PAH) (Maher, Strong and Elveback, 1971), but it currently represents the compound of choice for determination of ERPF.

It is essential to use a highly stable OIH compound. As the material ages, ionic iodide is released (Hotte and Ice, 1979), and the presence of free iodide greater than 2% would lead to erroneous clearance values (Chervu and Blaufox, 1982).

More recently OIH has been labelled with [123]I (half-life 13 hours, mono-energetic gamma ray emission of 159 keV) (Chisholm, Short and Glass, 1974; Hawkins *et al.*, 1982). The results for measurement of ERPF have been reported to be similar to those of ^{131}I-OIH and PAH (Stadalnik *et al.*, 1980). ^{123}I-OIH would certainly be the radiopharmaceutical of choice for renal studies and ERPF if its availability were to improve and the cost to decrease.

Radiopharmaceuticals used for renal imaging and renography

Mercurial compounds

Chlormerodrin, a mercurial diuretic, labelled with [203]Hg was the first agent used for renal scanning (McAfee and Wagner, 1960). This radionuclide has a long half-life (47 days) and was later replaced by [197]Hg (half-life 2.7 days) (Sodee, 1964).

Although this reduced the radiation dose to the kidneys by a factor of 10, the figure remained high at 8 mSv/MBq (30 rad/mCi).

All mercurial diuretics circulate bound to human serum albumin, and as a consequence they cannot be filtered by the glomeruli. Their extraction from blood is a function of the cells of the proximal renal tubules (Greif et al., 1955; Wagner, 1968). Because the accumulation of these compounds is mainly in the cortical tissue, their uptake is an expression of the functional capacity of the tubular mass, and their concentration in the renal medulla is low. Their excretion is very slow; in cases of normal renal function approximately 45% of the injected dose accumulates in the kidneys at 2 hours, and at 24 hours the activity in the kidneys is of the order of 16% (McAfee, 1970). Quantitative studies of renal function measuring the uptake of mercurial agents have been described (Raynaud, 1974), but these compounds have now been replaced by ^{99m}Tc agents.

Technetium-99m compounds

Many ^{99m}Tc-labelled radiopharmaceuticals are available for renal imaging, and it is important to know the physiological behaviour of those in common use.

^{99m}Tc-DTPA

Diethylenetriamine pentaacetic acid (DTPA) is completely filtered by the glomeruli and is not reabsorbed by the renal tubules. A maximum concentration in the kidneys of approximately 5% is reached at 5 minutes, and by 15 minutes this has fallen to 2%. Best images are therefore obtained during this period (Arnold et al., 1975). The fact that it is purely filtered makes imaging with this agent truly functional and permits simultaneous GFR measurement if desired (see p. 83). Because both physical and biological half-lives are short, comparatively large doses may be given safely in order to study renal perfusion by first circulation. Furthermore because of its rapid passage into the collecting system, good renograms may be derived, and it is particularly suitable for the study of excretory pathways as well. Since both technetium and the chemical are readily available, DTPA has become widely accepted as an all-purpose renal radiopharmaceutical.

^{99m}Tc-gluconate

This radiopharmaceutical, introduced by Charamaza and Budikova (1969), is also excreted by glomerular filtration, but it is then partially reabsorbed, chemically bound and retained in the cells of the proximal convoluted tubules. Approximately 15 minutes after injection 17–22% of the injected dose is in the renal cortex, making possible clear cortical images at an early stage. Another 20% of the injected dose is excreted in this first 15 minutes and 36% is in the urine by 1 hour, making visualization of the excretory pathways possible. Since it gives information on both cortical morphology and excretory pathways, it has been reported as an ideal agent for renal screening (Boyd et al., 1973). However, although it produces better and more durable images of the renal cortex than DTPA, it is not suitable for renography.

^{99m}Tc-DMSA

Dimercaptosuccinic acid (DMSA) was introduced by Lin, Khentigan and Winchell (1974) as a technetium chelate substitute for radiomercurial renal agents; work performed in rats demonstrated that at 1 hour after injection 54% of the dose is localized in the kidney, 7% in the urinary bladder, 5% in the liver and spleen and 19% in the blood. The compound is strongly bound to plasma proteins—in the order of 90% in rats (Yee, Lee and Blaufox, 1981). As a consequence glomerular filtration is minimal and the clearance from blood occurs mainly through tubular secretion. Auto-radiography studies in rats (Willis *et al.*, 1977) showed that ^{99m}Tc-DMSA concentrates in the renal tubules, proximal and distal with little activity going to the renal medulla, the glomeruli, collecting tubules and blood vessels. Studies of subcellular distribution of ^{99m}Tc-DMSA showed that the complex penetrates the kidney cells. It is bound mostly to soluble cytoplasmic proteins and mitochondria and to a lesser extent to microsomes and nuclei (Vanlic-Razumenic and Petrovic, 1981). Due to its high level of cortical renal fixation it is a very useful agent for imaging the renal parenchyma with no interference from pelvicalyceal activity. Good cortical images are obtained 2–3 hours after injection (Vanlic-Razumenic and Gorkic, 1976), with practically no activity in the medulla or pelvicalyceal system which appears as a medial 'cold area'. It is the agent of choice when studying patients suspected of having scarred kidneys. Morales, Evans and Gordon (1984) used DMSA to measure absolute uptake in a group of children. They showed that uptake of the tracer reached a plateau at 6 hours and remained constant for 24 hours. The uptake in each normal kidney measured at 6 hours was 17% of the dose injected.

DMSA must be used soon after preparation because it oxidizes. A delay in administration may result in decreased renal uptake and increased background and liver activity.

Ortho-iodohippurate

Mention has already been made of *o*-iodohippuric acid (OIH) as an analogue of *p*-aminohippuric acid for the determination of effective renal plasma flow. Labelled OIH has a significantly higher clearance than any other radiopharmaceutical yet developed and is eminently suitable for renography. It is eliminated mainly by tubular secretion. In patients with normally functioning kidneys, 85% of the OIH may be found in the urine 30 minutes after intravenous injection.

OIH was first labelled with ^{131}I by Tubis and colleagues (Tubis, Posnick and Nordyke, 1960) and for many years this was the only radiopharmaceutical for renography. ^{131}I has a half-life of 8 days and emits high-energy gamma rays (364 keV) in addition to beta particles. These physical characteristics were acceptable for probe studies when quantities of the order of 1–2 MBq (25–50 μCi) were administered, but they are far from ideal for gamma camera studies which demand a higher activity and a gamma ray emission of lower energy. The introduction of OIH labelled with ^{123}I, with its short physical half-life (13 hours) and its gamma emission of 159 keV has greatly improved the diagnostic potential of renal studies by combining the production of high-quality functional images with the ability to derive a renogram (O'Reilly *et al.*, 1977). The only factor limiting its widespread use is restricted availability and the expense involved in its cyclotron production.

^{67}Ga-gallium citrate

Gallium-67 is a cyclotron-produced radionuclide with a half-life of 78 hours and principal gamma ray emissions of 93 keV (38%), 185 keV (24%) and 300 keV (16%). After intravenous injection gallium citrate binds to serum proteins, especially to trans-ferrin. During the first 24 hours 10–15% of the dose injected is excreted by the kidneys, which are usually visualized during that period; thereafter the main route of elimination is via the faeces; about one-third is excreted in the first week. The compound is taken up by normal liver, spleen, bone and bone marrow, but its

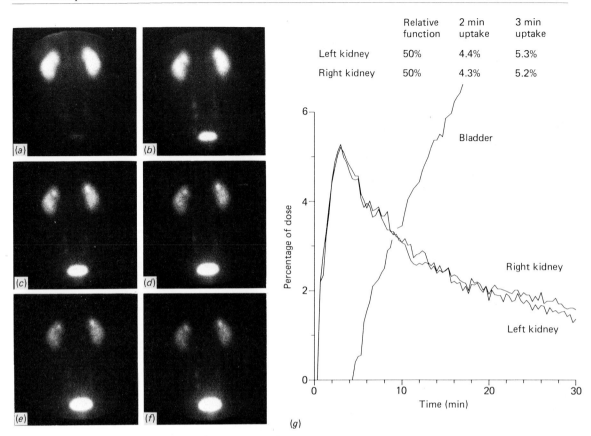

	Relative function	2 min uptake	3 min uptake
Left kidney	50%	4.4%	5.3%
Right kidney	50%	4.3%	5.2%

Figure 17.1A Gamma camera renogram performed with ^{99m}Tc-TDG in normal patient: (*a*) to (*f*) analogue images at 0–5, 5–10, 10–15, 15–20, 20–25 and 25–30 minutes; (*g*) derived renogram curves

introduction in clinical medicine was due to its unusual affinity for certain soft tissue tumours (Edwards and Hayes, 1969), and later by its high accumulation in abscess and infectious diseases. More recently gallium citrate has been used to study patients with pyelonephritis (Handmaker, 1982). The technique is simple: the patient is injected intravenously with 1–2 MBq/kg body weight (25–50 μCi/kg); images may be acquired as early as 6 hours in acute pyelonephritis (Mendez, Morillo and Alonso, 1980), but most workers prefer to start images at 24 hours and repeat if necessary at 48 and 72 hours; anterior, posterior and oblique views are usually obtained using a gamma camera.

It has been said that activity of gallium in the kidneys beyond 24 hours after injection suggests an inflammatory disease such as abscess (Hurwitz *et al.*, 1976; Raghavaiah, 1978), interstitial nephritis (Wood, Sharma and German, 1978; Linton, Clark and Driedger, 1980) or infection (Kumar and Coleman, 1976), but recent work has suggested that this criterion may be rather strict and a minimal amount of activity may be seen in the kidneys at 48 hours or later (Hauser and Alderson, 1978; Sherman and Byum, 1982).

Further evaluation of renal gallium studies may be necessary before their role in the investigation of renal disease is clearly defined (*see* also Chapter 11).

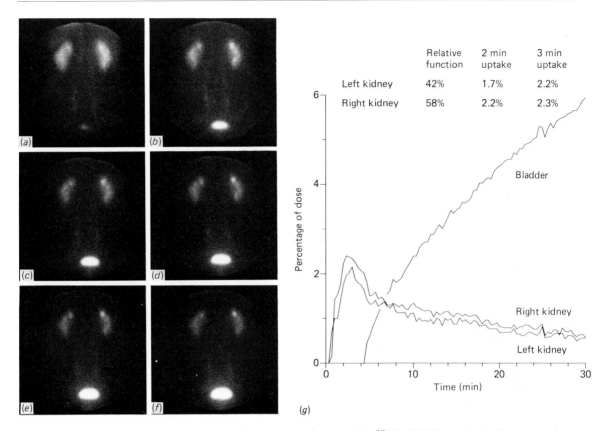

	Relative function	2 min uptake	3 min uptake
Left kidney	42%	1.7%	2.2%
Right kidney	58%	2.2%	2.3%

Figure 17.1B Same patient as *Figure 17.1A*. Renogram performed with ^{99m}Tc-DTPA under similar protocol

Developments in radiopharmaceuticals

With the exception of OIH most of the radiopharmaceuticals now used to investigate renal morphology and function are labelled with ^{99m}Tc. A great deal of effort has been put into the development of new agents labelled with ^{99m}Tc which would have the same physiological behaviour as OIH.

Thiodiglycolic acid (TDG) labelled with ^{99m}Tc was developed by Amersham International in 1982 as a new radiopharmaceutical for the study of renal function. In experiments performed in rats and rabbits TDG has shown physiological properties closely related to those of OIH. In studies performed in humans (Bevis *et al.*, 1983) the clearance of TDG was shown to be approximately twice that of DTPA and 40% of that of OIH. This represented a significant advance for a technetium-labelled agent. The images obtained with 75 MBq of ^{99m}Tc-TDG were found to be superior to those obtained with a similar quantity of ^{99m}Tc-DTPA in all cases, and comparison with images obtained using ^{123}I-OIH was favourable although it should be noted that only 12 MBq of ^{123}I was used. *Figure 17.1* shows an example of a gamma camera renogram performed in the same patient with TDG and DTPA and *Figure 17.2* a similar comparison between TDG and OIH. The mean ratio of kidney to background (K/B) values of TDG to DTPA for 20 normal kidneys was 1.6; this is presumably related to the greater clearance and higher uptake of TDG. The mean ratio of K/B values of OIH

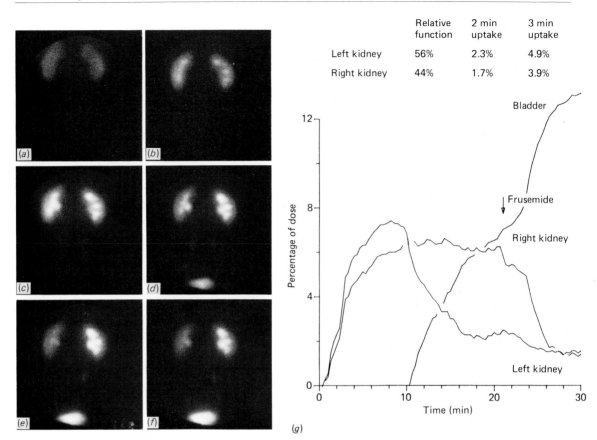

	Relative function	2 min uptake	3 min uptake
Left kidney	56%	2.3%	4.9%
Right kidney	44%	1.7%	3.9%

Figure 17.2A Diuresis renogram performed with ^{99m}Tc-TDG in patient with dilated right renal pelvis: (*a*) to (*f*) analogue images at 0–2½, 2½–5, 5–10, 10–15, 15–20, 20–25 minutes; (*g*) derived renogram curves

to TDG in six normal kidneys was 1.0. Since the clearance is lower than that of OIH, this suggests some fixation of the TDG in the renal cells. Mean transit times determined by deconvolution analysis of the renograms for the whole kidney were, 4.1, 3.9 and 3.1 minutes respectively for TDG, DTPA and OIH (Bevis *et al.*, 1984a). Comparisons carried out in patients with the suspicion of upper urinary tract obstruction suggested that TDG behaves similarly to OIH when the techniques of diuresis renography are applied (Bevis *et al.*, 1984b).

Other radiopharmaceuticals which have been investigated include ^{99m}Tc-N,N', bis(mercaptoacetamido)-ethylenediamine and ^{99m}Tc-N,N',bis(mercaptoacetyl)-2,3-diaminopropanoate (^{99m}Tc-DADS) (Fritzberg *et al.*, 1981, 1982). Biological studies using the ethylenediamine compound in mice, rats and rabbits indicated that this agent is cleared by the kidneys faster than ^{99m}Tc-DTPA and slower than ^{131}I-OIH. In a study in 11 patients with renal transplants the extraction efficiency was $(76 \pm 3)\%$ (mean $\pm$ sem) of that of ^{131}I-OIH, and the proportion of the injected dose found in the bladder at 30 minutes was $(25 \pm 4)\%$ that of OIH (Klingensmith *et al.*, 1982, 1984).

These new compounds have not yet been fully accepted, but one may look forward to a time when a ^{99m}Tc-labelled material will replace radioiodinated OIH.

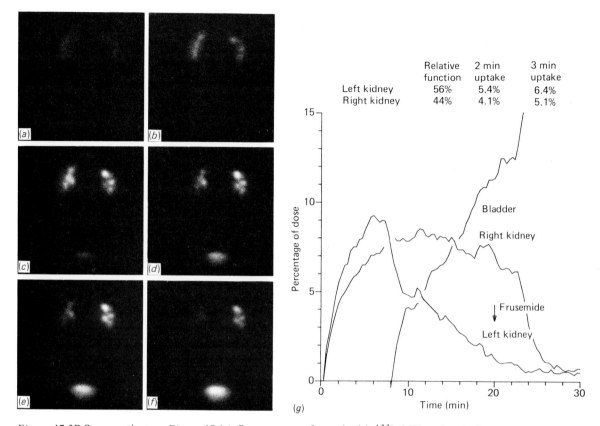

Figure 17.2B Same patient as *Figure 17.1A*. Renogram performed with ^{123}I-OIH under similar protocol

References

ARNOLD, R. W., SUBRAMANIAN, G., MCAFEE, J. G., BLAIR, R. J. and DEAVER, T. F. (1975) A comparison of ^{99m}Tc-complexes for renal imaging. *Journal of Nuclear Medicine*, **16**, 357–367

BENNETT, W. M. and PORTER, G. A. (1971) Endogenous creatinine clearance as a clinical measure of glomerular filtration rate. *British Medical Journal*, **4**, 84–86

BERLYNE, G. M., VARLEY, H., NILWARANGKUR *et al.* (1964) Endogenous creatinine clearance and glomerular filtration rate. *Lancet*, **2**, 874

BEVIS, C. R. A., LAWSON, R. S., SHIELDS, R. A. and TESTA, H. J. (1983) A new radiopharmaceutical for gamma camera renography. *Nuclear Medicine Communications*, **4**, 386–394

BEVIS, C. R. A., LAWSON, R. S., SHIELDS, R. A. and TESTA, H. J. (1984a) ^{99m}Tc-TDG renography with deconvolution analysis: A comparative study with ^{99m}Tc-DTPA and ^{123}I-hippuran. *Nuclear Medicine Communications*, **5**, 513–517

BEVIS, C. R. A., LAWSON, R. S., SHIELDS, R. A. and TESTA, H. J. (1984b) A comparison of ^{99m}Tc-thiodiglycolic acid (TDG) and ^{123}I-hippuran in the evaluation of upper urinary tract dilatation. *Nuclear Medicine Communications*, **4**, 212 (abstract)

BIANCHI, C. (1972) Measurement of the glomerular filtration rate. *Progress in Nuclear Medicine*, **2**, 21–53

BLAUFOX, M. D., CHERVU, L. R. and FREEMAN, L. M. (1975) Radiopharmaceuticals for quantitative study of renal function. In: *Radiopharmaceuticals*, G. Subramanian, B. A. Rhodes, J. F. Cooper and V. J. Sodd (eds.), New York: Society of Nuclear Medicine, pp. 389–392

BOYD, R. E., ROBSON, F., HUNT, F. C., SORBY, P. F., MURRAY, J. P. C. and MCKAY, W. J. (1973) ^{99m}Tc-gluconate complexes for renal scintigraphy. *British Journal of Radiology*, **46**, 604–612

CARLSEN, J. E., MOLLER, M. L., LUND, J. O. and TRAP-JENSEN, J. (1979) Comparison of four commercial Tc-99m(Sn)DTPA preparations used for the measurement of glomerular filtration rate. Concise communication. *Journal of Nuclear Medicine*, **21**(2), 126–129

CHANTLER, C., GARNETT, E. S., PARSONS, V. and VEALL, N. (1969) GFR measurements in man using the single injection method using ^{51}Cr EDTA. *Clinical Science*, **37**, 169–180

CHARAMAZA, O. and BUDIKOVA, M. (1969) Method of preparation of a ^{99m}Tc-complex for renal scintigraphy. *Nuclear Medicine*, **8**, 301

CHERVU, L. R., LEE, H. B., GOYAL, Q. and BLAUFOX, M. D. (1977) Use of ^{99m}Tc-Cu-DTPA complex as the renal function agent. *Journal of Nuclear Medicine*, **18**(1), 62–66

CHERVU, L. R. and BLAUFOX, M. D. (1982) Renal pharmaceuticals—an update. *Seminars in Nuclear Medicine*, **XII**(3), 224–243

CHISHOLM, G. D., SHORT, M. D. and GLASS, H. J. (1974) The measurement of renal plasma flow using ^{123}I-hippuran and the gamma camera. *British Journal of Urology*, **46**, 591–600

COTLOVE, E. (1955) ^{14}C-carboxy I-labelled inulin as a tracer for inulin. *Federation Proceedings*, **14**, 132 (abstract)

EDWARDS, C. L. and HAYES, R. L. (1969) Tumor scanning with ^{67}Ga citrate. *Journal of Nuclear Medicine*, **10**, 103–105

FRITZBERG, A. R., KLINGENSMITH III, W. C., WHITNEY, W. P. and KUNI, C. C. (1981) Chemical and biological studies of ^{99m}Tc N,N'-bis(mercaptoacetamido)-ethylenediamine: A potential replacement for ^{131}I iodohippurate. *Journal of Nuclear Medicine*, **22**, 258–263

FRITZBERG, A. R., KUNI, C. C., KLINGENSMITH III, W. C., STEVENS, J. and WHITNEY, W. P. (1982) Synthesis and biological evaluation of ^{99m}Tc, N,N'-bis(mercaptoacetyl)-2,3-diaminopropanoate. A potential replacement for (^{131}I) o-iodohippurate. *Journal of Nuclear Medicine*, **23**, 592–598

GARNETT, E. S., PARSONS, V. and VEALL, N. (1967) Measurement of GFR in man using a ^{51}Cr EDTA complex. *Lancet*, **1**, 818–819

GOLDRING, W., CLARKE, R. W. and SMITH, H. W. (1936) The phenol red clearance in normal man. *Journal of Clinical Investigation*, **15**, 221–228

GREIF, R., SULLIVAN, J., JACOBS, G. S. and PITTS, R. (1955) The use of radiomercury administered as chlormerodrin (neohydrin) in the kidneys of rats and dogs. *Journal of Clinical Investigation*, **35**, 38–43

HANDMAKER, H. (1982) Nuclear renal imaging in acute pyelonephritis. *Seminars in Nuclear Medicine*, **XII**, 246–253

HAUSER, W., ATKINS, H. L. and NELSON, K. G. (1970) ^{99m}Tc-DTPA—a new radiopharmaceutical for brain and kidney imaging. *Radiology*, **94**, 679–684

HAUSER, W. and ALDERSON, P. O. (1978) Gallium-67 imaging in abdominal disease. *Seminars in Nuclear Medicine*, **VIII**, 251–268

HAWKINS, L., ELLIOTT, A., SHIELDS, R. A. et al. (1982) A rapid quantitative method for the preparation of ^{123}I-iodo-hippuric acid. *European Journal of Nuclear Medicine*, **7**, 58–61

HILSON, A. J. W., MISTRY, R. D. and MAISEY, M. N. (1976) ^{99m}Tc-DTPA for the measurement of GFR. *British Journal of Radiology*, **49**, 794–796

HOTTE, C. E. and ICE, R. D. (1979) The in vitro stability of [^{131}I]o-iodohippurate. *Journal of Nuclear Medicine*, **20**(5), 441–447

HURWITZ, S. R., KESSLER, W. O., ALAZRAKI, N. P. and ASHBURN, W. L. (1976) Gallium-67 imaging to localize urinary tract infections. *British Journal of Radiology*, **49**, 156–160

KLINGENSMITH III, W. C., GERHOLD, J. P., FRITZBERG, A. R., SPITZER, V. M., KUNI, C. C., SINGER, C. J. and WEIL III, R. (1982) Clinical comparison of ^{99m}Tc N,N'-bis(mercaptoacetamide)-ethylenediamine and (^{131}I) ortho-iodohippurate for evaluation of renal tubular function. *Journal of Nuclear Medicine*, **23**, 377–380

KLINGENSMITH III, W. C., FRITZBERG, A. R., SPITZER, V. M. et al. (1984) Clinical evaluation of ^{99m}Tc N,N'-bis(mercaptoacetyl)-2,3-diaminopropanoate as a replacement for ^{131}I hippuran. *Journal of Nuclear Medicine*, **25**, 42–48

KUMAR, B. and COLEMAN, R. E. (1976) Significance of delayed ^{67}gallium localisation in the kidneys. *Journal of Nuclear Medicine*, **17**, 872–875

LIN, T. H., KHENTIGAN, A. and WINCHELL, H. S. (1974) A ^{99m}Tc chelate substitute for organoradiomercurial renal agents. *Journal of Nuclear Medicine*, **11**, 34–38

LINTON, A., CLARK, W. F. and DRIEDGER, A. A. (1980) Acute interstitial nephritis due to drugs. *Annals of Internal Medicine*, **93**, 735–741

MCAFEE, J. G. and WAGNER, H. N. (1960) Visualisation of renal parenchyma: scintiscanning with ^{203}Hg-neohydrin. *Radiology*, **75**, 820

MCAFEE, J. G. (1970) Problems in evaluating the radiation dose for radionuclides excreted by the kidney. In: *Medical Radionuclides: Radiation Dose and Effects*, R. J. Cloutier, C. C. Edwards and W. D. Snyder (eds.), Conf. 691212: USAEC

MAHER, F. T., STRONG, C. G. and ELVEBACK, L. R. (1971) Renal extraction ratios and plasma binding studies of radioiodinated ortho-iodohippurate and iodopyracet and of p-aminohippurate in man. *Mayo Clinic Proceedings*, **46**, 189–192

MATERSON, B. J., JOHNSON, A. E. and PEREZ-STABLE, E. C. (1969) Inulin labelled with chromium-51 for determination of glomerular filtration rate. *Journal of the American Medical Association*, **207**, 94

MENDEZ, G., MORILLO, G. and ALONSO, M. (1980) Gallium-67 radionuclide imaging in acute pyelonephritis. *American Journal of Roentgenology, Radium Therapy and Nuclear Medicine*, **134**, 17–22

MORALES, B., EVANS, K. and GORDON, I. (1984) Absolute quantitation of ^{99m}Tc-DMSA in paediatrics. *Nuclear Medicine Communications*, **5**, 212 (abstract)

NOLL, B., SEIFERT, S. and MUNZE, R. (1983) Preparation and characterisation of technetium (IV) complexes of diethylene-triaminepentaacetic acid and ethylenediaminetetraacetic acid as ligands. *International Journal of Applied Radiation and Isotopes*, **34**, 581–584

O'REILLY, P. H., HERMAN, K. J., LAWSON, R. S., SHIELDS, R. A. and TESTA, H. J. (1977) 123-Iodine: A new agent for functional renal scanning. *British Journal of Urology*, **49**, 15–21

PITTS, R. F. (1963) *Physiology of the Kidney and Body Fluids*, Chicago: Year Book Medical Publishers

RAGHAVAIAH, N. V. (1978) Gallium-67 scintigraphy in the diagnosis of renal cortical abscess. *Journal of Urology*, **120**, 237–238

RAYNAUD, C. (1974) A technique for the quantitative measurement of function of each kidney. *Seminars in Nuclear Medicine*, **4**, 51

RUSSELL, C. D. and SPEISER, A. D. (1980) Complexes of technetium with hydroxycarboxylic acid: Gluconic, glucoheptanoic, tartaric and citric. *Journal of Nuclear Medicine*, **21**, 1086–1090

RUSSELL, C. D., BISCHOFF, P. G., ROWELL, K. L. *et al.* (1983) Quality control of Tc-99m DTPA for measurement of glomerular filtration. *Journal of Nuclear Medicine*, **24**, 722–727

SAWYER, D. T. (1984) Metal-gluconate complexes. *Chemical Reviews*, **64**, 633–643

SHERMAN, R. A. and BYUM, K. (1982) Nuclear medicine in acute renal chronic renal failure. *Seminars in Nuclear Medicine*, **XII**, 265–279

SMITH, H. W. (1956) *Principles of Physiology*, New York: Oxford University Press

SODEE, D. B. (1964) A new scanning isotope, ^{197}Hg neohydrin. *Journal of Nuclear Medicine*, **5**, 1964

STADALNIK, R. C., VOGEL, J. M., JANSHOLT, A. L., KROHN, K. A., MATOLO, N. M., LAGUNAS-SOLAR, M. C. and SIELINSKI, F. W. (1980) Renal clearance and estimation parameters of ortho-iodohippurate (I-123) compared with OIH(I-131) and PAH. *Journal of Nuclear Medicine*, **21**, 168–170

TUBIS, M., POSNICK, E. and NORDYKE, R. A. (1960) Preparation and use of ^{131}I-labelled sodium iodohippurate in kidney function tests. *Proceedings of the Society for Experimental Biology and Medicine*, **103**, 497–498

VANLIC-RAZUMENIC, N. M. and GORKIC, D. A. (1976) Studies of chemical and biological properties of ^{99m}Tc DMSA—renal imaging agent. *European Journal of Nuclear Medicine*, **1**, 235–243

VANLIC-RAZUMENIC, N. and PETROVIC, J. (1981) Biochemical studies of the renal radiopharmaceutical compound dimercaptosuccinate. *European Journal of Nuclear Medicine*, **6**, 169–172

WAGNER, H. N. Jr (1968) *Principles of Nuclear Medicine*, Philadelphia: Saunders, p. 628

WILLIS, K. W., MARTINEZ, D. A. and HEDLEY-WHYTE, E. T. (1977) Renal localisation of ^{99m}Tc (Sn) dimercaptosuccinate in the rat by frozen section autoradiography. *Radiation Research*, **69**, 475

WOOD, B. C., SHARMA, J. N. and GERMAN, D. R. (1978) Gallium-67 citrate imaging in non infectious interstitial nephritis. *Annals of Internal Medicine*, **138**, 1665–1666

YEE, C. A., LEE, H. B. and BLAUFOX, M. D. (1981) ^{99m}Tc-DMSA renal uptake: Influence of biochemical and physiological factors. *Journal of Nuclear Medicine*, **22**, 1054–1058

18 Mathematics

R. S. Lawson

The compartmental model of renal clearance

One of the quantities which may be derived from a functional study of the kidney is the rate at which it can clear an appropriate tracer from the blood. This is important because the renal clearance rate may be equated to either glomerular filtration rate (GFR) or effective renal plasma flow (ERPF), depending on the tracer used. Renal clearance may be determined as part of a renography study in which the appearance of tracer in the kidneys is monitored by external counters or a gamma camera. In this case the function of left and right kidneys can be assessed individually. Alternatively, total clearance of both kidneys together can be measured by monitoring the disappearance of tracer from the blood or its appearance in the urine. These techniques are described in detail in Chapter 5.

With some of these methods it is possible to calculate the clearance rate directly from the measurements taken, without any assumptions about the precise shape of the plasma disappearance curve. In other cases, however, it is necessary to make some assumptions regarding the distribution of tracer in the body in order to calculate the renal clearance, and this is often done by reference to some model of the system.

Use of a particular model does not imply that this is a true physical representation of what the body is really like; in fact, the model may only be a mathematical concept and need not be capable of actually being built at all. The model must embody the essential features of the system that it represents in as simple a manner as possible and be capable of predicting the behaviour of the system in a manner which agrees with the observations of how it actually behaves. The simplest model that is consistent with the behaviour of the real system is the best, because it is the one most likely to yield a simple relationship between the observable quantities (e.g. variation of tracer concentration in blood) and the unobserved quantity to be determined (e.g. GFR or ERPF).

The type of model which is widely used in tracer studies of this sort is the *compartmental model*. The basic concept behind any compartmental model is that a tracer substance in the body can be thought of as being distributed through several pools or *compartments*. These compartments might correspond to particular organs in the body or to some definite fluid volume distributed throughout the body, such as the blood plasma. This equivalence is not necessary for the model to be valid, however, and quite often a compartment will not actually correspond to any anatomical or physical

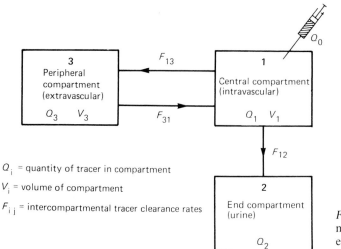

Q_i = quantity of tracer in compartment

V_i = volume of compartment

F_{ij} = intercompartmental tracer clearance rates

Figure 18.1 The three-compartment model of renal clearance. For explanation, *see* text

space in the body. The definition of a compartment is simply any space which maintains a uniform concentration of tracer throughout.

The simplest compartmental model for renal clearance would have only two compartments, one representing tracer in the blood and the other tracer that has been removed from the blood. Such a model would predict a single-exponential rate of decrease of tracer in the blood compartment. In practice, for most tracers this is found not to be the case.

The model is therefore usually extended to three compartments, and its predictions then agree well with what is found in practice. The compartments are arranged in what is called an *open mamillary system*, consisting of a *central compartment* with one (or more) *peripheral compartments* exchanging with it and an *end compartment* connected unidirectionally with the central compartment (*Figure 18.1*). This system has been analysed in detail by Matthews (1957), who applied it to protein turnover, and in connection with renal clearance by Sapirstein *et al.* (1955), Blaufox (1972), Van Stekelenburg, Kooman and Tertoolen (1976) and others.

The first, or central, compartment represents tracer which is exchangeable with proximal tubular cells in the kidney and is therefore referred to as the intravascular or blood plasma compartment. The end compartment (compartment 2) represents tracer that has been cleared via the kidney and is thus associated with urine in the kidney and in the bladder. It is the clearance rate from compartment 1 to compartment 2 that is to be determined. The third, peripheral, compartment represents all tracer that is not exchangeable into proximal tubular cells—i.e. mainly extravascular, extrarenal tracer, but it could include tracer in red blood cells or tracer bound to large protein molecules. It is possible for tracer to diffuse between compartments 1 and 3 in both directions, but between compartments 1 and 2 flow is only possible in the 1-to-2 direction.

If we inject a quantity of tracer into the central compartment via a peripheral vein, the assumption, implicit in the model, that tracer concentration is uniform throughout the compartment is not valid for the first few seconds after injection. During this time the concentration of tracer in the blood will be very high in some places and low in others, but this non-uniform distribution will rapidly even out as the blood circulates. Thus the graph of tracer concentration against time will show an initial rapid rise of activity, which then falls over the next few seconds. The magnitude of this initial mixing spike will be different for different parts of the body, and will also depend on the injection site and the speed of the injection. The compartmental model cannot predict

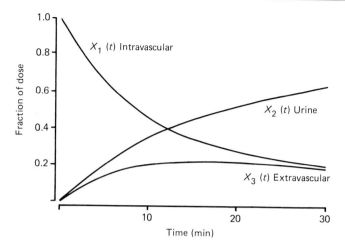

Figure 18.2 Compartmental model predictions for the fraction of tracer in each compartment

the details of this phase, since its basic assumptions of uniform distribution within each compartment are not satisfied.

After mixing, the quantity of tracer in compartment 1 starts to fall. This occurs for two reasons: first, uptake by the kidneys (represented by clearance F_{12} in *Figure 18.1*), and secondly, diffusion into extravascular space (clearance F_{13}). As the quantity of tracer in compartment 3 builds up, diffusion in the reverse direction becomes important (clearance F_{31}), and therefore after a while extravascular tracer reaches a maximum and then falls. Ultimately there will be no tracer left in compartments 1 and 3, and it will all end up in compartment 2. *Figure 18.2* shows the shapes of the curves expected for the variation of tracer in each compartment with time.

In order to derive the curves of *Figure 18.2* from the compartmental model the distribution volumes available to the tracer in compartments 1 and 3 are first defined. These are called V_1 and V_3 respectively. Here it is easy to fall into the trap of identifying V_1 with blood plasma volume. Typically, for OIH as the tracer, V_1 is measured to be about 9 litres (Blaufox, 1972), whereas blood plasma volume is only 3.5 litres. In this case V_1 should be interpreted as the initial dilution volume into which OIH is mixed before clearance begins. Blood plasma is obviously part of this volume, and therefore part of compartment 1, but not the whole of it. The volume V_3 is even less meaningful in physical terms.

Let the quantity of tracer in each of the three compartments be Q_1, Q_2 and Q_3 (measured in mg) and the intercompartmental clearance rates F_{12}, F_{13} and F_{31} (ml/minute). F_{12} is the renal clearance rate.

Now the rate (in mg/minute) at which tracer leaves compartment i and enters compartment j is equal to the clearance rate F_{ij} (number of ml from compartment i cleared each minute) multiplied by the concentration of tracer in compartment i (mg/ml). So

$$\text{Rate of tracer loss from } i \text{ to } j = F_{ij} \cdot \frac{Q_i}{V_i}$$

and the total rate of loss (or gain), dQ_i/dt, is equal to the sum of the losses (or gains) from all other compartments:

$$\frac{dQ_1}{dt} = F_{31}\frac{Q_3}{V_3} - F_{13}\frac{Q_1}{V_1} - F_{12}\frac{Q_1}{V_1} \tag{1a}$$

$$\frac{dQ_2}{dt} = F_{12}\frac{Q_1}{V_1} \tag{1b}$$

$$\frac{dQ_3}{dt} = F_{13}\frac{Q_1}{V_1} - F_{31}\frac{Q_3}{V_3} \tag{1c}$$

Now let the total quantity of tracer injected be Q_0 and put

$$\frac{Q_1}{Q_0} = X_1; \qquad \frac{Q_2}{Q_0} = X_2; \qquad \frac{Q_3}{Q_0} = X_3 \tag{2}$$

so that X_1, X_2 and X_3 are the fractions of injected tracer in the three compartments. In addition, put:

$$\frac{F_{12}}{V_1} = K_{12}; \qquad \frac{F_{13}}{V_1} = K_{13}; \qquad \frac{F_{31}}{V_3} = K_{31} \tag{3}$$

K_{12}, K_{13} and K_{31} are called *rate constants* and will have units of minute^{-1}. In fact, K_{ij} is the fraction of the total volume of compartment i which is cleared into compartment j per minute.

Substituting equations (2) and (3) into (1) gives:

$$\frac{dX_1}{dt} = K_{31}X_3 - K_{13}X_1 - K_{12}X_1 \tag{4a}$$

$$\frac{dX_2}{dt} = K_{12}X_1 \tag{4b}$$

$$\frac{dX_3}{dt} = K_{13}X_1 - K_{31}X_3 \tag{4c}$$

These three differential equations describe mathematically the behaviour of the model. They have a solution in which X_1, X_2 and X_3 vary in a biexponential manner with time

$$X_1(t) = A_1 e^{-\lambda_1 t} + A_2 e^{-\lambda_2 t} \tag{5a}$$

$$X_2(t) = 1 - A_3 e^{-\lambda_1 t} - A_4 e^{-\lambda_2 t} \tag{5b}$$

$$X_3(t) = -A_5(e^{-\lambda_1 t} - e^{-\lambda_2 t}) \tag{5c}$$

This is the most general solution of the differential equations which is consistent with the starting conditions (at $t = 0$ all the tracer is injected into compartment 1) and with the condition that eventually all the tracer must end up in compartment 2. These boundary conditions also require that:

$$A_1 + A_2 = 1; \qquad A_3 + A_4 = 1 \tag{6}$$

If equations (5) are substituted into equations (4), it is possible to find the values of all the coefficients A_1 to A_5 together with λ_1 and λ_2 in terms of the three rate constants.

Alternatively, the rate constants themselves may be evaluated as:

$$K_{12} = \frac{\lambda_1 \lambda_2}{A_1 \lambda_2 + A_2 \lambda_1} \tag{7a}$$

$$K_{13} = \frac{A_1 A_2 (\lambda_1 - \lambda_2)^2}{A_1 \lambda_2 + A_2 \lambda_1} \tag{7b}$$

$$K_{31} = A_1 \lambda_2 + A_2 \lambda_1 \tag{7c}$$

This shows that all the rate constants can be determined if A_1, A_2, λ_1 and λ_2 are measured. In practice, this might be done by measuring the concentration of tracer in blood plasma (part of compartment 1). If this concentration $P(t)$ is measured in mg/ml:

$$P(t) = \frac{\text{Tracer remaining in compartment 1}}{\text{Volume of compartment 1}} = \frac{Q_0 X_1(t)}{V_1}$$

Now it is known how $X_1(t)$ varies with time from equations (5), so $P(t)$ will vary in the same way. $P(t)$ can therefore be written:

$$P(t) = C_1 e^{-\lambda_1 t} + C_2 e^{-\lambda_2 t} \tag{8}$$

where C_1 and C_2 are proportional to A_1 and A_2, respectively. It is then easy to show that:

$$V_1 = \frac{Q_0}{C_1 + C_2} \tag{9}$$

and

$$F_{12} = V_1 K_{12} = \frac{Q_0 \lambda_1 \lambda_2}{C_1 \lambda_2 + C_2 \lambda_1} \tag{10}$$

The clearance rate F_{12} can therefore be measured by observing the biexponential fall of blood plasma concentration of tracer (equation 8) and determining C_1, C_2, λ_1 and λ_2. Together with the known amount of tracer injected, Q_0, these give F_{12} from equation (10).

In *Figure 18.2* the compartmental model predictions for the fraction of tracer remaining in each compartment as a function of time have been plotted for a typical case. The values assumed for the rate constants are:

$$K_{12} = 0.05 \text{ minute}^{-1}; \qquad K_{13} = 0.04 \text{ minute}^{-1}; \qquad K_{31} = 0.06 \text{ minute}^{-1}$$

These are typical values found for normal handling of OIH by Blaufox (1972). They correspond to:

$\lambda_1 = 0.13$ minute^{-1}; $\lambda_2 = 0.024$ minute^{-1}

$A_1 = 0.65$; $A_2 = 0.35$

One of the limitations of the compartmental model described so far is that compartment 2 comprises all tracer in the urine and does not distinguish between kidneys and bladder. This distinction is easily made, however, by extending the model slightly and subdividing compartment 2 into compartment 4 (renal tubules) and compartment 5 (bladder). The main effect of passage through the renal tubules is to introduce a fixed delay with hardly any mixing of tracer since the tubules are very narrow. However, mixing will occur in the renal calyces and pelvis and so the model can be refined further by adding compartment 6 (renal pelvis) to act as an intrarenal mixing chamber (*see Figure 18.3*).

If the usual substitutions are made:

$$\frac{Q_4}{Q_0} = X_4; \qquad \frac{Q_5}{Q_0} = X_5; \qquad \frac{Q_6}{Q_0} = X_6 \tag{11}$$

$$\frac{F_{65}}{V_6} = K_{65} \tag{12}$$

then the differential equations for rate of gain of tracer in compartments 5 and 6 are:

$$\frac{dX_5}{dt} = K_{65}X_6(t) \tag{13a}$$

$$\frac{dX_6}{dt} = 0 \qquad \text{for } t < t_0$$

$$= K_{12}X_1(t - t_0) - K_{65}X_6(t) \qquad \text{for } t \geqslant t_0 \tag{13b}$$

where t_0 is the delay introduced by compartment 4. This last equation results from the fact that tracer entering compartment 6 is just that which had entered compartment 4 a time t_0 previously.

The solution to these differential equations is a sum of three exponentials with a time lag:

$$X_6(t) = 0 \qquad \text{for } t < t_0$$

$$= A_7 e^{-\lambda_1(t - t_0)} + A_8 e^{-\lambda_2(t - t_0)} - A_9 e^{-\lambda_3(t - t_0)} \qquad \text{for } t \geqslant t_0 \tag{14a}$$

$$X_5(t) = 0 \qquad \text{for } t < t_0$$

$$= 1 - A_{10} e^{-\lambda_1(t - t_0)} - A_{11} e^{-\lambda_2(t - t_0)} + A_{12} e^{-\lambda_3(t - t_0)} \qquad \text{for } t \geqslant t_0 \tag{14b}$$

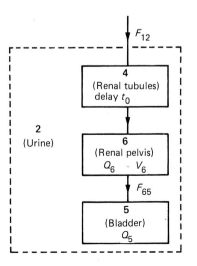

Figure 18.3 Subdivision of compartment 2 used in extended model of renal clearance. For explanation, *see* text

The boundary conditions, that X_5 and X_6 are both zero at time $t = t_0$, require that:

$$A_9 = A_7 + A_8; \qquad A_{12} = A_{10} + A_{11} - 1 \tag{15}$$

If equations (14) and (15) are substituted into equations (13) it is possible to find the values of the coefficients A_7 to A_{12} in terms of the rate constants. This analysis also gives a value for λ_3:

$$\lambda_3 = K_{65} = \frac{F_{65}}{V_6} = \frac{\text{Urine production rate}}{\text{Intrarenal mixing volume}} \tag{16}$$

Now all activity in the urine (compartment 2) at any time is made up of the activity previously in the urine at a time t_0 before, plus new activity which is still in the renal tubules (compartment 4). Therefore:

$$X_2(t) = X_2(t - t_0) + X_4(t) \tag{17}$$

from which an equation for $X_4(t)$ can be derived by making use of equation (5b) for $X_2(t)$

$$\begin{aligned} X_4(t) &= 1 - A_3 e^{-\lambda_1 t} - A_4 e^{-\lambda_2 t} \qquad \text{for } t < t_0 \\ &= A_3(1 - e^{-\lambda_1 t_0}) e^{-\lambda_2(t - t_0)} + A_4(1 - e^{-\lambda_2 t_0}) e^{-\lambda_2(t - t_0)} \qquad \text{for } t \geqslant t_0 \end{aligned} \tag{18}$$

Total renal activity at any time can be calculated from the sum of X_4 and X_6.

Figure 18.4 shows how the fraction of tracer in the kidneys and in the bladder vary with time according to this model. These have been calculated using equations (14) and (18), with values for the rate constants taken as above with, in addition, $t_0 = 2$ minutes and $K_{65} = 1$ minute^{-1}. These curves correspond quite well with what is observed in a normal renogram.

Background subtraction of the renogram

In renography the passage of a labelled tracer through the kidney is monitored by either an external scintillation counter probe or a gamma camera connected to a computer system. Ideally only tracer actually in the renal parenchyma (and in some cases in the renal pelvis as well) should be detected, but of course this is never possible in practice.

In gamma camera renography, non-renal areas surrounding the kidney are excluded from the calculation by the use of a region of interest drawn on the computer stored images, and, with care, the renal pelvis can be excluded or included as desired. Although the activity measured by this method is mainly due to tracer in the renal parenchyma,

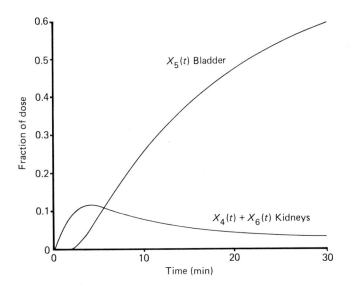

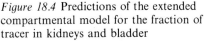

Figure 18.4 Predictions of the extended compartmental model for the fraction of tracer in kidneys and bladder

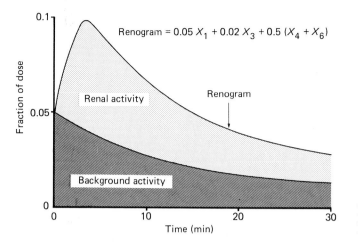

Figure 18.5 Compartmental model predictions for the total activity within a kidney region of interest

this is not the only source. There are contributions from non-renal tissue overlying the kidney and also from intravascular activity within the kidney itself. All these constitute a background on which the true renal activity is superimposed.

With a probe renography system, background contributions are even more extensive, because it is virtually impossible to use a collimator which is just the right size to include only the kidney in its field of view, due to the difficulty of knowing exactly where to position it before the test starts. Thus, any probe system will detect significant extrarenal activity, and it is impossible to exclude activity in the renal pelvis.

The background is not constant with time, nor does it change with time in the same way as does the renal activity. According to the predictions of the compartmental model, activity in the renal parenchyma will vary like $X_4(t)$ (equation 18). The background activity is partly intravascular and partly extravascular and therefore behaves as a sum of $X_1(t)$ and $X_3(t)$ (equation 5). A background curve of this form is shown in *Figure 18.5*, where it has been assumed that 5% of compartment 1 and 2% of compartment 3, together with 50% of compartments 4 and 6 are within the region of interest for one kidney. It is clear that not only does the background vary with time in a different way to the renal activity but also, since the background starts high and falls with time—contrasting renal activity which starts low and rises—the background can dominate the observed renogram over the first minute. The effect is most pronounced for poorly functioning kidneys and tracers with relatively low clearance, such as DTPA. It is therefore essential to take the background into account in some way when assessing the renogram. If the renogram is to be quantified, the background contribution must be measured and subtracted from the observed renogram to give the true renal activity. This is the process often referred to as blood background subtraction, although this is something of a misnomer, as much of the background activity is extravascular.

Background subtraction techniques are often validated by results obtained for nephrectomy sites. It should be noted, however, that removal of a kidney also removes one of the sources of background, namely intrarenal vascular activity. A nephrectomy site often looks 'colder' than the surrounding tissues on a gamma camera image whereas a non-functioning but perfused kidney may well appear 'hotter' than the surrounding tissues simply due to activity in the blood pool.

Background subtraction with gamma camera renography

In a patient with one kidney absent or known to be non-functioning the background contribution to the functioning kidney can easily be estimated by placing an identical region of interest over the contralateral side. In other patients some non-renal region must be used to obtain background measurements. Ideally this region should have the same blood and tissue distribution as the kidney, so that activity in it is related to the background activity in the kidney by some constant factor. Choice of a suitable background region is obviously limited to sites within the field of view of the gamma camera when it is positioned over the kidneys. The region must not include the kidneys, ureters or bladder, but even with these restrictions different workers prefer different sites, and there seems to be no general agreement as to which should be used.

However, assuming that a suitable background region has been chosen, the computer can be instructed to calculate the activity–time curve for this region. This may not yet be quite the proper background curve to use if the defined region of interest was not of the same size as the kidney region. This is corrected for by dividing the background curve by the area of the background region (to give the counts per unit area) and multiplying by the area of the kidney region to give the expected background activity in this region. This scaled background curve can be subtracted from the kidney curve to give the subtrated renogram.

The limitation of this method is that it assumes that the distribution of blood and tissue per unit area of the image is the same in the kidney region as in the background region. This assumption can be checked by comparing the curve from a background region with that from a nephrectomy site. Differences may show up in either the shapes of the curves or their amplitudes when normalized to the same area. Short, Glass and Vernon (1970) have done this, and observe that it is not possible to find a background area which exactly simulates the kidney region anywhere within the limited field of view of the gamma camera.

Kenny et al. (1975) have compared several background regions, and find that an area chosen between the two kidneys approximates most closely to a nephrectomy site in the shape of the curve but that the counts per unit area are greater. The background is therefore overestimated unless it is scaled down by a background subtraction factor. They find an average value of 0.79 ± 0.06 for the left subtraction factor and 0.87 ± 0.11 for the right. Even if these average factors are taken into account and applied to all normal patients, there will still be some uncertainty in the true background for any individual patient due to the variation among the population implied by the standard deviations quoted on the above figures. It would therefore seem that an uncertainty of the order of 10% in the background is inevitable when using this method.

At Manchester Royal Infirmary the normal procedure is to define a 'T'-shaped background region of interest extending between and above both kidneys. The area of this region should be approximately the same as either kidney region. The activity–time curve from the background region is scaled to correct for differences in the areas of the background and kidney regions, but no additional background subtraction factor is applied. This method is found to be adequate for most studies using ^{123}I-OIH where the background is not severe. However, when using ^{99m}Tc-DTPA with a poorly functioning kidney the method can overestimate the background, and small changes in the definition of the background region of interest can produce large changes in the subtracted curve. In order to cope with difficult cases like this and to make the results less operator-dependent, several alternative methods of background subtraction have been proposed.

Alternative methods of background subtraction

Brown (1982) has suggested an interpolative background subtraction technique which permits the background to vary across the kidney region. A rectangle is positioned round the kidney, and the background contribution to each pixel within the rectangle is estimated by linear interpolation between the corresponding edge pixels on the rectangle. This allows a dynamic sequence of background-corrected images to be produced, from which a background-corrected activity–time curve can be generated.

Two other techniques (Rutland, 1979; Thomson, Leach and Middleton, 1984), which are principally designed to calculate relative renal function, but which produce background subtraction factors at the same time, are discussed on page 256. Deconvolution of the renogram (page 257) also yields an alternative method of carrying out background subtraction.

Background subtraction with probe renography

When probe renography is performed there is a far wider choice of sites for background estimation than there is when a gamma camera is used, as the background probe can be placed almost anywhere over the body. The infraclavicular region gives the best approximation to a nephrectomy site (Hine *et al.*, 1963; Britton and Brown, 1971), although the heart and the head have been used.

A method of calculating the appropriate subtraction factor was first described by Hall and Monks (1966), and the technique has been developed and automated by Brown and Britton (1969). The method involves the use of a preliminary injection of an intravascular tracer, such as HSA, labelled with the same radionuclide as that used for the renal tracer. The ratio of the observed count rates in the kidney and background detectors gives the required background subtraction factor to be used when the renal tracer is injected.

After analysing the results of over 100 probe renograms reported independently from subtracted and unsubtracted curves, this author has concluded that an experienced observer can obtain all the available qualitative information from the raw renogram and the chest and bladder curves alone. The report on the test is not improved by the availability of the subtracted curves unless quantitative information on renal function is required. In order to quantify the renogram it is essential to allow for the background in some way, but nowadays this is more conveniently achieved using a gamma camera and computer system.

Calculation of relative renal function

The *relative function* of an individual kidney is defined as the kidney's individual renal clearance expressed as a percentage of the patient's total renal clearance. Now it can be shown that, for times less than the minimum kidney transit time, the background corrected kidney count rate is proportional to the individual renal clearance; therefore:

$$\text{Left kidney relative function} = \frac{\text{Left kidney counts}}{\text{Left + right kidney counts}} \times 100\% \tag{19}$$

with a similar expression for the right kidney.

In order to prove this result the relationships between the observed count rates and the amount of tracer in each compartment must be defined. Let $C'_K(t)$ be the background subtracted count rate from a kidney region of interest and $C_V(t)$ be the count rate from a vascular region of interest. If S_K and S_V are the sensitivities of detection for each region, defined as the count rate obtained for each unit of tracer uniformly distributed in kidney and blood respectively (units of, say, cps/mg), then:

$$C'_K(t) = S_K Q_0 X_4(t) \tag{20a}$$

and

$$C_V(t) = S_V Q_0 X_1(t) \tag{20b}$$

The equation (4b) is integrated to obtain:

$$X_2(t) = K_{12} \int_0^t X_1(\tau) \, d\tau \tag{21}$$

These three equations are combined—for times less than t_0 no urine has left the kidneys, so X_4 and X_2 are equal—to obtain:

$$C_K'(t) = UC \int_0^t C_V(\tau) \, d\tau \qquad \text{for } t < t_0 \tag{22}$$

where:

$$UC = \frac{S_K}{S_V} K_{12} = \frac{S_K}{S_V} \frac{F_{12}}{V_1} \tag{23}$$

UC is the kidney *uptake constant*. If this result is applied to each individual kidney—assuming that both kidneys are detected with equal sensitivity—then the uptake constant is proportional to the individual renal clearance. Therefore,

$$\text{Left relative function} = \frac{\text{Left uptake constant}}{\text{Left + right uptake constants}} \times 100\% \tag{24}$$

From equation (22) the background subtracted kidney count rate at any time before elimination starts is proportional to the corresponding kidney uptake constant and hence equation (19) is an alternative expression of (24).

The kidney counts in equation (19) are corrected for background and summed over any period up to the renogram peak, e.g. from 1 minute up to 20 seconds before the time of the renogram peak. Before 1 minute mixing is not complete and the background subtraction is not reliable. Twenty seconds before the peak time is an approximation to the time at which elimination begins. If the left and right renograms peak at different times the earlier time should be used, and if neither renogram peaks before 15 minutes the summation may be stopped at 15 minutes.

Ideally a correction should be applied to allow for the fact that, if the kidneys do not lie at exactly the same depth, they will not be detected with equal sensitivity. In extreme cases of ectopic kidneys this can be done by taking the geometric mean of results obtained from anterior and posterior views (p. 266). However, in most patients the discrepancy will be small and is usually ignored. Using ^{99m}Tc a difference in kidney depths of 10 mm will make a true relative function of 50% appear as 54%, and 20% appear as 22%. A difference in depths of 25 mm will make these same values appear as 59% and 27% respectively.

A more sophisticated way of quantifying the kidney uptake is to plot a graph of background-corrected kidney count rate against the integral of the count rate from a vascular region of interest (Britton and Brown, 1971). By equation (22), for times less than t_0, this can be fitted to a straight line with gradient UC. This method will give an uptake constant for each kidney which can be used to calculate relative renal function according to equation (24).

Rutland (1979) has extended this method to use the raw count rate from a kidney region of interest, $C_K(t)$, instead of the background-subtracted rate, $C_K'(t)$:

$$C_K'(t) = C_K(t) - b_1 C_V(t) \tag{25}$$

where b_1 is a background subtraction factor. This is combined with equation (22) to obtain:

$$\frac{C_K(t)}{C_V(t)} = b_1 + UC \frac{\int_0^t C_V(\tau) \, d\tau}{C_V(t)} \qquad \text{for } t < t_0 \tag{26}$$

So a graph of C_K/C_V against $\int C_V \, d\tau$ should be a straight line until time t_0. The gradient of this line gives the uptake constant and the intercept gives the background subtraction factor.

A further improvement of the method (Thomson, Leach and Middleton, 1984) utilizes two separate non-renal regions of interest to allow for the fact that the background is partly vascular and partly non-vascular. If $C_T(t)$ is the count rate from a non-vascular tissue background region then:

$$C_K'(t) = C_K(t) - b_1 C_V(t) - b_2 C_T(t) \tag{27}$$

This is combined with equation (22) to obtain:

$$\frac{C_K(t)}{C_V(t)} = b_1 + b_2 \frac{C_T(t)}{C_V(t)} + UC \frac{\int_0^t C_V(\tau)\,d\tau}{C_V(t)} \qquad \text{for } t < t_0 \tag{28}$$

A multiple linear regression will give the uptake constant and the values of the two background subtraction factors, b_1 and b_2. The advantage of this method is that it automatically allows for the correct proportions of intravascular and extravascular background and therefore produces results which are less dependent on the operator's skill in choosing a suitable single background region.

Calculation of absolute renal function

The most accurate method of measuring the absolute function of each kidney is to determine the overall renal clearance, using one of the methods described in Chapter 5, and to apportion this between the two kidneys according to the relative function determined from a renogram.

Calculation of absolute renal function from a renogram alone is never as accurate as the calculation of relative renal function, since it must involve a knowledge of the gamma camera sensitivity, including an allowance for kidney depth which reduces the count rate due to attenuation. An approximate but simple technique is to measure the camera sensitivity using a kidney phantom (e.g. a bag of saline) filled with a known quantity of tracer and placed in an attenuating medium (e.g. a bowl of water) at an average kidney depth. The counts in a region of interest over the image of such a phantom enable the sensitivity to be determined in counts per second per MBq. If the activity administered for any renogram is then measured before injection, the renogram count rate can be expressed as a percentage of the injected dose. The percentage of the dose in the kidney at a given time, say 2 minutes or 3 minutes, is then an approximate measure of the absolute function of the kidney.

The renal uptake constant (page 256) also gives a measure of absolute renal function. It has the units of a rate constant (minute^{-1}) but its value will depend on the imaging system used because of the ratio of sensitivities, S_K/S_V, in equation (23). The uptake constant can only be converted to a true clearance in ml/minute if the tracer distribution volume, V_1, is measured by taking a blood sample at some time during the test.

Deconvolution of the renogram

The purpose of deconvolution

The renogram curve, after corrections for blood and tissue background, is a representation of how the amount of OIH in the kidney is changing with time. This depends both on the rate at which OIH is entering the kidney and on the rate at which it is leaving the kidney via the ureter.

The rate at which OIH enters the kidney at any time will be called the input rate $I(t)$, measured in units of, say, mg/minute. The input rate at any time will be proportional to the ERPF (ml/minute), and the concentration of OIH in plasma in the renal artery at that time $P(t)$ (mg/ml):

$$I(t) = \text{ERPF} \cdot P(t) \tag{29}$$

Thus the subtracted renogram is the response of the kidney to an input which varies with time in the same way as the plasma concentration of OIH. From discussion of the compartmental model (page 247) it is known that the plasma concentration–time curve shows an initial spike which depends on the speed of injection and the site of injection and also on how quickly OIH mixes in the blood. After the initial spike the blood concentration of OIH continues to fall biexponentially, as determined by the rates of diffusion into extravascular space and removal by the kidneys. Thus the plasma concentration–time curve depends on many physiological parameters, some of which are not related to kidney function. It also depends on the manner in which the OIH was injected. In the extreme case of extravasation of tracer, the plasma concentration may even rise with time. Therefore it may not be easy to compare renograms from different patients or indeed from the same patient at different times, owing to differences in the plasma concentration–time curves and, hence, the input rate to the kidney.

Deconvolution is one way of overcoming this difficulty by calculating what the response of the kidney would have been to some standard input. It is convenient to refer to the so-called 'impulse input' for this purpose. Mathematically this is expressed by making $I(t)$ a delta function; a spike in the graph of input rate against time with unit area but infinitesimally narrow. In practice, of course, such an input rate can never be achieved, but it can be imagined as an idealized bolus injection of unit quantity of OIH straight into the renal artery with no recirculation.

The renogram that would be observed if such an input were possible is called the *impulse response* or the *impulse retention function* of the kidney. This will be denoted by $H(t)$ and defined as the fraction of the injected dose of OIH remaining in the kidney at any time after an ideal impulse input. Since $H(t)$ is a fraction, it has no units. It is possible to calculate it if the response of the kidney to some other known input is measured. This response, $R(t)$, is defined as the total amount of OIH in the kidney at any time following an input $I(t)$. $R(t)$ will be measured in units of, say, mg.

The ordinary background-subtracted renogram is, of course, a representation of $R(t)$ and from equation (29) the plasma concentration of OIH can be used as a representation of $I(t)$. The process of calculating $H(t)$ from a known $I(t)$ and $R(t)$ is called *deconvolution*; before considering how this can be done, the reverse process—*convolution*—should be examined.

Convolution

Convolution is the process of calculating the response of a system to a given input when the response of the system to an impulse input is already known.

To illustrate the principle first, suppose that discrete measurements of tracer input rate are made at 1-minute intervals. Since $I(t)$ is the amount of tracer entering the system per minute, the amount entering during the first minute may be called I_1, that during the second minute I_2, etc. In this discrete form an impulse input of unit quantity of tracer at the beginning of the first minute will be represented by $I_1 = 1$ and $I_2 = 0$, etc. In a similar manner discrete measurements can be taken of the quantity of tracer in the system after an impulse input. The quantity of tracer in the system expressed as a fraction of the injected dose and averaged over the first minute is called H_1, the average during the second minute H_2, etc.

Consider, as an example, a system of four pipes carrying a uniform flow of fluid past some detecting device (*Figure 18.6*). If a bolus of one unit of tracer is injected into the fluid in the pipe, the detector will measure its impulse response. Suppose that the flow divides equally between the four pipes, which are all of different lengths, so that the times for the bolus to pass through them are respectively, 3, 4, 5 and 6 minutes. The response of the detector will therefore represent 100% of the tracer in the system for the first 3 minutes ($H_1 = 1$; $H_2 = 1$; $H_3 = 1$), but at 3 minutes one-quarter of the tracer (that passing through the shortest pipe) will leave the field of view. Thus during the fourth minute only three-quarters of the tracer is in the system ($H_4 = \frac{3}{4}$). Similarly, at 4 minutes the tracer from the next-shortest pipe will leave the system and the response will drop again ($H_5 = \frac{1}{2}$). It will drop again at 5 minutes ($H_6 = \frac{1}{4}$) and finally drop to

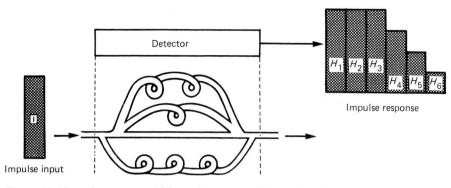

Figure 18.6 Impulse response of four-pipe system. For explanation, *see* text

zero at 6 minutes ($H_7 = 0$). The stepwise fall of the impulse response is an indication of the transit times through the various pipes in the system and of how much of the tracer flowed through each pipe.

It is now possible to calculate the response of the system to any other given input (*Figure 18.7*). Take an input, I, that shows an initial sudden rise followed by an exponential decrease, such as might be expected for the plasma OIH concentration in renography. If this input is thought of as being made up of a succession of impulse inputs I_1, I_2, I_3, etc., it is easy to calculate the response of the system to each input in turn. The impulse response, H, was the fraction of tracer in the system, so after an input I_1 the response will be I_1H. The response to I_2 will be I_2H, but since I_2 occurs 1 minute after I_1, the response will also start 1 minute later. The responses to I_3, I_4, etc., are

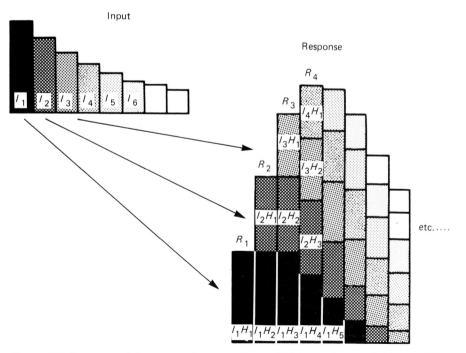

Figure 18.7 Response of the system shown in *Figure 18.6* to an exponential input. This is the process of convolution

constructed in the same way. The response of the system to the complete input can now be calculated by summing these individual responses. *Figure 18.7* shows that this response, R, is given by:

$$R_1 = I_1 H_1$$

$$R_2 = I_1 H_2 + I_2 H_1$$

$$R_3 = I_1 H_3 + I_2 H_2 + I_3 H_1$$

$$R_4 = I_1 H_4 + I_2 H_3 + I_3 H_2 + I_4 H_1$$

etc., or, in general,

$$R_i = \sum_{j=1}^{i} I_j \cdot H_{i-j+1} \Delta t \qquad i = 1, 2, 3, \text{ etc.} \tag{30}$$

where Δt is the time interval used for the discrete measurements.

If the time interval Δt is made smaller and smaller, so that the series of discrete measurements become continuous functions, the sum in equation (30) becomes an integral:

$$R(t) = \int_0^t I(\tau) H(t - \tau) \, d\tau \tag{31}$$

This is the convolution integral. It is sometimes written as:

$$R(t) = I(t) * H(t) \tag{32}$$

where the asterisk means 'convolved with', $H(t)$ is the response to an impulse input, and $R(t)$ is the response to the input $I(t)$.

The main assumption made in the above derivation is that the response of the system to a succession of impulse inputs is the sum of the individual responses. A system for which this is true is said to be a *linear system*. The quantities of OIH used in renography are very small, typically 0.3 mg, so the concentration in the tubules never reaches the point where tubular secretion becomes saturated. It is therefore reasonable to assume that the kidney is a linear system as far as OIH transport is concerned.

The other important assumption made is that, if a given input produces a certain response, then if the same input had been applied 1 minute later, the only difference in the response would be to shift it by 1 minute also. A system for which this is true is said to be *stationary*. In renography this means that, for convolution to be valid the ERPF, the GFR and the urine flow rate must all remain constant during the test. These conditions are unlikely to be strictly maintained in practice. For example, urine flow may not be a steady process but may fluctuate with changes in ureteric peristalsis. However, provided that the fluctuations are rapid enough to be averaged out in each time interval, Δt, so that the renogram remains smooth, they can reasonably be ignored. It is, however, not uncommon for excretion to occur in sudden, widely spaced bursts which show up as steps on the renogram. It is also possible for a sudden shock to alter renal blood flow temporarily and disturb the renogram. In these circumstances stationarity of the system is not maintained and deconvolution cannot safely be applied.

Discrete deconvolution

Deconvolution is the process of solving the convolution equations (30), (31) or (32) to find H if I and R are known. The simplest method of doing this is to use the discrete form of the convolution equation (30) and treat this as a set of simultaneous equations:

$$R_1 = I_1 H_1 \Delta t \tag{33a}$$

$$R_2 = (I_1 H_2 + I_2 H_1)\Delta t \tag{33b}$$

$$R_3 = (I_1 H_3 + I_2 H_2 + I_3 H_1)\Delta t \tag{33c}$$

$$R_4 = (I_1 H_4 + I_2 H_3 + I_3 H_2 + I_4 H_1)\Delta t \tag{33d}$$

etc. These equations may be rearranged to give the solution:

$$H_1 = \frac{1}{I_1}\left[\frac{R_1}{\Delta t}\right] \tag{34a}$$

$$H_2 = \frac{1}{I_1}\left[\frac{R_2}{\Delta t} - I_2 H_1\right] \tag{34b}$$

$$H_3 = \frac{1}{I_1}\left[\frac{R_3}{\Delta t} - (I_3 H_1 + I_2 H_2)\right] \tag{34c}$$

$$H_4 = \frac{1}{I_1}\left[\frac{R_4}{\Delta t} - (I_4 H_1 + I_3 H_2 + I_2 H_3)\right] \tag{34d}$$

etc., or, in general,

$$H_i = \frac{1}{I_1}\left[\frac{R_i}{\Delta t} - \sum_{j=1}^{i-1} I_{i-j+1} \cdot H_j\right] \tag{35}$$

If all the R_i and I_i are known, the H_i may be calculated one at a time using these equations.

The method will work perfectly if I and R are accurately known, but real data will always be subject to statistical uncertainties in the measurements. This means that a small error in R_1 or I_1 will produce a corresponding error in H_1. This error in H_1 will affect the value of H_2, and errors in H_1 and H_2 will affect H_3, and so on. The method is therefore very sensitive to errors in the first few values of R and I, since these propagate through the whole calculation of H.

This method of deconvolution is sometimes known as the *matrix algorithm*, because equation (33) can be written in matrix form as:

$$\mathbf{R} = \mathbf{I} \cdot \mathbf{H}\Delta t \tag{36}$$

which has a solution:

$$\mathbf{H} = \frac{1}{\Delta t}\mathbf{I}^{-1} \cdot \mathbf{R} \tag{37}$$

where $\mathbf{I}^{-1}$ is the inverse of the matrix $\mathbf{I}$. All that is needed is to calculate $\mathbf{I}^{-1}$ to find $\mathbf{H}$. $\mathbf{I}$ is a triangular matrix which is readily inverted; the process already described is really doing just this.

Other methods of deconvolution
If the renogram is treated as a continuously measured curve, rather than a set of discrete measurements, the integral form of the convolution equation (equation 31) is the appropriate one to use. This can be solved by making use of the Fourier transform. It can be shown that the Fourier transform of a convolution integral is just the product of the Fourier transforms of the two functions. So, by taking the Fourier transform of equation (31), we get:

$$\mathscr{F}(R(t)) = \mathscr{F}(I(t)) \cdot \mathscr{F}(H(t)) \tag{38}$$

This can be solved for $H(t)$ by dividing $\mathscr{F}(R(t))$ by $\mathscr{F}(I(t))$ and taking the inverse Fourier transform.

To apply this method in practice the renogram curve $R(t)$ and the input function $I(t)$ are both analysed into their frequency components by Fourier transformation at a series of frequencies up to some maximum which is determined by the sampling of the original data. Rapid fluctuations from one sampling point to the next are mainly due to statistical variations, or 'noise', and not to real changes in the data. These rapid fluctuations appear as high-frequency components in the Fourier transformed data, and so the high frequencies are usually artificially reduced in amplitude by filtering, or, equivalently, the original data are smoothed.

A slight variation of this method is to use the Laplace transform, which is very similar to the Fourier transform and has the same useful property when applied to the convolution integral.

None of the methods of deconvolution discussed so far relies on the assumptions of any particular model of renal function. There are, however, some simplifications which can be made to the calculations if certain models for the handling of OIH are used. One such approach is that suggested by Fleming and Goddard (1974), which assumes that the concentration of OIH in blood plasma can be described by a biexponential curve, as predicted by the compartmental model. The Laplace transform of the input function can then be evaluated analytically, and when it is used to calculate $H(t)$ by the method described above, it yields an expression which is easy to evaluate at any value of t. While this method has the advantage that it is amenable to easy calculation, it is only applicable if the blood clearance curve is satisfactorily described by a biexponential. It will not work if, for example, the injection is extravasated, whereas the more general methods will still apply. Van Stekelenburg (1978) has applied the same technique to a blood clearance curve which is the sum of three exponentials.

Practical considerations

The preceding discussion of deconvolution has assumed that the amount of tracer in the kidney, $R(t)$ (in mg), and the input rate to the kidney, $I(t)$ (in mg/min), are known and that these are used to calculate the impulse response, $H(t)$. In practice these quantities are not known directly, and so it is necessary to use instead the count rates (in cps) from suitable regions of interest on a gamma camera renogram, or from appropriately placed detectors during a probe renogram. The background-subtracted count rate from a kidney region of interest, $C'_K(t)$, will be proportional to $R(t)$ and the count rate from a vascular region of interest, such as the heart, $C_V(t)$, will be proportional to plasma concentration of tracer and hence to $I(t)$. In practical terms therefore, when deconvolution is performed using these count rate curves, a result, $G(t)$, is obtained that is proportional to $H(t)$ but not equal to it. This presents no problem, however, since it is the shape of the curve rather than its absolute value which contains all the useful information. In fact $G(t)$ is actually a more useful function than $H(t)$, as, although at $t = 0$ $H(0)$ must be 1 by definition it can be shown that $G(0)$ is equal to the kidney uptake constant (p. 256) and so is proportional to the individual kidney clearance.

To prove this the sensitivities defined on page 255 are used to write equations analogous to (20):

$$C'_K(t) = S_K R(t) \tag{39a}$$

and

$$C_V(t) = S_V V_1 P(t) = \frac{S_V V_1}{\text{ERPF}} I(t) \tag{39b}$$

where the latter result makes use of equation (29).

Now the convolution equation for $G(t)$ that is analogous to equation (32) is:

$$C'_K(t) = C_V(t) * G(t) \tag{40}$$

so substituting equations (39) into (40) and using (32) and (23)

$$G(t) = \frac{S_K}{S_V} \frac{\text{ERPF}}{V_1} H(t) = UCH(t) \tag{41}$$

since $H(0)$ is 1 this gives:

$$G(0) = UC \tag{42}$$

The calculations involved in the deconvolution of a renogram are rather long and tedious but are easily carried out on even a small computer. Deconvolution routines are available for several nuclear medicine computer systems, either as a standard feature or through user group programs. The matrix algorithm of deconvolution is in fact sufficiently straightforward for any competent programmer to implement in FORTRAN or even in BASIC. The skill in performing deconvolution really lies in the acquisition of the correct data in the first place and in the application of the correct amount of smoothing.

In this context, choice of the acquisition time per frame, which determines the time interval Δt, between successive data points, is important. If Δt is too long then the detailed shape of the curve is lost and the deconvolution procedure is inaccurate; if it is too short, then the counts in each image are low and the statistical uncertainty of each data point is large. In principle it is better to have a short Δt and then smooth the data rather than to have a long Δt, but there are practical limitations to the number of images which can reasonably be handled. In common with most other workers we have found an acquisition time of 20 seconds per frame to be a reasonable compromise. Using a dose of 12 MBq ^{123}I-OIH with the gamma camera 100 cps may be obtained typically in a renal region of interest and so in 20 seconds 2000 counts are accumulated. This will be subject to a statistical error of 45 counts which is 2.2%, and this seems to be an acceptable value for the raw data. However, before deconvolution analysis can be satisfactorily applied it is necessary to reduce the effects of statistical variations or 'noise' in the data until it accounts for less than about 0.5% of the actual number of counts. This is necessary because deconvolution is particularly susceptible to noise in the data. If the 'matrix algorithm' for discrete deconvolution is used (equation 34), it is easy to see how an error in one of the values of I_i or R_i will propagate through the rest of the calculation. If the Fourier transform method is used, spurious high-frequency components are produced. These two methods are, in fact, equivalent and equally sensitive to noise. When any method of deconvolution is applied it is necessary to reduce the noise in some way to a level below that present in the raw data.

In the Fourier transform method noise reduction can be achieved by reducing the amplitudes of the high-frequency components of the transformed data. Any frequency filtering of this type has an exactly equivalent smoothing operation which can be applied to the original data. It simply involves replacing each point in the activity–time curve by some appropriate weighted average of itself and its immediate neighbours. A convenient set of weights sometimes used for three-point smoothing is the ratio 1:2:1 for previous point:this point:next point. Other sets of weights can be used which are equivalent to fitting a polynomial through groups of points (Savitzky and Golay, 1964). These smoothing processes can be applied several times over to reduce noise even further.

Other methods of reducing the contributions from noise that have been applied in renography are data bounding (Diffey and Corfield, 1976) and spline fitting (Reinsch, 1967). The relative merits of these various methods of noise reduction have been compared by Fleming and Kenny (1977). With any of the methods, the amount of noise reduction selected must be appropriate for the particular acquisition parameters, such as frame time, administered activity and camera sensitivity, that are encountered in a particular department. Too little noise reduction may result in a wildly oscillating impulse retention function. Too much smoothing will tend to lose real changes in the data and will prolong the retention function, leading to an overestimate of the calculated mean and maximum transit times and the range of transit times (Lawson *et al.*, 1979).

The other important criterion for successful deconvolution is the selection of appropriate regions of interest. The kidney region may include the renal pelvis if 'whole kidney' transit times are under investigation but should exclude the renal pelvis and calyces if parenchymal transit times are to be calculated. In the latter case, in order to obtain an accurate transit time, it is more important to define a region that is 'pure' parenchyma than to try to include all parenchyma, even though this may underestimate renal uptake. Relative renal function is best determined from whole kidney regions of interest. The vascular region of interest is usually taken over the heart. However, if there is a significant time delay (comparable with Δt) between appearance of tracer in the vascular region and first appearance in the kidney, erroneous results will be produced. In these cases it may be necessary to select a different vascular region or to delay the vascular curve appropriately. Because of practical problems such as this there will always be a percentage of studies which are not amenable to deconvolution, particularly in cases of reduced renal function and in renal transplantation.

Deconvolution and background subtraction

In the discussion in the previous section it was assumed that the kidney count rate, $C'_K(t)$, used in practical deconvolution has already had blood and tissue background subtracted from it, so that it represents only tracer in the tubules and renal pelvis. If the unsubtracted count rate is used instead, then the retention function calculated by deconvolution will include the retention of tracer by blood and non-renal tissues. *Figure 18.8* illustrates how the observed retention function will be made up of two distinct components. After an impulse input, tracer would wash out of blood and non-renal tissues very rapidly, whereas it would be retained for several minutes in the renal parenchyma. In the resultant combined retention function the effect of tissue background would be concentrated at the very beginning. In practice, therefore, the background may be subtracted without making any assumptions or measurements of background-subtraction factors, by extrapolating the plateau of the observed retention function backwards.

In this way the impulse response can be obtained by deconvolution from the unsubtracted renogram just as easily as from the subtracted curve. The subtracted curve can be obtained by reconvolving G with C_V, using an equation similar to equation (30).

This provides an independent method of correcting for blood and tissue background. In effect the background, which is superimposed on all points in the ordinary renogram curve, is all concentrated in the first few points of the impulse response renogram.

Interpretation of results

The impulse response is nothing more than the renogram that would have been obtained if an ideal, sharp bolus injection were made straight into the aorta proximal to the renal arteries and if recirculation of any OIH not taken up in the first passage of blood were somehow eliminated.

The qualitative information obtained from the impulse response renogram is no different from that which can be deduced by an experienced observer reading the standard renogram, provided the shape of the blood clearance curve is always borne in mind. The impulse response renogram, however, is more useful when it comes to quantifying the results. As we have already observed, the initial height of the curve is equal to the kidney uptake constant and so can be used to calculate relative renal function according to equation (24). The duration of the impulse retention function is a

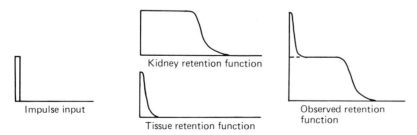

Impulse input

Kidney retention function

Tissue retention function

Observed retention function

Figure 18.8 The impulse retention function of kidney and tissue background together. Background subtraction can be performed on the combined retention function by extrapolation of the plateau

measure of the transit time for OIH transport through the kidney. This may be quantified by the *minimum transit time* (when the retention function first falls from the initial plateau), the *maximum transit time* (when the retention function reaches zero) or the time to any convenient intermediate amplitude. However, in a comparison of six deconvolution procedures in use at different hospitals, these parameters, and particularly those close to the maximum transit time, were found to be more dependent on the individual technique than the *mean transit time* (Lawson et al., 1979).

In order to quantify the elimination of OIH from the kidney, the rate of fall of the impulse response curve is required. It is convenient to define another function, $h(t)$, where:

$$h(t) = -\frac{dH(t)}{dt} \tag{43}$$

$h(t)$ is just the rate at which the OIH leaves the kidney after the ideal impulse input. It could be called the impulse output function, but it also represents the probability of OIH having a transit time near to t, and so it is usually called the *transit time spectrum*. The mean transit time can be calculated from $h(t)$ or from $H(t)$, using:

$$\bar{t} = \frac{\int_0^\infty t \cdot h(t)\,dt}{\int_0^\infty h(t)\,dt} = \frac{\int_0^\infty H(t)\,dt}{H(t=0)} \tag{44}$$

where the final expression results from substituting equation (43) and integrating by parts. Note that the denominator in these expressions is equal to 1 if $h(t)$ and $H(t)$ are properly normalized. In the same way the mean square transit time is calculated as:

$$\overline{t^2} = \frac{\int_0^\infty t^2 \cdot h(t)\,dt}{\int_0^\infty h(t)\,dt} = \frac{2\int_0^\infty t \cdot H(t)\,dt}{H(t=0)} \tag{45}$$

A convenient measure of the range of transit times is the width of the $h(t)$ distribution. This can be expressed mathematically by the root mean square deviation from the mean transit time, σ:

$$\sigma^2 = \overline{t^2} - (\bar{t})^2 \tag{46}$$

Deconvolution has been used to quantify probe renograms using ^{131}I-OIH (Britton and Brown, 1971) and gamma camera renograms using ^{123}I-OIH (Kenny et al., 1975; Gruenewald et al., 1981), ^{99m}Tc-DTPA (Diffey, Hall and Corfield, 1976; Piepsz et al., 1982) and the experimental agent ^{99m}Tc-TDG (Bevis et al., 1984).

Renal blood flow: first-pass studies

The compartmental model described earlier in this chapter was not able to analyse the mixing phase during the first few seconds after the injection of a radiopharmaceutical. The passage of a tracer bolus can, however, yield useful information on the blood flow through individual organs. This is most conveniently measured in terms of the mean transit time $\bar{t}$ defined by:

$$\bar{t} = \frac{V}{F} \tag{47}$$

where V is the volume of distribution of tracer within the organ (in ml) and F the flow rate through the organ (in ml/min). The reciprocal of mean transit time for an intravascular tracer is therefore a measure of the organ blood flow per unit volume.

If several parts of the vascular system receive their blood supply in series such that the flow through them all is the same, then it follows from equation (47) that the total mean transit time will be equal to the sum of the individual mean transit times. For example, if the mean transit time from an injection site to the renal artery is $\bar{t}_A$ and the mean transit time through the renal vascular system is $\bar{t}$ then the mean transit time from injection site to renal vein will be:

$$\bar{t}_V = \bar{t}_A + \bar{t} \tag{48}$$

so $\bar{t}$ can be deduced if $\bar{t}_A$ and $\bar{t}_V$ are measured.

This is the basis of one method for measuring the mean transit time of blood through the kidney. The renal artery mean transit time is calculated using an equation similar to (44):

$$\bar{t}_A = \frac{\int_0^\infty t \cdot C_A(t)\,dt}{\int_0^\infty C_A(t)\,dt} \tag{49}$$

where $C_A(t)$ is the count rate measured from a region of interest over the aorta during the first passage of a bolus injection of a tracer such as ^{99m}Tc-DTPA. A similar equation would allow $\bar{t}_V$ to be calculated from the count rate over the renal vein, but since this is not practicable the count rate over the kidney itself must be used, giving:

$$\bar{t}_K = \frac{\int_0^\infty t \cdot C_K(t)\,dt}{\int_0^\infty C_K(t)\,dt} \tag{50}$$

The transit time index given by the difference of these two values is then only an approximation to $\bar{t}$ and it can be shown that in fact:

$$\text{Transit time index} = \bar{t}_K - \bar{t}_A = \frac{1}{2}\left[\bar{t} + \frac{\sigma^2}{\bar{t}}\right] \tag{51}$$

where σ^2 is the mean square deviation of transit times.

A further practical difficulty arises because of tracer recirculating in the blood as well as tracer which is taken up by the kidney. The effects of this are removed from the activity–time curves by extrapolation of the initial portion of the downslope of the curve by fitting to an exponential or a function based on the shape of a gamma distribution (Davenport, 1983).

The most direct method of calculating the mean transit time of renal blood flow would be by deconvolution in a manner similar to that used for OIH transit through the tubules using the renogram. However, this is difficult to carry out in practice due to the poor counting statistics and time lags between the curves.

Alternative indices of renal perfusion that have been applied to transplanted kidneys are based on the ratio of the initial upslopes of the kidney and aorta curves (Kirchner et al., 1978) or the area under the curves up to their peak (Hilson et al., 1978).

Geometric mean count rate

Suppose that a point source of activity, A, is situated at a distance, d, from the midline of a uniform block of attenuating material with thickness, t, and attenuation coefficient μ (Figure 18.9). If a detector with geometrical efficiency, g, views the source from the posterior side it will detect a count rate:

$$C_P = g \cdot A\, e^{-\mu(t/2 - d)} \tag{52}$$

However, if the same detector views the source from the anterior side it will observe a lower count rate due to the greater thickness of intervening medium:

$$C_A = g \cdot A\, e^{-\mu(t/2 + d)} \tag{53}$$

The geometric mean of the anterior and posterior count rates is defined by:

$$C_{GM} = \sqrt{C_A C_P} = g \cdot A\, e^{-\mu t/2} \tag{54}$$

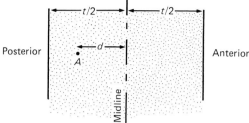

Figure 18.9 A point source in a uniform block of attenuating material

The geometric mean count rate is therefore independent of d, the position of the source in the material, and is proportional to the activity of the source attenuated by half the total thickness of material. It turns out that this result is still true even if the material is non-uniform, as in the human body. Of course if we are to apply the result to kidney studies we must allow for the fact that the kidney is not actually a point source but an extended, and probably non-uniform, distribution of activity. If a detailed analysis is carried out equation (54) becomes modified to:

$$C_{GM} = g \cdot A\, e^{-\mu t/2} \cdot S \tag{55}$$

where S is a shape factor that depends only on the size and activity distribution of the source. It is independent of the source position within the material.

The shape factor for a point source is one. For an extended source the shape factor increases as the size of the source increases. For a uniform distribution of activity with extent s, the shape factor is:

$$S = \frac{\sqrt{2}}{\mu s} [\cosh(\mu s) - 1]^{1/2} \tag{56}$$

and for the extreme case of two equal point sources separated by a distance s:

$$S = \frac{1}{\sqrt{2}} [\cosh(\mu s) + 1]^{1/2} \tag{57}$$

The adult kidney has an A–P diameter of 30–40 mm (ICRP, 1975) and for 140 keV gamma rays in tissue $\mu = 0.015\,\text{mm}^{-1}$. For these values the above equations give shape factors of 1.015 and 1.045 respectively, and so, for any arbitrary distribution of activity within the kidney, we would not expect a correction of more than 5% due to the shape factor. It is thus a reasonable approximation to assume that the shape factors for all kidneys are the same and approximately equal to one. Therefore the geometric mean count rate should be directly proportional to kidney activity irrespective of kidney depth.

The geometric mean count rate can be used, therefore, to calculate a depth-corrected relative function in a similar manner to equation (19):

$$\text{Left kidney relative function} = \frac{C_{GM}(\text{left}) \times 100\%}{C_{GM}(\text{left}) + f \cdot C_{GM}(\text{right})} \tag{58}$$

where

$$f = e^{\mu(t_R - t_L)/2} \tag{59}$$

and $(t_R - t_L)$ is the difference in patient thickness at the two kidney sites. If this difference is less than 15 mm, f will lie between 0.9 and 1.1 and may reasonably be ignored. Larger differences may easily be determined from external patient measurements and an appropriate correction applied.

Summary of symbols used in mathematical analysis of renography

Compartmental model

Compartment 1 = central compartment (intravascular)
Compartment 3 = peripheral compartment (extravascular)
Compartment 2 = end compartment (urine)
        subdivided into:
        Compartment 4 = urine in renal tubules
        Compartment 5 = urine in bladder
        Compartment 6 = urine in renal pelvis

Q_0	= total quantity of tracer injected (mg)
$Q_i(t)$	= quantity of tracer in compartment i (mg)
$X_i(t)$	= fraction of injected tracer in compartment i (dimensionless)
V_i	= volume of compartment i (ml)
F_{ij}	= clearance rate from compartment i to compartment j (ml/min)
K_{ij}	= rate constant = fractional clearance rate (minute^{-1})
$\lambda_1, \lambda_2, \lambda_3$	= rate constants of exponentials describing $X_i(t)$ (minute^{-1})
$A_1 - A_{12}$	= constants multiplying exponentials in $X_i(t)$ (dimensionless)
C_1, C_2	= constants multiplying exponentials in $P(t)$ (mg/ml)
$P(t)$	= blood plasma concentration of tracer = $Q_1(t)/V_1$ (mg/ml)
t_0	= transit time for urine through renal tubules (minute)
t_v	= time before bladder is voided (minute)

Renal function

$C_K(t)$	= count rate from kidney region (cps)
$C_K'(t)$	= background-corrected count rate from kidney region (cps)
$C_V(t)$	= count rate from vascular region (cps)
$C_T(t)$	= count rate from tissue region (cps)
S_K	= sensitivity of detection in kidney region to tracer in the kidney (cps/mg)
S_V	= sensitivity of detection in vascular region to tracer uniformly distributed in blood (cps/mg)
UC	= kidney uptake constant (minute^{-1})
b_1	= background subtraction factor for vascular background
b_2	= background subtraction factor for tissue background

Deconvolution

$I(t)$	= input rate of tracer to kidney (mg/minute)
$R(t)$	= total quantity of tracer in kidney (mg)
$H(t)$	= fraction of tracer in kidney after impulse input
	= impulse retention function (dimensionless)
$h(t)$	= fractional rate at which tracer leaves the kidney after impulse input
	= transit time spectrum = $-\mathrm{d}H/\mathrm{d}t$ (minute^{-1})
Δt	= time interval between renogram curve points (minute)
$\bar{t}$	= mean transit time for tracer through kidney (minute)
$\overline{t^2}$	= mean square transit time (minute^2)
σ	= root mean square deviation of transit time from $\bar{t}$ (minute)
$G(t)$	= H calculated using C_K' instead of R and C_V instead of I (minute^{-1})

Renal blood-flow

$\bar{t}$	= mean transit time of blood through kidney (seconds)
$\bar{t}_A$	= mean transit time from injection site to renal artery (seconds)
$\bar{t}_V$	= mean transit time from injection site to renal vein (seconds)
$\bar{t}_K$	= approximation to $\bar{t}_V$ using kidney counts (seconds)
σ	= root mean square deviation of transit time from $\bar{t}$ (seconds)
$C_A(t)$	= count rate from aorta region of interest (cps)
$C_K(t)$	= count rate from kidney region of interest (cps)

Geometric mean count rate

μ	= linear attenuation coefficient of tissue (mm^{-1})
t	= total thickness of patient at kidney site (mm)
d	= displacement of kidney from midline (mm)
A	= activity in kidney (MBq)
g	= geometrical efficiency of gamma camera (cps/MBq)
C_P	= count rate from posterior view (cps)
C_A	= count rate from anterior view (cps)
C_{GM}	= geometric mean count rate (cps)
S	= correction factor which depends on kidney shape (dimensionless)
s	= anterior–posterior size of kidney (mm)

References

BEVIS, C. R. A., LAWSON, R. S., SHIELDS, R. A. and TESTA, H. J. (1984) ^{99m}Tc-TDG renography with deconvolution analysis: A comparative study with ^{99m}Tc-DTPA and ^{123}I-hippuran. *Nuclear Medicine Communications*, **5**, 513–517

BLAUFOX, M. D. (1972) Compartment analysis of the radiorenogram and kinetics of ^{131}I-hippuran. *Progress in Nuclear Medicine*, **2**, 107–124

BRITTON, K. E. and BROWN, N. J. G. (1971) *Clinical Renography*, London: Lloyd Luke

BROWN, N. J. G. and BRITTON, K. E. (1969) The renogram and its quantitation. *British Journal of Urology*, **41**, Suppl. 15

BROWN, N. J. G. (1982) The application of interpolative background subtraction to Tc-99m DTPA gamma camera renography data. In: *Radionuclides in Nephrology*, A. M. Joekes, A. R. Constable, N. J. G. Brown and W. N. Tauxe (eds.), London: Academic Press, pp. 113–118

DAVENPORT, R. (1983) The derivation of the gamma variate relationship for tracer dilution curves. *Journal of Nuclear Medicine*, **24**, 945–948

DIFFEY, B. L. and CORFIELD, J. R. (1976) The data bounding technique in discrete deconvolution. *Medical and Biological Engineering*, **14**, 478

DIFFEY, B. L., HALL, F. M. and CORFIELD, J. R. (1976) The ^{99m}Tc-DTPA dynamic renal scan with deconvolution analysis. *Journal of Nuclear Medicine*, **17**, 352–355

FLEMING, J. S. and GODDARD, B. A. (1974) A technique for the deconvolution of the renogram. *Physics in Medicine and Biology*, **19**, 546–549

FLEMING, J. S. and KENNY, R. W. (1977) A comparison of techniques for the filtering of noise in the renogram. *Physics in Medicine and Biology*, **22**, 359–364

GRUENEWALD, S. M., NIMMON, C. C., NAWAZ, M. K. and BRITTON, K. E. (1981) A non-invasive gamma camera technique for the measurement of intrarenal flow distribution in man. *Clinical Science*, **61**, 385–389

HALL, F. M. and MONKS, G. K. (1966) The renogram: A method of separating vascular and renal components. *Investigative Radiology*, **1**, 220–224

HILSON, A. J. W., MAISEY, M. N., BROWN, C. B., OGG, C. S. and BESWICK, M. S. (1978) Dynamic renal transplant imaging with Tc 99m DTPA (Sn) supplemented by a transplant perfusion index in the management of renal transplants. *Journal of Nuclear Medicine*, **19**, 994–1000

HINE, G. J., FARMELANT, M. H., CARDARELLI, J. A. and BURROWS, B. A. (1963) Four channel magnetic tape recording and digital analysis of radio-hippuran renal function tests in normal subjects. *Journal of Nuclear Medicine*, **4**, 371–381

I.C.R.P. (1975) International Commission on Radiological Protection Publication 23, *Reference Man: Anatomical, Physiological and Metabolic Characteristics*, Oxford: Pergamon Press

KENNY, R. W., ACKERY, D. M., FLEMING, J. S., GODDARD, B. A. and GRANT, R. W. (1975) Deconvolution analysis of the scintillation camera renogram. *British Journal of Radiology*, **48**, 481–486

KIRCHNER, P. T., GOLDMAN, M. H., LEAPMAN, S. B. and KIEPFER, R. F. (1978) Clinical application of the kidney to aortic blood flow index (K/A ratio). *Contributions to Nephrology*, **11**, 120–126

LAWSON, R. S., BROWN, N. J. G., DANCE, D. R., DIFFEY, B. L., ERBSMANN, F., FLEMING, J. S., HOUSTON, A. S. and TOFTS, P. S. (1979) A multicentre comparison of techniques for deconvolution of the renogram. Paper presented at the 7th BNMS Annual Meeting, London, April 1979

MATTHEWS, C. M. E. (1957) The theory of tracer experiments with ^{131}I-labelled plasma proteins. *Physics in Medicine and Biology*, **2**, 36–53

PIEPSZ, A., HAM, H. R., ERBSMANN, F., DIFFEY, D. L., COGGIN, M. J., HALL, F. M., MILLAR, J. A., LUMBROSO, J., BAZIN, J. P., DI PAOLA, M. and FRIES, D. (1982) A cooperative study on the clinical value of dynamic renal scanning with deconvolution analysis. *British Journal of Radiology*, **55**, 419–433

REEVE, J. and CRAWLEY, J. C. W. (1974) Quantitative radioisotope renography: The derivation of physiologica data, by deconvolution analysis using a single injection technique. *Clinical Science and Molecular Medicine*, **47**, 317–330

REINSCH, C. H. (1967) Smoothing by spline functions. *Numerische Mathematik*, **10**, 177–183

RUTLAND, M. D. (1979) A single injection technique for subtraction of blood background in ^{131}I hippuran renograms. *British Journal of Radiology*, **52**, 134–137

SAPIRSTEIN, L. A., VIDT, D. G., MANDEL, M. J. and HANUSEK, G. (1955) Volumes of distribution and clearances of intravenously injected creatinine in the dog. *American Journal of Physiology*, **181**, 330–336

SAVITSKY, A. and GOLAY, J. R. (1964) Smoothing and differentiation of data by simplified least squares procedures. *Analytical Chemistry*, **36**, 1627–1639

SHORT, M. D., GLASS, H. I. and VERNON, P. (1970) Use of gamma camera for ^{131}I renography: A case study on a nephrectomised patient. *Journal of Nuclear Medicine*, **11**, 758–760

THOMSON, W. H., LEACH, K. G. and MIDDLETON, G. M. (1984) A new technique for accurate blood background subtraction in renography—validation and comparison with other methods. *Nuclear Medicine Communications*, **5**, 222 (abstract of a paper presented at 12th BNMS Annual Meeting, London, April 1984)

VAN STEKELENBURG, L. H. M., AL, N., KOOMAN, A. and TERTOOLEN, J. F. W. (1976) A three compartment model for the transport and distribution of hippuran. *Physics in Medicine and Biology*, **21**, 74–84

VAN STEKELENBURG, L. H. M. (1978) Hippuran transit times in the kidney: A new approach. *Physics in Medicine and Biology*, **23**, 291–301

Further reading

INGRAM, D. and BLOCH, R. (eds.) (1984) *Mathematical Methods in Medicine*, Chichester: John Wiley and Sons

19 Radiation dosimetry

R. S. Lawson

The damaging effects of radiation on biological tissue are due to ionization produced by the primary radiation or by secondary electrons. Such ionization occurring within a living cell may result in its death, or it may produce a change in the nucleus which is passed on to future generations of the cell, possibly giving rise to malignant growth.

However, although ionization can have harmful effects, it does provide a useful means of detecting radiation and measuring its intensity. Thus a quantity called *exposure*, which is a measure of the intensity of X or gamma radiation and the time for which it has been acting, has traditionally been measured by the amount of ionization that is produced in air. This can be determined by the total electric charge liberated as ions in a given quantity of air. The SI unit of exposure is therefore the coulomb per kilogram, but the traditional unit of the *röntgen* (R), equal to one electrostatic unit of charge per cm^3, is still sometimes encountered. The relationship between the two units is:

$$1 C kg^{-1} = 3876 R$$

The intensity of an X or gamma ray beam is measured by its *exposure rate* in $C kg^{-1} s^{-1}$ (or $R s^{-1}$).

However, the biological effect of radiation depends not just on its intensity but more on how much of its energy is absorbed by tissue. Hence, the quantity *absorbed dose* is defined as the energy absorbed per unit mass of material. The SI unit of absorbed dose is the *gray* (Gy), which is equal to one joule per kilogram, although the traditional unit is the *rad* (from röntgen-absorbed dose), equal to 100 erg/g. The conversion between old and new units is therefore:

$$1 Gy = 100 rad$$

The biological effect of radiation on tissue depends primarily on the absorbed dose, but also on other factors such as how quickly this dose was delivered, how uniformly it was distributed and the type of radiation involved. To take account of this a third quantity, the *dose equivalent* is used. This is defined by:

$$\text{Dose equivalent} = \text{Absorbed dose} \times \text{Modifying factors} \tag{1}$$

The SI unit of dose equivalent is the *sievert* (Sv), and the traditional unit is the *rem* (from röntgen equivalent in man):

$$1 Sv = 100 rem$$

The most important of the modifying factors in equation (1) is the *quality factor* which allows for the different densities of ionization produced by different types of radiation. All X-rays and gamma rays and most beta particles are assigned a quality factor of 1 but alpha particles, which produce very dense ionization, have a quality factor of 20 (IRCP, 1977a). This is the main reason why alpha-emitting radionuclides are not used in nuclear medicine. For all X-rays, gamma rays and beta particles at the energies and dose rates usually encountered in nuclear medicine, the modifying factors may all be taken as equal to 1, so that dose equivalent and absorbed dose are numerically equal although they really measure physically distinct quantities.

The harmful effects of ionizing radiation may be classified as either *stochastic* or *non-stochastic*. Non-stochastic effects, such as cataract of the lens of the eye or haematological deficiencies due to bone marrow cell damage, vary in severity with the size of the dose equivalent received. However, there appears to be a threshold dose below which none of these effects is observed. The International Commission on Radiological Protection (ICRP) has therefore recommended that, to prevent non-stochastic effects, radiation workers should not receive a dose of more than 150 mSv in a year to the lens of the eye (ICRP, 1980) and 500 mSv in a year to any other tissues (ICRP, 1977a). It is extremely unlikely that these limits would ever be exceeded, even by patients, in diagnostic nuclear medicine investigations.

The stochastic effects of radiation include carcinogenesis, particularly breast cancer, lung cancer and leukaemia, and genetic damage which only becomes manifest in subsequent generations. These effects cannot be measured by their severity because either they appear or they do not appear. Instead it is the probability of the effect occurring which varies with the dose. Reducing the dose reduces the likelihood of a stochastic effect occurring, but there is no threshold level which is completely risk-free. In order to keep the radiation risk at an acceptable level that is no worse than the risk from other occupations or in everyday life, the ICRP has set an occupational limit of 50 mSv per year and a limit of 5 mSv per year for members of the public (ICRP, 1977a). This dose equivalent limit applies to uniform irradiation of the whole body. If the dose distribution is non-uniform—as it usually is in nuclear medicine—the different susceptibilities of each organ must be allowed for by taking a weighted sum over all irradiated organs. This sum defines the *effective dose equivalent*—the uniformly distributed dose which would involve the same overall risk.

$$\text{Effective dose equivalent} = \sum_{\text{all tissues}} \text{Weighting factor} \times \text{Dose equivalent} \qquad (2)$$

The appropriate weighting factors for different tissues are shown in *Table 19.1*.

Although the concept of effective dose equivalent was originally devised for assessment of occupational risk, it now provides a convenient index for comparing the risk to a patient from a diagnostic nuclear medicine investigation with the risk from

Table 19.1. Weighting factors recommended for calculating effective dose equivalent (ICRP, 1977a)

Tissue	Weighting factor
Whole body (uniform)	1.00
Gonads	0.25
Breast	0.15
Red bone marrow	0.12
Lung	0.12
Thyroid	0.03
Bone surfaces	0.03
Any other organ (up to 5 organs)	0.06

possible alternative procedures. Most nuclear medicine studies involve an effective dose equivalent of less than 5 mSv. By comparison, in the United Kingdom, the mean effective dose equivalent from naturally occurring background radiation is about 2 mSv per year (NRPB, 1984). The effective dose equivalent of a plain abdominal X-ray is about 1 mSv and that from an intravenous urogram ranges from 1 to 27 mSv with a mean of about 2 mSv (B. F. Wall, personal communication). The probability of a fatal cancer in the irradiated individual or severe hereditary effects in the next two generations is believed to be about $1.7 \times 10^{-2} \, Sv^{-1}$ (ICRP, 1977b) so an effective dose equivalent of 1 mSv would entail a risk of about 1 in 60 000. This is about the same as the risk of death from smoking a packet of 20 cigarettes or travelling 500 miles by car (Brill, 1982).

There is no specific dose limit for patients undergoing diagnostic investigations since the risks involved must be weighed against the potential benefits to the patient. However, as a general principle, the dose must be kept as low as reasonably achievable (the ALARA principle) consistent with the need to obtain reliable results that will benefit the patient's management. Special precautions should be taken with regard to women of reproductive age, avoiding in particular non-urgent investigations in pregnancy which might involve a significant dose to the fetus. The ICRP has published guidance on the protection of patients in radionuclide investigations (ICRP, 1969), and an updated report from the task group on protection of the patient in nuclear medicine is currently in preparation. In Britain the Department of Health and Social Security has issued guidance prepared by the Administration of Radioactive Substances Advisory Committee (DHSS, 1984) and all doctors carrying out radio-isotope investigations must obtain a certificate from the UK Health Ministers, or work under the direction of someone who holds a certificate.

Method of calculating absorbed dose

From the foregoing definition of absorbed dose it follows that:

$$\text{Absorbed dose} = \frac{\text{Total energy absorbed}}{\text{Mass of absorbing organ}} \qquad (3)$$

Therefore the process of calculating the absorbed dose for a particular organ is really one of calculating the total energy absorbed by that organ.

Following the administration of a radiopharmaceutical to a patient, the radio-activity will be distributed throughout various organs of the body in a manner dependent on the biological handling of the particular pharmaceutical. The organs containing radioactivity may be thought of as *source organs* emitting radiation in all directions but, in particular, towards the *target organ* for which the radiation dose is to be calculated. In general, any target organ will receive radiation from several source organs, so that the absorbed dose must be calculated from each and the results combined. The largest contribution is very often from activity within the target organ itself.

The absorbed dose to a given target organ due to radiation from a particular source organ depends on many factors:

1. The energy of the radiation;
2. The type of radiation—in particular, the numbers of gamma rays, beta particles and X-rays emitted on average from each disintegration of the radionuclide. This is important, since beta particles and low-energy X-rays will not penetrate out of the source organ and so can be ignored if source and target organs are separate, but they

may be the major factor in calculating the dose to an organ from a radio-pharmaceutical within itself;

3. Source and target organ shapes, source-to-target distance and the nature of the intervening material. These factors determine what fraction of the gamma rays originating within a source organ is absorbed within it and what fraction is absorbed within a remote target organ. The greater the distance between the two organs the lower the dose that one contributes to the other;

4. Target organ mass. This is needed in the denominator of equation (3);

5. Administered dose of radiopharmaceutical;

6. Physical half-life of decay of the radionuclide; and

7. Physiological handling of the radiopharmaceutical—i.e. the uptake by the source organ and the rate of biological elimination.

These last three factors between them govern the total activity in the source organ and the length of time that it remains there. These factors therefore determine a quantity, $\tilde{A}$, called the *cumulated activity*, measured in units such as $MBq \cdot s$ (or $\mu Ci\,h$). Since this depends largely on physiological data which may not be accurately known, it is the major source of uncertainty in the calculation of absorbed dose.

On the other hand, the first two factors in the above list relate only to the physical process of the radioactive decay, and their values are well known and tabulated (Dillman and Von der Lage, 1975). The third and fourth factors relate to organ size and position and are thus not precisely defined, but they may be described in terms of a suitable anatomical model. These first four factors together determine a quantity, S, called the *absorbed dose per unit cumulated activity*. This would be measured in units of $\mu Gy/MBq \cdot s$ (or $rad/\mu Ci\,h$). Since it depends only on physical and anatomical data, for a given target organ and source organ, S will only depend on the radionuclide used and the size of the patient. It can, in principle, be accurately calculated but generally this requires a computer and often simplifying approximations are made.

The calculation of absorbed dose is split into two parts

$$\text{Absorbed dose to target organ} = \sum_{\substack{\text{sum over all} \\ \text{source organs}}} S \cdot \tilde{A} \qquad (4)$$

$\tilde{A}$ is equal to the activity in the source organ multiplied by the time that it remains there or, if the activity is varying continuously with time,

$$\tilde{A} = \int_0^\infty A(t)\,dt \qquad (5)$$

where $A(t)$ is the activity in the source organ at any time t. This only depends on factors (5) to (7) above.

As has already been remarked, the quantity S, which depends on factors (1) to (4), can be calculated from purely physical and anatomical data. This has been done by Snyder *et al.* and published in a report by the Medical Internal Radiation Dose Committee (MIRD) of the Society of Nuclear Medicine (Snyder *et al.*, 1975). They have tabulated S for 20 different source organs and 20 target organs of a standard adult human phantom for a range of radionuclides likely to be encountered in nuclear medicine. One of the limitations of their method is that it only gives the average dose to an organ, and, in cases where the activity is not distributed uniformly throughout the organ, this will underestimate the local dose. This will be the case, for example, with any radiopharmaceutical that concentrates in the kidney cortex and not in other renal tissues. The method also does not distinguish between renal parenchyma and renal pelvis as separate source organs. Another important limitation of the method is that it assumes a constant bladder volume and does not allow for a changing S as the bladder fills.

However, if the limitations are borne in mind, these tabulated values for S can be used, together with the appropriate physiological data for $A(t)$, to compute the absorbed dose for any particular examination using equations (4) and (5).

Estimation of the dose equivalent for various renal studies in adults

Radiation dosimetry calculations are not precise and can only give an estimate of the dose from any particular nuclear medicine investigation. A wide range of results can therefore be found in the literature.

Variations between different authors' results for the radiation dose from the same test are usually due to the fact that they have made different, but equally plausible, assumptions about the biological handling of the radiopharmaceutical. The range of variation found in the physiological assumptions made often only reflects different opinions as to normality, whereas many patients undergoing investigation will have abnormal physiological function.

In order to compare several different tests, it is useful to know the radiation dose from each under the same physiological conditions, but, unfortunately, it is not always possible to find such data published. For this reason we have estimated the dose equivalent to adults for a variety of renal studies and for several radiopharmaceuticals, under two consistent sets of physiological assumptions, representing normal and abnormal function. The range of these results is therefore a guide to the variation that might be expected from patient to patient, while, for a given set of physiological data, they allow an intercomparison of several tests and different radiopharmaceuticals.

The method uses a simplified version of the compartmental model described in Chapter 18 to represent the handling of compounds that are excreted by the kidneys. It is assumed that tracer is initially injected into an intravascular compartment, from where it can exchange with extravascular space. Tracer is cleared from the intravascular compartment by the kidneys and passes to the bladder.

In order to estimate the absorbed radiation dose we have considered the accumulation of activity in four source organs: whole body, kidneys, bladder and thyroid. The intravascular and extravascular compartments are assumed to be uniformly distributed throughout the body. No distinction has been made between activity in the renal tubules and the renal pelvis because S factors are not available for these organs separately. It has been assumed that the bladder is empty initially and thereafter is voided at regular intervals.

The activity in the thyroid has been estimated using another simple compartmental model. It is assumed that a fraction of the administered activity is in the form of free iodide and that this is eliminated via the kidneys with a rate constant K_E and taken up by the thyroid with a rate constant K_T. Secretion of activity from the thyroid as thyroid hormone takes place at a rate K_S, and it is assumed that this is rapidly degraded into free iodide again.

The cumulated activity in each of the source organs has been calculated using the predictions of these compartmental models (see Chapter 18) and allowing for radioactive decay. The absorbed dose to various target organs—kidneys, bladder wall, whole body, thyroid and gonads—has then been calculated using the methods described above. The dose equivalent to each organ and the effective dose equivalent to the whole body have then been calculated using equations (1) and (2).

The values assumed for the various parameters used in the calculations are shown in Table 19.2, and the physical data for each nuclide appear in Table 15.1. The renal model parameters K_{12}, K_{13}, K_{31} and V_1 have the same meaning as in Chapter 18 and the renal transit time is equivalent to the sum of tubular transit time and mean transit time

TABLE 19.2. Parameters used in radiation dosimetry estimations

Renal model parameters	Hippuran	EDTA	DTPA gluconate and DMSA	MDP
Renal uptake, K_{12} (min^{-1})				
Normal	0.05	0.02	0.02	0.007
Abnormal	0.005	0.002	0.002	0.0007
Exchange with EVS				
K_{13} (min^{-1})	0.04	0.05	0.05	0.003
K_{31} (min^{-1})	0.06	0.01	0.01	0.0002
Renal transit time (min)				
Normal	4	5	5*	5
Abnormal	20	20	20*	20
Bladder voiding interval (h)				
Normal	2	2	2	2
Abnormal	5	5	5	5
Equivalent clearance (ml/min)				
Normal	450	120	120	40
Abnormal	45	12	12	4
Volume of dilution, V_1 (litres)	9	6	6	6

Thyroid iodide model parameters:

Renal excretion of iodide, K_E (h^{-1})				
Normal		0.08		
Abnormal		0.008		
Thyroid uptake rate, K_T (h^{-1})		0.04		
Thyroid hormone secretion rate, K_s (h^{-1})		0.0006		
Equivalent 24 h thyroid uptake		30%		

	^{123}I	^{125}I	^{131}I
Free iodide content of OIH		0.5%	1%

All ^{99m}Tc pharmaceuticals assumed to contain 5% free pertechnetate

Isotopic purity:
^{123}I assumed to contain 0.2% ^{125}I impurity

* Transit times shown are for DTPA; 15% of gluconate and 50% of DMSA assumed to have infinite transit time

through the renal pelvis. DMSA and, to a lesser extent, gluconate, are known to be partially bound in the renal cortex (Arnold *et al.*, 1975), and so a fraction of these compounds has been assumed to have an infinite renal transit time. The rate constants for thyroid iodine metabolism are based on figures used by the MIRD Committee (MIRD, 1975). The distribution of pertechnetate is not fitted adequately by the three-compartment model, and dose estimates have been taken directly from the MIRD Committee report (MIRD, 1976).

The results of these radiation dose estimates for adults are shown in *Table 19.3*, assuming typical administered activities for each test. The first value in each case represents the physiological assumptions that correspond to normal renal function and the second value represents a worst-case estimate based on poor renal function or urinary obstruction or both.

The effective dose equivalent for a GFR measurement using ^{51}Cr-EDTA is insignificant, being less than the dose received from natural background radiation in 1 week. The radiation dose for an ERPF measurement using ^{125}I-OIH is also small, but in this case, as with most other OIH studies, the largest contribution to the effective dose equivalent is from the dose to the thyroid, which arises from free iodide in the radiopharmaceutical. It is therefore desirable to keep the free iodide

TABLE 19.3. Dose equivalent (mSv) to adults for various renal studies: normal renal function and worst-case estimates

Test	Administered activity (MBq)	Dose equivalent (mSv) to						Effective dose equivalent (mSv)
		Kidneys	Bladder wall	Thyroid	Whole body	Testes	Ovaries	
^{51}Cr-EDTA clearance for GFR	3	0.006	0.04	0.002	0.002	0.003	0.004	0.01
		0.036	0.11	0.019	0.020	0.021	0.026	0.03
^{125}I-OIH clearance for ERPF	2	0.01	0.2	3	0.003	0.001	0.002	0.1
		0.05	0.5	11	0.014	0.006	0.008	0.4
^{131}I-OIH probe renogram	1	0.03	0.5	5	0.006	0.01	0.01	0.2
		0.15	1.4	12	0.026	0.03	0.03	0.5
^{131}I-OIH gamma camera renogram	3	0.09	1.5	14	0.02	0.02	0.03	0.5
		0.45	4.3	40	0.08	0.08	0.10	1.4
^{123}I-OIH gamma camera renogram	12	0.08	1.3	3	0.02	0.03	0.05	0.2
		0.35	3.3	6	0.07	0.08	0.12	0.4
^{99m}Tc-DTPA gamma camera renogram	75	0.3	3	0.2	0.16	0.2	0.3	0.4
		0.9	6	0.4	0.32	0.3	0.4	0.7
^{99m}Tc-DTPA renal imaging	400	1.8	14	1	0.8	0.9	1.5	2.1
		5.0	32	2	1.7	1.5	2.3	3.8
^{99m}Tc-gluconate renal imaging	400	18	12	1	1.0	0.9	1.5	3.2
		7*	27	2	1.7	1.5	2.2	4.5
^{99m}Tc-DMSA renal imaging	70	10	1	0.2	0.2	0.1	0.3	1.0
		3*	3	0.3	0.3	0.3	0.4	1.1
^{99m}Tc-MDP bone scan	550	2.5	17	1.7	1.3	1.4	2.1	3.7
		6.5	40	2.6	2.4	2.1	3.2	6.0

* Dose to the kidneys from gluconate and DMSA reduces for decreasing renal function
Units: To convert mSv to mrem, multiply by 100
     To convert MBq to μCi, multiply by 27

content as low as possible or to block the thyroid with a prior administration of potassium perchlorate or iodide solution. However, thyroid blocking is not normally considered necessary for any of the studies discussed here. Unfortunately some published figures for OIH radiation dosimetry fail to take free iodide into account. The assumptions regarding free iodide content of the radiopharmaceuticals that have been used in these calculations are included in *Table 19.2*.

^{131}I-OIH can be used satisfactorily for probe renograms with a low radiation dose, but for gamma camera studies the radiation dose limits the activity that can reasonably be administered. However, using ^{123}I-OIH sufficient activity may be administered to give a high quality study for an effective dose equivalent that is about one-tenth of that for an IVU. A much smaller radiation dose is given by ^{123}I-OIH than the same activity of ^{131}I because of its shorter half-life and greatly reduced electron emission (*see Table 15.1*). The results presented here for ^{123}I assume a 0.2% impurity of ^{125}I. This is the quality of material supplied by AERE (Harwell) using proton bombardment of an iodine target. An alternative method, using alpha particle bombardment of an antimony target, produces significant ^{124}I contamination which can treble the radiation dose.

The use of high activities of technetium agents for gamma camera imaging of the kidneys involves a higher radiation dose despite the short half-life of ^{99m}Tc. However, the use of a bolus injection of 400 MBq (10 mCi) of the agent gives information on the vascularity of the kidney as well as its function for an effective dose equivalent comparable with an IVU and much less than for angiography. The use of gluconate and DMSA involves a higher radiation dose to the kidneys than DTPA because a fraction of these agents is bound in the kidney rather than being excreted. For this reason the dose equivalent to the kidneys from these agents reduces with decreasing renal function. For several ^{99m}Tc radiopharmaceuticals the most important contribution to the effective dose equivalent is from the bladder dose and this can be kept to a minimum by frequent voiding.

The ^{99m}Tc-labelled phosphate agents used for bone scanning also follow a urinary excretory pathway, and a three-compartment model has been used to describe the kinetics of ^{99m}Tc-MDP. The rate constants shown in *Table 19.2* have been derived to fit the urinary excretion data observed by Subramanian *et al.* (1975), and, hence, the cumulated activities and organ doses have been calculated as for renal imaging agents. This method does not give a dose equivalent to the bones, but this has been estimated by Subramanian *et al.* to be 5.7 mSv to the skeleton and 3.7 mSv to the red bone marrow for a 550-MBq administered dose. This contribution to the effective dose equivalent has been included in *Table 19.3*.

All the results presented here are subject to the limitations of the method discussed on page 274. The method also assumes organ masses and sizes appropriate to a standard man, and so the results are only applicable to adults.

Radiation dosimetry in children

When performing nuclear medicine investigations in children, the activity of radio-pharmaceutical used in usually reduced compared with that which would be appropriate for an adult. However, this can be done without reducing the quality of the information obtained. If a clearance measurement is being performed, the administered activity may be reduced in direct proportion to body weight, and the same count rate per millilitre of plasma will be obtained as for an adult. If gamma camera images are being acquired, the information density depends on the counts per unit area in the image. Since the image size will be smaller for children the same information density can be obtained by reducing the administered activity in proportion to body surface area or the two-thirds power of body weight. This latter method of scaling would result in a somewhat higher administered activity than the former method, but in practice the activity is often scaled in direct proportion to body weight even for imaging studies. To some extent the reduced gamma ray attenuation in a child compensates for the reduced activity, and the imaging time need be extended only slightly to obtain the same count density.

Since the radiation dose to an organ is defined as the energy absorbed divided by the mass of the organ (equation 3) the radiation dose to a child will be greater than that to an adult administered with the same activity. The mass of many individual organs remains a nearly constant proportion of the total body weight from birth to maturity (NCRP, 1983), with the notable exception of the testes which remain disproportionately small in boys until puberty. Apart from the testes, it is therefore approximately true that the radiation dose per MBq of activity administered is inversely proportional to the total body weight. The effective dose equivalent per test for children can thus be kept to the same sort of levels as for adults by scaling down the administered activity in proportion to body weight. However, for some tests there may be an absolute minimum activity required to obtain a meaningful result. Careful consideration must be given to the balance between the dose received and the potential benefits of the information obtained.

An exact calculation of the radiation dose to a child of a given age requires a knowledge of both the appropriate physiological information and the correct *S* factors.

It may be safe to assume that some adult physiological data still apply to children, provided that fractional rate constants are used rather than absolute clearance rates, but this assumption is not always valid. For example, thyroid uptake of iodide may be as high as 70% in a newborn child, but this falls to a more normal 30% after a few days (Morrison *et al.*, 1963).

S factors for children of any size can be calculated by scaling the values of *S* from the standard adult phantom to allow for the following changes:

1. The reduced mass of each target organ leads to a proportionately increased dose;
2. Non-penetrating radiation (beta particles and low energy X-rays) will still be absorbed locally in the source organ;
3. Penetrating radiation (gamma rays) is less likely to be absorbed within smaller organs;
4. Since organs are closer together more penetrating radiation will be received from adjacent source organs;
5. Gamma rays will be attenuated less due to shorter paths through body tissues.

Yamaguchi, Kato and Shiragai (1975) have given details of a calculation which allows for all of these effects.

Alternatively, *S* factors for standard phantoms of children of various ages can be calculated by the same Monte Carlo method that has been used for an adult phantom. Results of this type have been reported by Poston (1976), and a selection of values for a few radionuclides have been published by the National Council on Radiation Protection and Measurements (NCRP, 1983).

Because of the infinite variation in physique among children calculations with standard phantoms cannot be expected to give anything more than a general indication of how the radiation dose will change with age of the patient. Due to the inevitable uncertainties in the physiological data it is not even worth attempting to carry out an accurate calculation for every individual patient. Therefore, in this context, the simple rule of thumb may as well be used—that the effective dose equivalent will remain roughly the same as for an adult, provided that the administered activity is scaled down in proportion to body weight.

References

ARNOLD, R. W., SUBRAMANIAN, G., MCAFEE, J. G., BLAIR, R. J. and THOMAS, F. D. (1975) Comparison of 99mTc complexes for renal imaging. *Journal of Nuclear Medicine*, **16**, 357–367
BRILL, A. B. (1982) *Low-level Radiation Effects: A Fact Book*, New York: The Society of Nuclear Medicine
DHSS (1984) *Notes for Guidance on the Administration of Radioactive Substances to Persons for Purposes of Diagnosis, Treatment or Research*, HN(84)5, London: Department of Health and Social Security
DILLMAN, L. T. and VON DER LAGE, F. C. (1975) *Radionuclide Decay Schemes and Nuclear Parameters for Use in Radiation Dose Estimation*, MIRD Pamphlet No. 10, New York: Society of Nuclear Medicine
ICRP (1969) Publication 17: *Protection of the Patient in Radionuclide Investigations*, Oxford: Pergamon Press
ICRP (1977a) Publication 26: Recommendations of the International Commission on Radiological Protection. *Annals of the ICRP*, **1**, 3
ICRP (1977b) Publication 27: Problems involved in developing an index of harm. *Annals of the ICRP*, **1**, 4
ICRP (1980) Statement and recommendations of the International Commission on Radiological Protection from its 1980 meeting. *British Journal of Radiology*, **53**, 816–818
MIRD (1975) Dose Estimate Report No. 5. *Journal of Nuclear Medicine*, **16**, 857–860
MIRD (1976) Dose Estimate Report No. 8. *Journal of Nuclear Medicine*, **17**, 74–77
MORRISON, R. T., BIRKBECK, J. A., EVANS, T. C. and ROUTH, J. I. (1963) Radioiodine uptake studies in newborn infants. *Journal of Nuclear Medicine*, **4**, 162–166
NCRP (1983) *Protection in Nuclear Medicine and Ultrasound Diagnostic Procedures in Children*, NCRP report No. 73, Bethesda, Maryland: National Council on Radiation Protection and Measurements
NRPB (1984) *The Radiation Exposure of the UK Population—1984 Review*, London: HMSO
POSTON, J. W. (1976) The effect of body and organ size on absorbed dose: There is no standard patient. In: *Radiopharmaceutical Dosimetry Symposium* (Proc. Conf. Oak Ridge), R. J. Cloutier, J. L. Coffey, W. S.

Snyder, E. E. Watson and D. R. Hamilton (eds.), HEW publication (FDA) 76-8044, p. 92, Springfield, Virginia: National Technical Information Service

SNYDER, W. S., FORD, M. R., WARNER, G. G. and WATSON, S. B. (1975) 'S' *Absorbed Dose per Unit Cumulated Activity for Selected Radionuclides and Organs*, MIRD pamphlet No. 11, New York: Society of Nuclear Medicine

SUBRAMANIAN, G., MCAFEE, J. G., BLAIR, R. J., KALLFELZ, F. A. and THOMAS, F. D. (1975) Technetium 99m methylene diphosphonate—a superior agent for skeletal imaging: Comparison with other technetium complexes. *Journal of Nuclear Medicine*, **16**, 744–755

YAMAGUCHI, H., KATO, Y. and SHIRAGAI, A. (1975) The transformation method for the MIRD absorbed fraction as applied to various physiques. *Physics in Medicine and Biology*, **20**, 593–601

20 Current developments

P. H. O'Reilly, R. A. Shields and H. J. Testa

The development of nuclear medicine depends upon advances which may be considered under three headings: radiopharmaceuticals, instrumentation and clinical application. To a certain extent these are interdependent, the stimulus for advances to be made in one arising from a development in another. During recent years there has been significant progress in all three areas, and we may expect to see further developments having a similar impact on future practice in diagnostic nephrourology.

Radiopharmaceuticals

In spite of much useful work achieved in some centres with ^{123}I, it must be admitted that ^{99m}Tc is the radionuclide of choice because of its cost, availability and physical characteristics. It remains a matter of concern, therefore, that there is no pharmaceutical agent excreted by active tubular secretion which can be labelled with ^{99m}Tc. Such an agent is necessary for the determination of renal plasma flow, and is highly desirable for renography. For both these applications ortho-iodohippurate (OIH) reigns supreme, but OIH cannot be labelled with ^{99m}Tc. Most renal imaging agents which have been developed (^{99m}Tc-DTPA, ^{99m}Tc-gluconate, etc.) are excreted by glomerular filtration and exhibit a clearance rate from plasma of up to 120 ml/min. There is a quantum leap between this type of clearance and the 600 ml/min exhibited by OIH.

Some progress has been made towards the technetium-labelled OIH analogue. Both ^{99m}Tc-DADS and ^{99m}Tc-TDG (*see* p. 241) have been shown to have clearances approximately twice that of DTPA, but still under half that of OIH. Clearly some combination of excretory mechanisms is involved, and this has been cited as a disadvantage of such compounds. Traditionally it was considered that an ideal renal radiopharmaceutical should be handled by a single physiological process; for example, glomerular filtration, tubular secretion. Indeed, this approach is highly desirable since its implication is that it will be possible to differentiate between glomerular disease and tubular disease; within this context a step in the right direction is the work of van Luijk *et al.* (1984) which suggests that ^{99m}Tc-DMSA seems to be an indicator of proximal tubular function. However, one should bear in mind the intact nephron hypothesis (Bricker, Morrin and Kime, 1960) which suggests that any aspect of its function may indicate the function of the whole, and that a deterioration in one aspect will rarely be found in isolation. If this is true, it does not really matter which physiological function the radiopharmaceutical follows, and the main consideration for renographic studies is the target-to-background ratio of the compound. Inevitably a compound secreted by the tubules will be ideal; there is no doubt that research will continue in the search for a high-clearance ^{99m}Tc-labelled compound.

Instrumentation

During the last decade it has been possible to look to the latest developments in gamma camera technology for advances in spatial resolution and, hence, improved detail in images.

It is probably now true to say that the intrinsic spatial resolution of the detectors is so high that it is the resolution of the collimator which determines the quality of the image, and the latter is generally subject to the constraint that improvement can be gained only at the expense of loss of sensitivity. In the search for higher quality of images it should not be forgotten, however, that small organs can be imaged with remarkable resolution if a pinhole collimator is used to throw a magnified image of photon distribution onto the detector.

Each of the nuclear medicine images shown in this book has been, in fact, a projection of a three-dimensional distribution onto a two-dimensional plane. The posterior view of a kidney, for example, is composed of information from planes at all depths in the organ superimposed; furthermore, activity in tissues underlying or overlying the organ will also make a contribution. Better images showing finer detail at improved contrast might be obtained if tomographic techniques were employed to reproduce cross-sectional distributions. Instrumentation is now generally available for *single photon emission computed tomography* (*SPECT*). The gamma camera rotates about a supine patient, sets of projection images are acquired, and the distribution in transverse cross-sections is computed. Other cross-sections may also be computed and, whilst evaluation of the technique is still underway, it may be said that the longitudinal (both sagittal and coronal) sections through the kidney show promise for the enhancement of visualization of renal distributions (*Figure 20.1*).

Looking further to the future, we may see the exploitation of multiwire proportional chambers (Bateman and Connolly, 1977; Lacy *et al.*, 1984) in completely new types of imaging detection system which offer not only high-resolution gamma imaging but also the potential to bring positron emission tomography within the capabilities of the hospital nuclear medicine department.

Clinical application

The shape of a renogram curve is determined by several factors, and much effort has been expended in attempting to distinguish between them when interpreting abnormal results. It is generally acknowledged that the uptake during the first few minutes may be used to measure *relative function* and that the elimination shown during the third phase may be used to assess degree of obstruction. Impairment of one may, however, influence the other and it is to be hoped that developments in the application of the theory may still help to separate them. It is also desirable that the diagnostic information obtained include a measure of the *absolute* renal function in addition to the relative.

One approach to the assessment of obstruction is that of diuresis renography, and this is also affected by the difficulty referred to above. A brisk response to frusemide

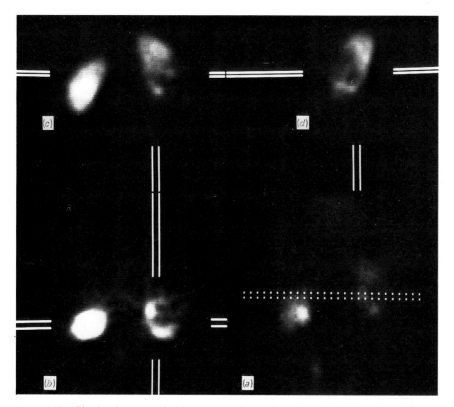

Figure 20.1 Single photon emission computed tomography (SPECT) study of the kidneys using 600 MBq ^{99m}Tc-gluconate. Sixty-four projection images were acquired for 15 seconds each during a 360-degree rotation. (*a*) The anterior projection image with double dotted line indicating the level selected for display of a transverse section cut. (*b*) Transverse cross-sectional image with horizontal lines indicating the position selected for display of a coronal section. (*c*) Coronal section with vertical lines indicating the position selected for display of a saggital section. (*d*) Sagittal section through the right kidney. The study clearly demonstrates a normal left kidney and a large space-occupying lesion in the lower pole of the right kidney

may well be observed on a renogram in which good renal function has produced a good initial curve, but how does one assess the response to frusemide when uptake is poor?

Clinicians have been gratified by the unequivocal results found in the majority of cases but frustrated by equivocal curves. This has stimulated attention to the physiological and pathophysiological determinants of the various responses. Already, several British and European centres are looking independently into the diuretic response in patients with indwelling percutaneous nephrostomy tubes to observe the effect of the diuresis on resting pressures and its correlation with both the curve forms and subsequent perfusion pressure flow studies.

A further potential aid to diuresis renogram interpretation might be found in exploration of the diuresis excretion index (DEI) to quantify the effect of the diuretic (whatever the time of its administration) on retained radiopharmaceutical. We found the original DEI useful in probe renography, and the same principle may be applied to gamma camera results. In the majority of cases interpretation continues to rely on visual inspection of the curve forms, and some method of quantification might be useful.

Frusemide is, of course, only one kind of intervention which can modify, and greatly enhance, the application of the renogram. Another new technique, which merits further evaluation, is the application of captopril to stimulate changes in the function of kidneys with renal artery stenosis (Wenting *et al.*, 1984; Fommei *et al.*, 1985). In this test renal function is measured by performing renography and clearance studies both before and after the oral administration of captopril. A kidney which suffers from impaired blood supply may react to the drug by exhibiting a marked deterioration of function, whereas a well supplied kidney should be unaffected. Preliminary results indicate that this may be a promising diagnostic tool for the investigation of unilateral renovascular hypertension.

There is little doubt that radionuclide studies are going to play a vital role in the evaluation of new techniques for the management of renal stone disease. This has undergone revolutionary changes in the last 5 years. Percutaneous nephrolithotomy (PCN) involves the introduction of a nephroscope through a preformed percutaneous transparenchymal nephrostomy track to allow the extraction of small stones from the renal pelvis and calyces. Large stones can be electrohydraulically or ultrasonically disrupted into smaller fragments for extraction. Major surgery is thus avoided.

Even more spectacular is the arrival of extracorporeal shock wave lithotripsy (ESWL), first introduced in the form of the Dornier lithotripter. This technique depends on the fact that the electrical shock wave emitted from the source has an ellipsoid form which passes through fluid and soft tissue without damaging the environment until it concentrates at the second focal point of the ellipsoid; at this point it is capable of shattering a hard object such as a renal calculus into small fragments. In clinical practice, general or regional anaesthesia is used, the patient is lowered into a water bath for treatment, and the stone is localized by two X-ray beams orientated at right angles. The resulting stone fragments are passed from the kidney via the ureter to the exterior in a stream of dust and fragments of varying sizes (the *steinstrasse*). This process may take a few days or, in the case of large stones, up to 3 months. It is during this time that strict urological supervision is required with plain abdominal radiographs, ultrasound and radionuclide techniques to monitor the *steinstrasse*, proximal dilatation and renal function. Intervention by percutaneous or endoureteric surgery may be required in infective or obstructive complications.

The success of such techniques can only be judged after several years, when the results of the procedure and its problems have been identified. Radionuclides will play a most important role in such investigations (Bomanji *et al.*, 1985) and in the evaluation of the second-generation lithotripters which are already in development and which will be closely scrutinized in terms of their effect on renal function and drainage after treatment.

References

BATEMAN, J. E. and CONNOLLY, J. F. (1977) A multi-wire proportional gamma camera for imaging ^{99m}Tc radionuclide distributions. RL-77-031/8. Rutherford Laboratory, Chilton, Oxon

BOMANJI, J., MAJEED, F., BRITTON, K. E., NIMMON, C. C., CARROLL, M. J. and WHITFIELD, H. N. (1985) A radionuclide evaluation pre and post extracorporeal shock wave lithotripsy (ESWL) for renal calculus. Presented to the European Nuclear Medicine Congress, London, September 1985

BRICKER, J. S., MORRIN, B. A. F. and KIME, S. W. (1960) The pathological physiology of chronic Bright's disease. An exposition of the intact nephron hypothesis. *American Journal of Medicine*, **28**, 77–98

FOMMEI, E., GHCONE, S., PALLA, L. *et al.* (1985) Validity of kidney scintography after captopril as a screening test for renovascular hypertension. Presented to the European Nuclear Medicine Congress, London, September 1985

LACY, J. L., LeBLANC, A. D., BABICH, J. W. *et al.* (1984) A gamma camera for medical applications, using a multi-wire proportional counter. *Journal of Nuclear Medicine*, **25**, 1003–1012

van LUCIJK, W. H. J., ENSING, G. J., MEIJER, S., DONKER, A. J. M. and PIERS, D. A. (1984) Is the relative ^{99m}Tc-DMSA clearance a useful marker of proximal tubular dysfunction? *European Journal of Nuclear Medicine*, **9**, 439–442

WENTING, G. J., TAN-TJIONG, H. L., DERKX, F. H. M., DE BRUYN, J. H. B., MAN IN'T VELD, A. J. and SCHALEKAMP, M. A. D. H. (1984) Split renal function after captopril in unilateral renal artery stenosis. *British Medical Journal*, **288**, 886–890

Index